Urological Cancer Management

Urological Cancer Management

Editor: Klara Walker

AMERICAN
MEDICAL PUBLISHERS
www.americanmedicalpublishers.com

AMERICAN
MEDICAL PUBLISHERS
www.americanmedicalpublishers.com

Cataloging-in-Publication Data

Urological cancer management / edited by Klara Walker.
p. cm.
Includes bibliographical references and index.
ISBN 978-1-63927-820-6
1. Urinary organs--Cancer--Treatment. 2. Genitourinary organs--Cancer--Treatment.
3. Urinary organs--Cancer. 4. Genitourinary organs--Cancer. 5. Oncology. I. Walker, Klara.
RC280.U74 U76 2023
616.994 6--dc23

American Medical Publishers,
41 Flatbush Avenue,
1st Floor, New York,
NY 11217, USA

ISBN 978-1-63927-820-6 (Hardback)

Contents

Preface

Urological cancer refers to a type of cancer which affects the structures and organs of female and male urinary systems, as well as the male reproductive system. It is classified into five types, including testicular cancer, bladder cancer, urethral cancer, kidney cancer and penile cancer. Blood in the urine is a sign of penile, bladder and kidney cancer. It can also lead to pelvic and back pain in the later stages. Those suffering from penile or testicular cancer may develop a visible lesion on the skin, as well as swelling or other skin abnormalities. The consumption of tobacco is a major risk factor for all types of urological cancers. The diagnosis is done through lab tests, biopsies, ureteroscopy or cystoscopy, and imaging techniques such as ultrasound, MRI, X-ray, angiogram or CT scan. The treatments of this disease rely on the stage and grade of tumor as well as on the choices of patients, and include radiation therapy, surgery and chemotherapy. This book unravels the recent studies on urological cancer. It strives to provide a fair idea about the latest advances in the clinical management of this disease. Those in search of information to further their knowledge will be greatly assisted by this book.

After months of intensive research and writing, this book is the end result of all who devoted their time and efforts in the initiation and progress of this book. It will surely be a source of reference in enhancing the required knowledge of the new developments in the area. During the course of developing this book, certain measures such as accuracy, authenticity and research focused analytical studies were given preference in order to produce a comprehensive book in the area of study.

This book would not have been possible without the efforts of the authors and the publisher. I extend my sincere thanks to them. Secondly, I express my gratitude to my family and well-wishers. And most importantly, I thank my students for constantly expressing their willingness and curiosity in enhancing their knowledge in the field, which encourages me to take up further research projects for the advancement of the area.

Editor

1

Dysregulation of Type II Transmembrane Serine Proteases and Ligand-Dependent Activation of MET in Urological Cancers

Shoichiro Mukai [1,*], Koji Yamasaki [1], Masato Fujii [1], Takahiro Nagai [1], Naoki Terada [1], Hiroaki Kataoka [2] and Toshiyuki Kamoto [1]

1 Department of Urology, Faculty of Medicine, University of Miyazaki, Miyazaki 889-1692, Japan; koji_yamasaki@med.miyazaki-u.ac.jp (K.Y.); masato_fujii@med.miyazaki-u.ac.jp (M.F.); takahiro_nagai@med.miyazaki-u.ac.jp (T.N.); naoki_terada@med.miyazaki-u.ac.jp (N.T.); tkampro@med.miyazaki-u.ac.jp (T.K.)

2 Oncopathology and Regenerative Biology Section, Faculty of Medicine, University of Miyazaki, Miyazaki 889-1692, Japan; mejina@med.miyazaki-u.ac.jp

* Correspondence: syoichiro_mukai@med.miyazaki-u.ac.jp

Abstract: Unlike in normal epithelium, dysregulated overactivation of various proteases have been reported in cancers. Degradation of pericancerous extracellular matrix leading to cancer cell invasion by matrix metalloproteases is well known evidence. On the other hand, several cell-surface proteases, including type II transmembrane serine proteases (TTSPs), also induce progression through activation of growth factors, protease activating receptors and other proteases. Hepatocyte growth factor (HGF) known as a multifunctional growth factor that upregulates cancer cell motility, invasiveness, proliferative, and anti-apoptotic activities through phosphorylation of MET (a specific receptor of HGF). HGF secreted as inactive zymogen (pro-HGF) from cancer associated stromal fibroblasts, and the proteolytic activation by several TTSPs including matriptase and hepsin is required. The activation is strictly regulated by HGF activator inhibitors (HAIs) in physiological condition. However, downregulation is frequently observed in cancers. Indeed, overactivation of MET by upregulation of matriptase and hepsin accompanied by the downregulation of HAIs in urological cancers (prostate cancer, renal cell carcinoma, and bladder cancer) are also reported, a phenomenon observed in cancer cells with malignant phenotype, and correlated with poor prognosis. In this review, we summarized current reports focusing on TTSPs, HAIs, and MET signaling axis in urological cancers.

Keywords: matriptase; hepsin; hepatocyte growth factor (HGF); MET; prostate cancer; renal cell carcinoma; bladder cancer; HGF activator inhibitor (HAI)

---

1. Introduction

The interaction between cancer cells and stromal cells in the pericellular microenvironment has been fully discussed in the literature [1,2]. On the cancer cell surface, a variety of receptors for cytokines, growth factors, and protease activating-type receptor are widely expressed. The corresponding ligands (such as cytokines and growth factors) are provided from blood cells, stromal cells, and cancer cells in various situations. Among these, several growth factors must be proteolytically activated to achieve the biological activities. Recently, the activating process has been clarified. For example, hepatocyte growth factor (HGF) is secreted as an inactive zymogen (pro-HGF) by stromal fibroblasts and converted to active mature form by proteolytic cleavage [2–4]. HGF activator (HGFA) was initially identified and considered to be the single major activator in serum [3–7]. Indeed, coagulation cascade is initiated in pericancerous lesion, and then HGFA changes to the active form by thrombin-induced proteolytic activation [3–7]. Subsequently, several cell-surface transmembrane-type activators, including hepsin and matriptase, were identified [8–12]. These proteases may also be candidates for major activators considering HGF behavior (the so-called sticky protein) and the functional location (MET is located on the cell membrane). In physiological condition, the activation is tightly regulated by specific cell-surface protease inhibitors such as HGFA inhibitors (HAIs). However, dysregulated overactivation of pro-HGF has been reported to aggressively induce cancer invasion and metastasis through increased phosphorylation of MET [10–12]. This review focuses on the cell-surface pro-HGF activation system in urological cancers, including prostate cancer (PC), renal cell carcinoma (RCC), and urothelial carcinoma (UC) of bladder, and summarizes its significance in the progression of cancer.

2. HGF/MET and the Related Molecules

2.1. HGF and MET in Cancer

2.1.1. HGF/MET Signaling Axis

MET, encoded by *Met* proto-oncogene located on chromosome 7q31, is a tyrosine kinase-type specific receptor of HGF, which forms disulfide-inked heterodimer consisting of an extracellular alpha chain and single-pass transmembrane beta chain [3,13–15]. As shown in Figure 1, the intracellular domain of the beta chain comprises a juxtamembrane domain and catalytic kinase domain containing an activation loop and carboxy-terminal multifunctional docking site. The juxtamembrane domain downregulates the kinase activity by phosphorylation of Ser975, while the catalytic kinase domain upregulates the activity by phosphorylation of Tyr1234 and Tyr1235. The multifunctional docking sites contain Tyr1349 and Tyr1356, which lead to downstream signaling through several intracellular adaptor proteins [3,13–16]. Increased expression of MET with worse prognosis has been reported in various cancer cells, and phosphorylation (activation) potently promotes invasion and metastasis [16–19]. Activation of HGF/MET signaling axis in cancer cells also plays a significant role in proliferation, angiogenesis, epithelial-mesenchymal transition (EMT), and drug resistance [3,13,14]. Activation is introduced by: 1) ligand (HGF)-dependent activation, 2) reciprocal activation by overexpression-induced MET oligomerization, 3) activating point mutation of tyrosine kinase domain, and 4) transactivation by heterodimerization with another receptor tyrosine kinase [3,13,14]. In the ligand-dependent activation, proteolytic activation of pro-HGF is necessary. As mentioned above, two major activating protease families were reported: 1) a serum serine protease, HGFA; and 2) type II transmembrane serine proteases (TTSPs) such as matriptase, hepsin, and transmembrane protease/serine (TMPRSS) 2 [3,10–12]. Although these pro-HGF activating proteases are tightly regulated by two transmembrane serine protease inhibitors, HAI-1 and HAI-2, downregulation of HAIs has been observed in several cancers and has been shown to induce progression [11,12].

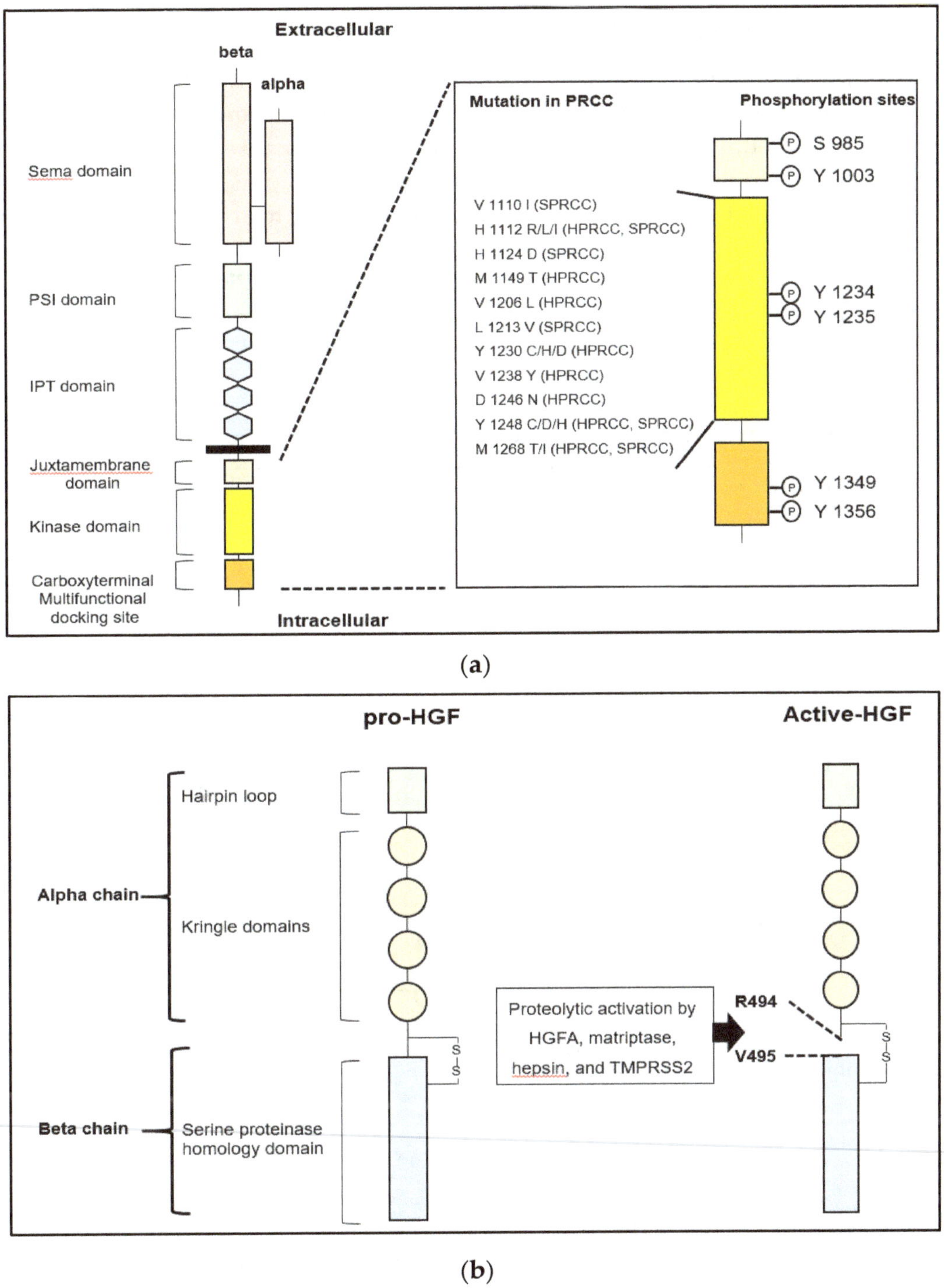

Figure 1. (**a**) Left: The structure of human MET is shown. MET consists of extracellular alpha and single-pass transmembrane beta chain, which are disulfide-linked heterodimer. The beta chain is composed of six major domains including Sema (semaphorin), PSI (plexin, semaphorin, integrin), IPT (immunoglobulin-like regions in plexins and transcription factors), juxtamembrane, tyrosine kinase domain, and multifunctional docking site. Right: Sites of point mutation in hereditary and sporadic papillary renal cell carcinoma (HPRCC and SPRCC) and conventional phosphorylation sites in intracellular domains are shown. (**b**) Left: The structure of human pro-hepatocyte growth factor (HGF) is shown. HGF consists of four Kringle domains and a serine proteinase homology domain. Right: The active form of HGF is shown. HGFA, hepsin, matriptase, and TMPRSS2 proteolytically cleave between Arg 494 and Val 495 to convert to a two-chain heterodimeric active form. One-letter abbreviation of amino acids is used.

2.2. Cell Surface pro-HGF Activating Enzymes and the Regulators

2.2.1. Type-II Transmembrane Serine Proteases (TTSP) in Cancers

The TTSP family in humans consists of 17 serine proteases [3,10,17]. The structures are specified as a single-pass hydrophobic transmembrane domain near the N-terminus with a short intracellular domain and a large extracellular portion including a carboxy-terminal serine protease domain [3,10,17]. All TTSPs are divided into the four subfamilies of hepsin, matriptase, human airway trypsin-like protease (HAT) and corin (Table 1) [3,10,17]. All TTSPs belong to the S1 peptidase family (noted in MEROPS as clan PA, family S1), and a catalytic triad consists of serine, aspartate, and histidine residues, as shown in Figure 2 [20,21]. Hepsin, matriptase and TMPRSS2 shows a strong cleavage preference for substrate with arginine in the P1 position [20,21]. In urogenital cancers, the expression of matriptase, hepsin and TMPRSS2 has been reported (Figure 2). Therefore, we focused on these TTSPs in this review.

Table 1. Type II transmembrane serine protease (TTSP) family content.

Subfamily	Protease
HAT/DESC	HAT DESC1 TMPRSS 11A HAT-like 4 HAT-like 5
Hepsin/TMPRSS	Hepsin (TMPRSS1) TMPRSS 2 TMPRSS 3 TMPRSS 4 TMPRSS 13 Enteropeptidase Spinesin
Matriptase	Matriptase Matriptase 2 Matriptase 3 Polyserase
Corin	Corin

TTSP: type II transmembrane serine protease; HAT: human airway trypsin-like protease; DESC: differentially expressed in squamous cell carcinoma; TMPRSS: transmembrane protease, serine.

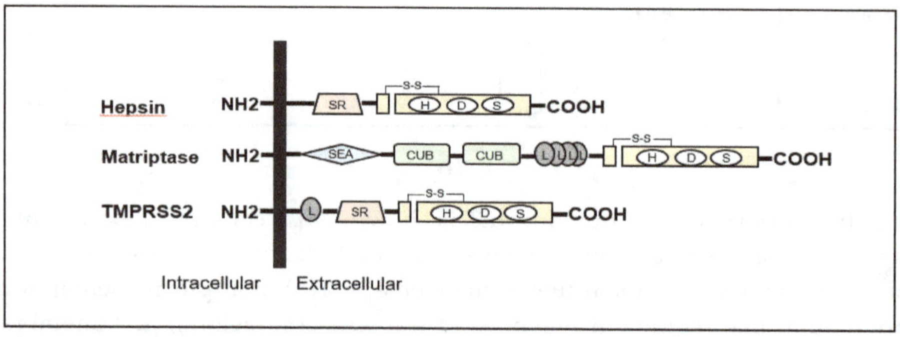

Figure 2. Structures of hepsin, matriptase and transmembrane protease serine (TMPRSS) 2 are shown. All type II transmembrane serine proteases (TTSPs) show single-pass transmembrane proteins with intracellular NH2-terminus and extracellular carboxy-terminal serine protease domains. Hepsin is composed of scavenger receptor (SR) and serine protease domains. Matriptase contains sea urchin sperm protein/enteropeptidase/agrin (SEA) domain, Cls/Cls, urchin embryonic growth factor, bone morphologic protein-1 (CUB) domain, four low-density lipoprotein receptor (L) domains class A and serine protease domains. TMPRSS2 is consists of an L domain, SR, and serine protease domains.

2.2.2. Matriptase

Matriptase (MT-ST1, ST14) gene is located on human chromosome 11q24-25, and 855 amino acids are encoded in the gene [3,10,17,18]. The molecular weight of matriptase is 80–90-kda. Matriptase was first discovered in breast cancer cell line (T-47D) and purified from human milk [3,10,17,18]. It is expressed in human epithelial cells of various organs to maintain the formation of epithelial barrier formation [3,10–12,19]. In addition, the major enzymatic functions are reported as follows: 1) activation of hepatocyte growth factor zymogen (pro-HGF), pro-platelet-derived growth factor (PDGF)-C, -D, and pro-macrophage stimulating protein (MSP); 2) activation of protease-activated receptor (PAR)-2; 3) activation of urokinase-type plasminogen activator; 4) degradation of extracellular matrix; and 5) activation of prostasin, which is a glycosylphosphatidylinositol (GPI)-anchored protease known to activate epithelial sodium channel (ENaC) [3,10,17,18]. Among TTSPs, matriptase has been reported as the most efficient activator of pro-HGF [3,10–12]. HAIs are major regulators of matriptase, and deregulation of matriptase activity facilitates cancer progression [3,10–12]. Indeed, matriptase expression is reported to be upregulated in various cancers (breast, ovarian, uterine, colon, cervical, skin, pancreatic, esophageal, head and neck, prostate, bladder and renal cell carcinoma: RCC) with poor prognosis [3,10–12,22].

2.2.3. Hepsin

Hepsin (*HPN, TMPRSS1*) gene is located on human chromosome 19q13.11, and 417 amino acids are encoded [3,10,17,18]. The molecular weight of hepsin protein is 45-kda. Although mRNA is highly expressed in liver and kidney, ubiquitous expression of the protein is reported [3,10,23]. The functions are reported as follows: 1) activation of pro-HGF; 2) activation of pro-MSP; 3) activation of pro-urokinase-type plasminogen activator; and 4) cleavage of laminin-332 [24]. Similar to matriptase, the catalytic activities of hepsin are regulated by HAI-1 and HAI-2 [3,10–12]. In cancer, overexpression of hepsin mRNA is reported in prostate, ovary, kidney, and breast [3,10,17,18]. Increased expression of the protein is also reported in prostate, ovarian, breast, and endometrial cancer [3,10,17,18].

2.2.4. Regulators of TTSPs—HAIs

HAI-1 (*SPINT-1*) gene is located at 15q 15.1 and *HAI-2* (*SPINT-2*) is located at 19q 13.2 [3,11,12]. Both proteins were initially identified in conditioned medium of human gastric cancer cell line MKN45 [3,11,12,25,26]. HAI-2 was also purified as placental bikunin from placenta [3,11,12,27]. The proteins have two specific extracellular Kunitz-type serine protease inhibitor domains, (KD)-1 and KD-2, except for a splicing variant of HAI-2 (isoform B has single KD) (Figure 3), which can inhibit several trypsin-like serine proteases, including all pro-HGF-activating enzymes [3,11,12,28,29]. Whereas, HAIs were initially discovered as HGFA inhibitors, they also inhibit matriptase and hepsin [3,11,12]. In addition, HAIs are required for intracellular transport and cell surface localization of matriptase in several types of cells [3,10–12]. HAI-1 is reported to express in the majority of normal epithelial cells [3,11,12,30]. In physiological condition, HAI-1 maintains epithelial integrity through regulation of matriptase activity [3,11,12,30]. HAI-1 is also required for placental differentiation, embryonic development and postnatal survival [11,12,31]. However, it has been reported that insufficient expression revealed dysregulation of pro-HGF activating enzymes in various cancers leading to progression [11,12]. Indeed, decreased expression of HAI-1 induced carcinogenesis (skin, intestine) and progression with worse prognosis (gastrointestinal, breast, ovarian, endometrial cancers and RCC) [11,12,32–42]. In addition, HAI-1 is also known as a suppressor of epithelial mesenchymal transition (EMT) [43].

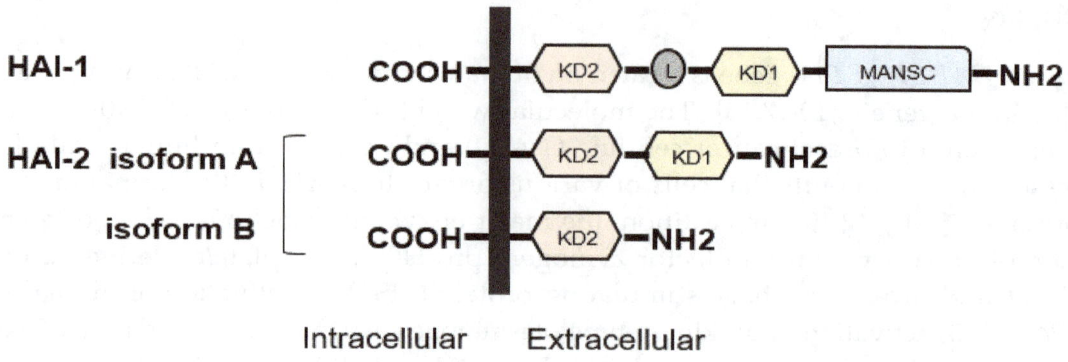

Figure 3. Structures of hepatocyte growth factor activator inhibitor (HAI)-1 and HAI-2 are shown. HAIs show single-pass transmembrane protein with intracellular carboxy-terminus and extracellular specific protease inhibitor domains, the so-called Kunitz domain (KD). HAI-1 is composed of two KDs, L domain, and motif at N terminus with seven cysteines (MANSC) domains. There are two isoforms in HAI-2. Similar to HAI1, HAI-2 isoform A has two KDs, whereas isoform B has a single KD.

HAI-2 is ubiquitously expressed in normal cells, including epithelial, mesenchymal, blood cells and trophoblasts [12]. HAI-2 is reported to maintain the integrity of intestinal epithelium through regulation of matriptase-induced epithelial cell adhesion molecule (EpCAM) cleavage [44]. Downregulation by hypermethylation of *SPINT2* gene has been reported in several cancers, including hepatocellular carcinoma, RCC, melanoma, gastric carcinoma, and esophageal squamous cell carcinoma [45–48]. Expression of HAI-2 is also decreased in PC. However, no apparent *SPINT2* promoter methylation has been observed in either clinical samples or cell lines [49]. In this report, the authors suggest that posttranslational regulation of HAI-2 expression is essential in prostate cancer. The regulatory role of HAI-2 in the activation of pro-HGF by inhibiting the activating proteases (including matriptase), which induces HGF/MET signaling axis, has been considered a major suppressive function in cancer progression [11,12]. Additionally, an alternative function such as the activation of caspase 3 in esophageal squamous cell carcinoma leading to the promotion of apoptosis and inhibition of proliferation was also reported [47,50]. However, HAI-2 has also been reported to be required for invasive growth in oral squamous cell carcinoma, which suggests that the role of HAI-2 may be tissue or cell-type specific and dependent on targeting TTSPs [51].

3. TTSPs and HAIs in Urological Cancers

3.1. Prostate Cancer

3.1.1. HGF/MET Signaling and Hepsin

Increased expression of MET and phosphorylation in proliferative inflammatory atrophy (PIA) and prostatic intraepithelial neoplasia (PIN), which are known precancerous findings, have been reported [52,53]. Regarding carcinogenesis, two interesting phenomena were reported in mouse models: 1) conditional *MET* overexpression in prostatic luminal cells revealed development of PIN by administration of HGF, however, the conditional transgenic mouse did not produce PC [54] and 2) Conditional overexpression of hepsin in prostate epithelium revealed disruption of basement membrane in vivo [55]. These results suggested that the single expression of an HGF-related molecule may be insufficient for carcinogenesis because co-existence of MET with PTEN loss or expression of hepsin with Myc in normal prostate epithelium revealed development of cancer [54–56]. However, expression of MET in PC induced aggressive metastatic phenotype with sarcomatoid features [54], and expression of hepsin in localized cancer promoted metastatic cancer with differentiation to neuroendocrine phenotype [55]. Therefore, HGF/MET signaling and hepsin may have a significant role in the progression of PC [57–59]. Indeed, upregulation of MET was observed in metastatic lesion compared with primary site [60]. In addition, overexpression of MET is reported in patients with metastatic PC and positively correlated with progression [3,53,61]. Furthermore, inhibition of hepsin by small molecule inhibitor has been reported to reduce bone metastasis of PC [58].

In the normal prostate, expression of MET is observed in basal cells, but not in luminal cells [52]. Androgen receptor (AR) is, however, expressed in luminal cells [52]. Of interest, the inverse expression of MET and AR has also been reported in PC [62,63]. For example, MET is highly expressed in AR-negative prostate cancer cell lines such as PC3 and DU145, however, it is downregulated in AR-positive cell lines (LNCaP, LAPC-4, CWR22, and LuCaP) [62,63]. In addition, the degree of MET expression in CWR22 cell line is reported to continue increasing during the process to become androgen independent phenotype (CWR22R), and downregulation of AR induced upregulation of MET with the signaling system is observed [62,63].

Despite this, AR signaling remains in the majority of CRPC. This is explained by the clinical efficacy of AR signaling-targeted agents (abiraterone and enzalutamide) for CRPC, and a recent clinical phase III trial of cabozantinib (dual inhibitor of MET and vascular endothelial growth factor receptor for CRPC revealed insufficient results [64]. The reported efficacy of combined therapy targeting both AR and MET suggests the coexistence of AR-positive cells and MET-positive cells in CRPC [65].

3.1.2. Matriptase and HAIs

Inhibition of matriptase by synthetic small molecule inhibitor and analysis of downregulation using hammerhead ribozyme revealed reduced invasiveness and motility of PC cell lines [66]. The significant role of matriptase in cancers has been discussed along with the ratio of HAIs activity. Several studies revealed that overexpression and functional upregulation of matriptase rather than HAIs leads to cancer progression [67,68]. In PC, increased expression of matriptase with concomitant loss of HAI-1 was observed [67]. In addition, a correlation between downregulation of HAI-2 with upregulation of matriptase and increasing PC tumor grade has been reported [49,69]. However, the following evidence suggests that HAI-2 is a main regulator of matriptase [49,50,68–70]. The role of HAI-2 in invasiveness and metastatic potential of PC cells was analyzed using human prostate cancer progression model cell lines and the xenograft model [49,68,69]. As a result, the expression of HAI-2 but not HAI-1 in cancer cells was gradually downregulated depending on increasing invasiveness accompanying matriptase upregulation. In additional analyses, the authors confirmed that matriptase induced upregulation of PC cell motility as well as the fact that invasive and metastatic capabilities were negatively regulated by HAI-2. This phenomenon was also confirmed by the inhibition of matriptase using recombinant protein consisting of HAI-2-Kunitz domains [68,69].

3.1.3. TMPRSS2 in PC

As noted above, TMPRSS2 is a member of the TTSP family. In the pathogenesis of viral infection, TMPRSS2 is known to proteolytically activate spike glycoprotein of emerging coronaviruses, including severe acute respiratory syndrome (SARS) coronavirus (CoV), SARS-CoV-2 (COVID-19), human CoV-229E, and Middle East Respiratory Syndrome CoV (CoV-EMC), which is required for virus-cell membrane fusions [71–73]. The proteolytic cleavage and activation of hemagglutinin protein are also essential for the viral infectivity of influenza A virus (strains of H1N1, H3N2, and H7N9) [73,74]. Recent studies revealed that a gene fusion of TMPRSS2 to erythroblast transformation-specific (ETS) transcription factors is commonly observed in prostate cancer tissues [75,76]. Among these, fusion of *TMPRSS2* and *ERG* is the most common (approximately 50%) chromosomal rearrangement [75,76]. However, no apparent proteolytic activity in this fusion protein has been reported (the protein mainly acts as a transcription factor). Expression of TMPRSS2 is positively regulated by androgens and expressed in both primary and metastatic sites of hormone sensitive PC [77,78]. Expression is reported to be increased in higher Gleason pattern [77,78]. As substrates, components of extracellular matrix (nidogen-1, laminin β1), matriptase zymogen, and pro-HGF were reported [78]. Ko et al. reported that androgen-induced TMPRSS2 can initiate a pericellular proteolytic cascade to activate matriptase, which promotes cancer cell invasion [79]. In addition, the correlation between increased expression of

TMPRSS2 and increased matriptase activation in PC tissue was also confirmed. They concluded that TMPRSS2 can promote PC progression through increased matriptase activation and degradation of nidogen-1 and laminin β1 [79].

The evidences of Sections 3.1.1–3.1.3 are summarized in Figure 4.

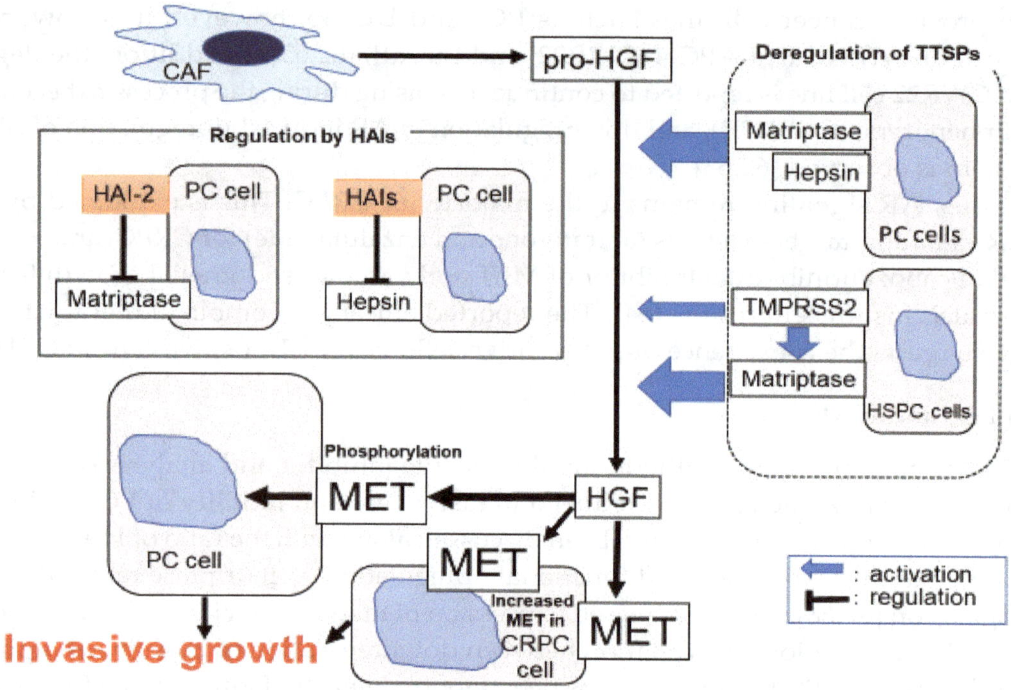

Figure 4. Hypothetical model of pericellular activation of hepatocyte growth factor zymogen (pro-HGF) in prostate cancer (PC) is shown. Downregulation of HAIs induced dysregulated overactivation of matriptase, hepsin, and TMPRSS2, leading to HGF-dependent phosphorylation of MET.

3.2. Renal Cell Carcinoma

3.2.1. HGF/MET Signaling

The most common histological subtype is clear cell RCC (approximately 80%–90% of RCC), followed by papillary RCC (10%–15%) [80]. Since expression of MET is observed in all subtypes, activating germline point mutations of MET are well known as the major cause of hereditary papillary RCC (PRCC) type-1 [15,16]. The mutation occurs at the tyrosine kinase (TK) domain and induces continuous ligand-independent phosphorylation of MET [15,16]. Although the mutation is observed only in 10%–46% of sporadic PRCC, overexpression including amplification of MET is common [81]. Of interest, phosphorylation of MET with auto-activating mutation was enhanced to a significant degree by HGF stimulation [82].

Inactivation of von Hippel-Lindau (*VHL*) tumor suppressor gene is the most common genetic abnormality of clear cell RCC [83,84]. Inactivation occurs not only in VHL patients (germline mutation) but also in patients with sporadic clear cell RCC (somatic abnormality) by deletion, mutation and epigenetic hypermethylation [83,84]. Deficiency of VHL protein in clear cell RCC causes progression of angiogenesis through activation of hypoxia inducible factor (HIF) 1α and 2α, which are major transcription factors of vascular endothelial growth factor (VEGF) and platelet-derived growth factor (PDGF) [83]. Of interest, HIF-1α is also reported to activate transcription of MET [3,84]. Indeed, overexpression of MET with worsening prognosis has been reported in patients with cc RCC. In addition, a significant body of evidence has revealed that activation of MET in RCC cells promotes proliferation, invasive activity, motility, antiapoptotic activity, and angiogenesis [3,42,84–88]. In addition, CD105+/CD24− cancer stem cells of RCC also expressed MET, and inhibition reduced development of bone metastasis [89].

Phase III METEOR(NCT01865747) trial revealed that cavozantinib, a novel TK inhibitor of VEGF receptor and MET, has demonstrated favorable efficacy for progression-free survival (PFS), overall survival (OS), and objective response rate (ORR) in patients with metastatic RCC in a second- or third-line treatment setting [90]. In addition, subgroup analysis of the METEOR trial demonstrated that treatment has clinical benefits in PFS, OS, and ORR for RCC patients with bone metastases associated with poor prognosis [91].

3.2.2. HAIs and TTSPs in RCC

Increased expression of matriptase and hepsin was reported to be correlated with poor prognosis [3,42,92]. In addition, decreased expression of HAI-1 and HAI-2 also revealed worse prognosis in patients with RCC [3,42,45,93]. As mentioned above, hypermethylation of *SPINT2* gene in RCC has been reported [45]. Morris et al. reported that *SPINT2* promoter methylation was observed in approximately 30% of ccRCC and 40% of pRCC patients with sporadic type, and they concluded that epigenetic inactivation caused loss of tumor suppressor activities in RCC [45].

3.2.3. MET and Matriptase/HAI-2 in Bone Metastasis

Approximately 30% of advanced RCC patients have bone metastasis [91,94]. Osteolytic metastasis affects patient quality of life through skeletal-related events. As mentioned above, bone metastasis is reported to be a negative prognostic factor and shows resistance to multimodal treatment, including surgery, radiation, and recent VEGFR-targeted medicines [91,94]. Interestingly, immunohistochemical analysis has revealed a significant increase in the expression of MET and matriptase in bone metastasis compared with primary site [87]. In analysis of mouse model of bone metastasis using human RCC cell line (786-O), expression of HGF, matriptase and decreased expression of HAI-2 were observed in bone metastasis compared with control [88]. Furthermore, increased phosphorylation of MET was also observed in bone metastasis [88]. These reports suggested that the HGF-dependent MET signaling axis plays a significant role in RCC bone metastasis.

The evidences of Sections 3.2.1–3.2.3 are summarized in Figure 5.

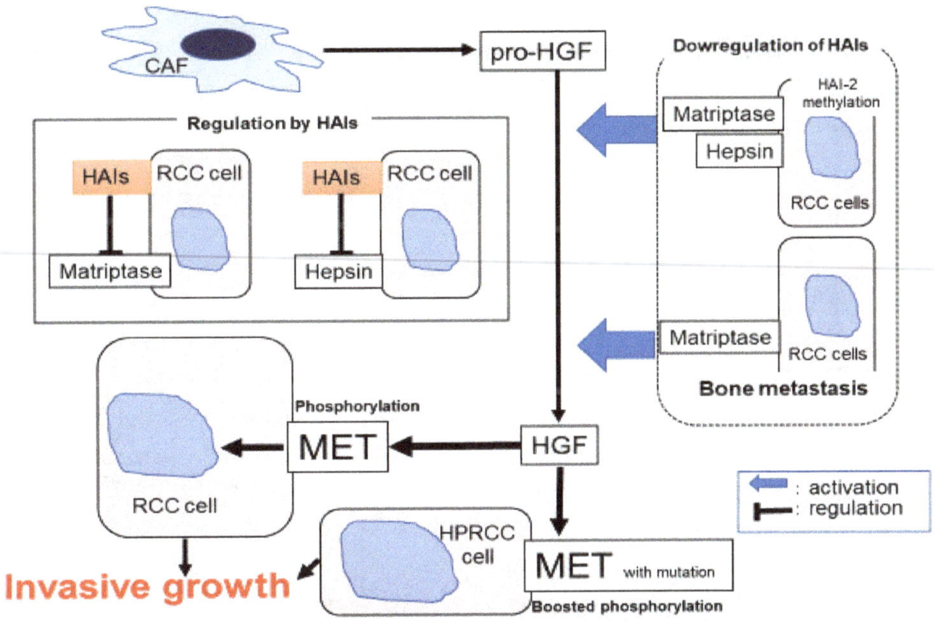

Figure 5. Hypothetical model of pericellular activation of pro-HGF in renal cell carcinoma (RCC) is shown. Downregulation of HAIs including HAI-2 methylation induced overactivation of matriptase and hepsin. In bone metastasis, increased expression of matriptase and downregulation of HAI-2 leads to the upregulation of HGF activation. In addition, phosphorylation of MET with auto-activating mutation was enhanced by HGF stimulation.

3.3. Bladder Cancer

3.3.1. Significance of HGF-dependent MET Activation in Muscle Invasive Bladder Cancer

Pathological analysis shows that approximately 90% of bladder cancers are UC and that 5% are squamous cell carcinoma [95]. Several studies reported a positive correlation between increased expression of MET and high tumor grade, pathological staging, and survival [96–100]. Phosphorylation was also analyzed by immunohistochemistry [97,98]. Increased phosphorylation of Tyr1234/1235 (at activation loop) and Tyr1349 (at multi-docking site) was positively correlated with pT stage, and multivariate analysis prompted the authors to conclude that phosphorylated Tyr1349 was a significant predictive factor of pT stage only. In addition, phosphorylated Tyr1349 was correlated with expression of matrix metalloprotease (MMP)-2, MMP-7, and E-cadherin [97]. Furthermore, the relationship between increased phosphorylation of Tyr 1235 in MET and worse cancer-specific survival in patients with muscle invasive bladder cancer (MIBC) was reported by Yamasaki et al. In this study, increased expression of matriptase and decreased expression of HAI-1 were also correlated with poor prognosis [98]. Interestingly, the area of HAI expression and MET phosphorylation presented reciprocally in spite of the strong expression of both total MET and matriptase (Figure 6b) [98]. These findings suggested that HAI-1 may regulate the ligand-dependent activation of MET in patients with MIBC. As a biomarker, the utility of urinary soluble MET concentration to detect bladder cancer and MIBC was reported [101,102]. In vitro analysis, efficient suppression of invasion and proliferation by cabozantinib (dual inhibitor of MET and VEGFR) was observed in invasive UC cell lines (5637, T24) [103]. HGF/MET signaling-induced expression of MMP-1 was also suppressed by cabozantinib in the same cell lines. HGF/MET signaling-induced EMT is a major phenomenon in various cancer cells [103]. Recently, it has been reported that HGF/MET signaling-induced inhibition of SMURF2 yielded stabilization of TGF-β receptor, and that upregulation of TGF-β signaling axis leads to EMT of UC cell line [104]. However, compared with PC and RCC, the function of TTSPs and HAIs in UC is not well known. Therefore, further analysis is required.

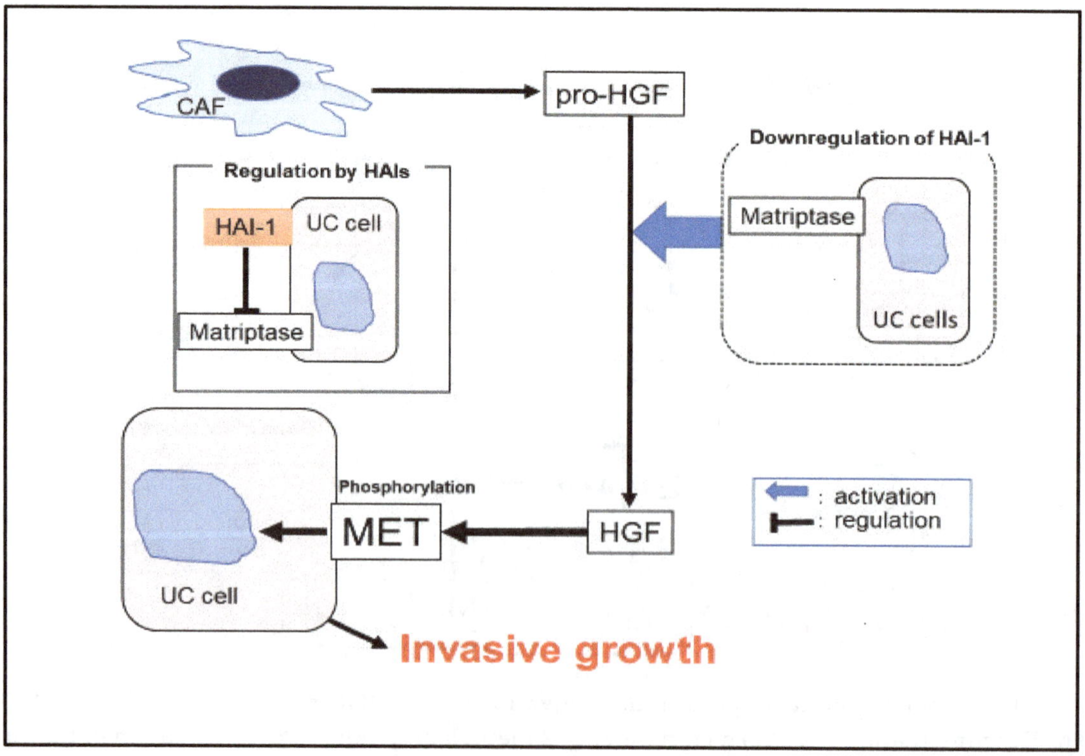

(a)

Figure 6. *Cont.*

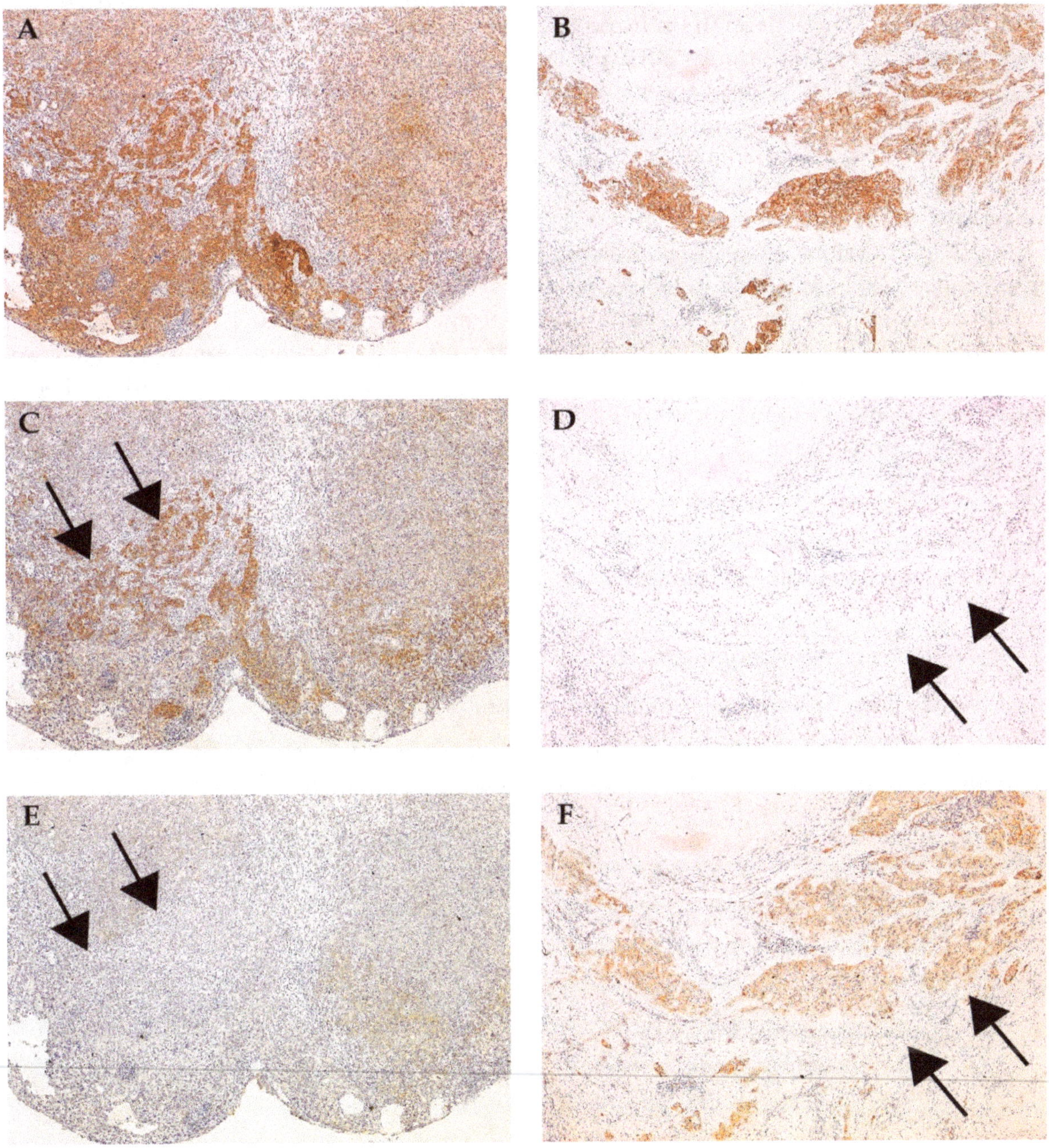

(b)

Figure 6. Hypothetical model of pericellular activation of pro-HGF in bladder urothelial carcinoma (UC) (**a**) is shown. Downregulation of HAI-1 induced overactivation of matriptase, which leads to upregulation of HGF-dependent MET phosphorylation (**a**). Immunohistochemical appearances are shown (**b**). Expression of MET (A–B), phosphorylated MET (C–D) and HAI-1 (E–F) is analyzed (case 1: A, C, and E; case 2: B, D, and F). Expression of MET is observed in both case 1 and case 2 (A and B). Whereas, increased phosphorylation of MET is observed in areas where expression of HAI-1 is decreased (C and E, arrows). On the other hand, phosphorylation is downregulated in areas where HAI-1 expressed (D and F, allows). The results suggested regulation of MET phosphorylation by HAI-1 may have a significant role in UC.

The evidence of Section 3.3.1 is summerized in Figure 6a.

4. Conclusions

In this review, we summarized the significance of pericellular pro-HGF activation in PC, RCC, and bladder cancer. Overactivation (induced by increased HGF-activating TTSPs or decreased HAIs) revealed cancer progression through MET phosphorylation.

Amplification of *MET* in lung cancer is a well-known mechanism of resistance to epidermal growth factor receptor-targeted tyrosine kinase inhibitors (EGFR-TKIs) [105–107]. In addition, overexpression of HGF is observed in approximately 61% of patients with EGFR-TKIs-resistant lung cancer and is known as a cause of acquired resistance [106,107]. The MET-signaling pathway is a major target in these patients. However, resistance to anti-MET therapy is also promoted by high amounts of pericellular HGF [106,107]. Therefore, the pro-HGF- activation system is significant in cancer progression. In urological cancers, several small molecule inhibitors targeting MET have been used in PC and RCC in clinical trials, and cavozantinib is used as a major agent targeting MET and VEGFR in patients with advanced RCC [90,91,108,109]. In addition, the efficacy of several agents for HGF and the activating TTSPs, including anti-HGF antibody, antibodies and small molecule inhibitors of hepsin and matriptase, has been reported [3,40,110–113]. Unfortunately, however, no such specific inhibitors have been verified in clinical trials [3,10]. Both matriptase and hepsin have other independent functions besides HGF-activation [114]. Therefore, inhibition of these TTSPs may yield additional therapeutic benefits in cancer treatment. As a candidate, the inhibitor domain of HAIs (KD1) shows significant inhibition for matriptase, hepsin, and HGFA [3,11,12,69]. Therefore, we believe KD1 has favorable therapeutic potential in urological cancers.

Author Contributions: The authors contributed in the following ways: S.M., conception of this review, reference selection and interpretation, and manuscript writing; K.Y., M.F., and T.N., review of literatures; H.K., conception of this review, review of literatures; N.T. and T.K., review of literatures and financial support. All authors have read and agreed to the published version of the manuscript.

Acknowledgments: The authors would like to thank Ms. Junko Kurogi of Oncopathology and Regenerative Biology Section, Faculty of Medicine, University of Miyazaki for technical support of immunohistochemistry.

Abbreviations

HGF	hepatocyte growth factor
HGFA	hepatocyte growth factor activator
HAI	hepatocyte growth factor activator inhibitor
PC	prostate cancer
RCC	renal cell carcinoma
EMT	epithelial-mesenchymal transition
TTSP	type II transmembrane serine protease
TMPRSS	transmembrane protease, serine
PRCC	papillary renal cell carcinoma
PDGF	platelet-derived growth factor
PAR	protease activated receptor
ENaC	epithelial sodium channel
RNA	ribonucleic acid
KD	Kunitz-type serine protease inhibitor domain
EPCAM	epithelial cell adhesion molecules
PIN	prostatic intraepithelial neoplasia
AR	androgen receptor
CRPC	castration resistant prostate cancer
TK	tyrosine kinase
VHL	von Hippel-Lindau
MMP	matrix metalloprotease
UC	urothelial carcinoma
SMURF	SMAD specific E3 ubiquitin protein ligase 2
TGF	transforming growth factor

References

1. Turk, B.; Turk, D.; Turk, V. Protease signalling: the cutting edge. *EMBO J.* **2012**, *4*, 1630–1643. [CrossRef] [PubMed]
2. Kataoka, H.; Tanaka, H.; Nagaike, K.; Uchiyama, S.; Itoh, H. Role of cancer cell-stroma interaction in invasive growth of cancer cells. *Hum. Cell.* **2003**, *16*, 1–14. [CrossRef] [PubMed]
3. Janetka, W.J.; Benson, M.R. *Extracellular Targeting of Cell Signaling in Cancer*; Strategies Directed at MET and RON Receptor Tyrosine Kinase Pathways; Wiley: Hoboken, NJ, USA, 2018; pp. 1–154.
4. Kataoka, H.; Miyata, S.; Uchinokura, S.; Itoh, H. Roles of hepatocyte growth factor (HGF) activator and HGF activator inhibitor in the pericellular activation of HGF/scatter factor. *Cancer Metastasis Rev.* **2003**, *22*, 223–236. [CrossRef]
5. Miyazawa, K.; Shimomura, T.; Kitamura, N. Activation of hepatocyte growth factor in the injured tissues is mediated by hepatocyte growth factor activator. *J. Biol. Chem.* **1996**, *16*, 3615–3618. [CrossRef] [PubMed]
6. Shimomura, T.; Kondo, J.; Ochiai, M.; Naka, D.; Miyazawa, K.; Morimoto, Y.; Kitamura, N. Activation of the zymogen of hepatocyte growth factor activator by thrombin. *J. Biol. Chem.* **1993**, *25*, 22927–22932.
7. Kataoka, H.; Kawaguchi, M. Hepatocyte growth factor activator (HGFA): pathophysiological functions in vivo. *FEBS J.* **2010**, *277*, 2230–2237. [CrossRef]
8. Kirchhofer, D.; Peek, M.; Lipari, M.T.; Billeci, K.; Fan, B.; Moran, P. Hepsin activates pro-hepatocyte growth factor and is inhibited by hepatocyte growth factor activator inhibitor-1B (HAI-1B) and HAI-2. *FEBS Lett.* **2005**, *28*, 1945–1950. [CrossRef]
9. Owen, K.A.; Qiu, D.; Alves, J.; Schumacher, A.M.; Kilpatrick, L.M.; Li, J.; Harris, J.L.; Ellis, V. Pericellular activation of hepatocyte growth factor by the transmembrane serine proteases matriptase and hepsin, but not by the membrane-associated protease uPA. *Biochem. J.* **2010**, *426*, 219–228. [CrossRef]
10. Martin, C.E.; List, K. Cell surface-anchored serine proteases in cancer progression and metastasis. *Cancer Metastasis Rev.* **2019**, *38*, 357–387. [CrossRef]
11. Kawaguchi, M.; Kataoka, H. Mechanisms of hepatocyte growth factor activation in cancer tissues. *Cancers (Basel)* **2014**, *29*, 1890–1904. [CrossRef]
12. Kataoka, H.; Kawaguchi, M.; Fukushima, T.; Shimomura, T. Hepatocyte growth factor activator inhibitors (HAI-1 and HAI-2): Emerging key players in epithelial integrity and cancer. *Pathol. Int.* **2018**, *68*, 145–158. [CrossRef] [PubMed]
13. Gentile, A.; Trusolino, L.; Comoglio, P.M. The Met tyrosine kinase receptor in development and cancer. *Cancer Metastasis Rev.* **2008**, *27*, 85–94. [CrossRef] [PubMed]
14. Trusolino, L.; Bertotti, A.; Comoglio, P.M. MET signalling: Principles and functions in development, organ regeneration and cancer. *Nat. Rev. Mol. Cell Biol.* **2010**, *11*, 834–848. [CrossRef] [PubMed]
15. Ma, P.C.; Maulik, G.; Christensen, J.; Salgia, R. c-Met: structure, functions and potential for therapeutic inhibition. *Cancer Metastasis Rev.* **2003**, *22*, 309–325. [CrossRef] [PubMed]
16. Tovar, E.A.; Graveel, C.R. MET in human cancer: germline and somatic mutations. *Ann. Transl. Med.* **2017**, *5*, 205. [CrossRef]
17. Tanabe, L.M.; List, K. The role of type II transmembrane serine protease-mediated signaling in cancer. *FEBS J.* **2017**, *284*, 1421–1436. [CrossRef]
18. List, K.; Bugge, T.H.; Szabo, R. Matriptase: potent proteolysis on the cell surface. *Mol. Med.* **2006**, *12*, 1–7. [CrossRef]
19. Wu, C.J.; Feng, X.; Lu, M.; Morimura, S.; Udey, M.C. Matriptase-mediated cleavage of EpCAM destabilizes claudins and dysregulates intestinal epithelial homeostasis. *J. Clin. Investig.* **2017**, *127*, 623–634. [CrossRef]
20. Szabo, R.; Bugge, T.H. Membrane-anchored serine proteases in vertebrate cell and developmental biology. *Annu. Rev. Cell Dev. Biol.* **2011**, *27*, 213–235. [CrossRef]
21. Rawlings, N.D.; Barrett, A.J.; Thomas, P.D.; Huang, X.; Bateman, A.; Finn, R.D. The MEROPS database of proteolytic enzymes, their substrates and inhibitors in 2017 and a comparison with peptidases in the PANTHER database. *Nucleic Acids Res.* **2018**, *46*, D624–D632. [CrossRef]
22. Cheng, M.F.; Huang, M.S.; Lin, C.S.; Lin, L.H.; Lee, H.S.; Jiang, J.C.; Hsia, K.T. Expression of matriptase correlates with tumour progression and clinical prognosis in oral squamous cell carcinoma. *Histopathology* **2014**, *65*, 24–34. [PubMed]

23. Tsuji, A.; Torres-Rosado, A.; Arai, T.; Le Beau, M.M.; Lemons, R.S.; Chou, S.H.; Kurachi, K. Hepsin, a cell membrane-associated protease. Characterization, tissue distribution, and gene localization. *J. Biol. Chem.* **1991**, *5*, 16948–16953.
24. Tripathi, M.; Nandana, S.; Yamashita, H.; Ganesan, R.; Kirchhofer, D.; Quaranta, V. Laminin-332 is a substrate for hepsin, a protease associated with prostate cancer progression. *J. Biol. Chem.* **2008**, *7*, 30576–30584.
25. Shimomura, T.; Denda, K.; Kitamura, A.; Kawaguchi, T.; Kito, M.; Kondo, J.; Kagaya, S.; Qin, L.; Takata, H.; Miyazawa, K.; et al. Hepatocyte growth factor activator inhibitor, a novel Kunitz-type serine protease inhibitor. *J. Biol. Chem.* **1997**, *272*, 6370–6376.
26. Kawaguchi, T.; Qin, L.; Shimomura, T.; Kondo, J.; Matsumoto, K.; Denda, K.; Kitamura, N. Purification and cloning of hepatocyte growth factor activator inhibitor type 2, a Kunitz-type serine protease inhibitor. *J. Biol. Chem.* **1997**, *272*, 27558–27564. [PubMed]
27. Marlor, C.W.; Delaria, K.A.; Davis, G.; Muller, D.K.; Greve, J.M.; Tamburini, P.P. Identification and cloning of human placental bikunin, a novel serine protease inhibitor containing two Kunitz domains. *J. Biol. Chem.* **1997**, *272*, 12202–12208.
28. Kataoka, H.; Itoh, H.; Nuki, Y.; Hamasuna, R.; Naganuma, S.; Kitamura, N.; Shimomura, T. Mouse hepatocyte growth factor (HGF) activator inhibitor type 2 lacking the first Kunitz domain potently inhibits the HGF activator. *Biochem. Biophy. Res. Commun.* **2002**, *290*, 1096–1100.
29. Kataoka, H.; Shimomura, T.; Kawaguchi, T.; Hamasuna, R.; Itoh, H.; Kitamura, N.; Miyazawa, K.; Koono, M. Hepatocyte growth factor activator inhibitor type 1 is a specific cell surface binding protein of hepatocyte growth factor activator (HGFA) and regulates HGFA activity in the pericellular microenvironment. *J. Biol. Chem.* **2000**, *275*, 40453–40462.
30. Kawaguchi, M.; Takeda, N.; Hoshiko, S.; Yorita, K.; Baba, T.; Sawaguchi, A.; Nezu, Y.; Yoshikawa, T.; Fukushima, T.; Kataoka, H. Membrane-bound serine protease inhibitor HAI-1 is required for maintenance of intestinal epithelial integrity. *Am. J. Pathol.* **2011**, *179*, 1815–1826.
31. Tanaka, H.; Nagaike, K.; Takeda, N.; Itoh, H.; Kohama, K.; Fukushima, T.; Miyata, S.; Uchiyama, S.; Uchinokura, S.; Shimomura, T.; et al. Hepatocyte growth factor activator inhibitor type 1 (HAI-1) is required for branching morphogenesis in the chorioallantoic placenta. *Mol. Cell Biol.* **2005**, *25*, 5687–5698.
32. Hoshiko, S.; Kawaguchi, M.; Fukushima, T.; Haruyama, Y.; Yorita, K.; Tanaka, H.; Seiki, M.; Inatsu, H.; Kitamura, K.; Kataoka, H. Hepatocyte growth factor activator inhibitor type 1 is a suppressor of intestinal tumorigenesis. *Cancer Res.* **2013**, *73*, 2659–2670. [CrossRef] [PubMed]
33. Baba, T.; Kawaguchi, M.; Fukushima, T.; Sato, Y.; Orikawa, H.; Yorita, K.; Tanaka, H.; Lin, C.Y.; Sakoda, S.; Kataoka, H. Loss of membrane-bound serine protease inhibitor HAI-1 induces oral squamous cell carcinoma cells' invasiveness. *J. Pathol.* **2012**, *228*, 181–192. [PubMed]
34. Ning, T.; Zhang, H.; Wang, X.; Li, S.; Zhang, L.; Deng, T.; Zhou, L.; Wang, X.; Liu, R.; Bai, M.; et al. miR-221 and miR-222 synergistically regulate hepatocyte growth factor activator inhibitor type 1 to promote cell proliferation and migration in gastric cancer. *Tumour. Biol.* **2017**, *39*, 1010428317701636. [CrossRef] [PubMed]
35. Ye, J.; Kawaguchi, M.; Haruyama, Y.; Kanemaru, A.; Fukushima, T.; Yamamoto, K.; Lin, C.Y.; Kataoka, H. Loss of hepatocyte growth factor activator inhibitor type 1 participates in metastatic spreading of human pancreatic cancer cells in a mouse orthotopic transplantation model. *Cancer Sci.* **2014**, *105*, 44–51. [CrossRef] [PubMed]
36. Oberst, M.D.; Johnson, M.D.; Dickson, R.B.; Lin, C.Y.; Singh, B.; Stewart, M.; Williams, A.; al-Nafussi, A.; Smyth, J.F.; Gabra, H.; et al. Expression of the serine protease matriptase and its inhibitor HAI-1 in epithelial ovarian cancer: Correlation with clinical outcome and tumor clinicopathological parameters. *Clin. Cancer Res.* **2002**, *8*, 1101–1107. [PubMed]
37. Nakamura, K.; Abarzua, F.; Hongo, A.; Kodama, J.; Nasu, Y.; Kumon, H.; Hiramatsu, Y. The role of hepatocyte growth factor activator inhibitor-1 (HAI-1) as a prognostic indicator in cervical cancer. *Int. J. Oncol.* **2009**, *35*, 239–248. [CrossRef]
38. Nakamura, K.; Hongo, A.; Kodama, J.; Hiramatsu, Y. The role of hepatocyte growth factor activator inhibitor (HAI)-1 and HAI-2 in endometrial cancer. *Int. J. Cancer* **2011**, *128*, 2613–2624.
39. Hamasuna, R.; Kataoka, H.; Meng, J.Y.; Itoh, H.; Moriyama, T.; Wakisaka, S.; Koono, M. Reduced expression of hepatocyte growth factor activator inhibitor type-2/placental bikunin (HAI-2/PB) in human glioblastomas: Implication for anti-invasive role of HAI-2/PB in glioblastoma cells. *Int. J. Cancer* **2001**, *93*, 339–345. [CrossRef]

40. Li, W.; Wang, B.E.; Moran, P.; Lipari, T.; Ganesan, R.; Corpuz, R.; Ludlam, M.J.; Gogineni, A.; Koeppen, H.; Bunting, S.; et al. Pegylated Kunitz domain inhibitor suppresses hepsin-mediated invasive tumor growth and metastasis. *Cancer Res.* **2009**, *69*, 8395–8402. [CrossRef]
41. Fukushima, T.; Kawaguchi, M.; Yamasaki, M.; Tanaka, H.; Yorita, K.; Kataoka, H. Hepatocyte growth factor activator inhibitor type 1 suppresses metastatic pulmonary colonization of pancreatic carcinoma cells. *Cancer Sci.* **2011**, *102*, 407–413. [CrossRef]
42. Betsunoh, H.; Mukai, S.; Akiyama, Y.; Fukushima, T.; Minamiguchi, N.; Hasui, Y.; Osada, Y.; Kataoka, H. Clinical relevance of hepsin and hepatocyte growth factor activator inhibitor type 2 expression in renal cell carcinoma. *Cancer Sci.* **2007**, *98*, 491–498. [CrossRef] [PubMed]
43. Cheng, H.; Fukushima, T.; Takahashi, N.; Tanaka, H.; Kataoka, H. Hepatocyte growth factor activator inhibitor type 1 regulates epithelial to mesenchymal transition through membrane-bound serine proteinases. *Cancer Res.* **2009**, *69*, 1828–1835. [CrossRef] [PubMed]
44. Kawaguchi, M.; Yamamoto, K.; Takeda, N.; Fukushima, T.; Yamashita, F.; Sato, K.; Kitamura, K.; Hippo, Y.; Janetka, J.W.; Kataoka, H. Hepatocyte growth factor activator inhibitor-2 stabilizes Epcam and maintains epithelial organization in the mouse intestine. *Commun. Biol.* **2019**, *2*, 11. [CrossRef] [PubMed]
45. Morris, M.R.; Gentle, D.; Abdulrahman, M.; Maina, E.N.; Gupta, K.; Banks, R.E.; Wiesener, M.S.; Kishida, T.; Yao, M.; The, B.; et al. Tumor suppressor activity and epigenetic inactivation of hepatocyte growth factor activator inhibitor type 2/SPINT2 in papillary and clear cell renal cell carcinoma. *Cancer Res.* **2005**, *65*, 4598–4606. [CrossRef]
46. Hwang, S.; Kim, H.E.; Min, M.; Raghunathan, R.; Panova, I.P.; Munshi, R.; Ryu, B. Epigenetic silencing of SPINT2 promotes cancer cell motility via HGF-MET pathway activation in Melanoma. *J. Investig. Dermatol.* **2015**, *135*, 2283–2291. [CrossRef]
47. Yue, D.; Fan, Q.; Chen, X.; Li, F.; Wang, L.; Huang, L.; Dong, W.; Chen, X.; Zhang, Z.; Liu, J.; et al. Epigenetic inactivation of SPINT2 is associated with tumor suppressive function in esophageal squamous cell carcinoma. *Exp. Cell Res.* **2014**, *322*, 149–158. [CrossRef]
48. Dong, W.; Chen, X.; Xie, J.; Sun, P.; Wu, Y. Epigenetic inactivation and tumor suppressor activity of HAI-2/SPINT2 in gastric cancer. *Int. J. Cancer* **2010**, *127*, 1526–1534. [CrossRef]
49. Tsai, C.H.; Teng, C.H.; Tu, Y.T.; Cheng, T.S.; Wu, S.R.; Ko, C.J.; Shyu, H.Y.; Lan, S.W.; Huang, H.P.; Tzeng, S.F.; et al. HAI-2 suppresses the invasive growth and metastasis of prostate cancer through regulation of matriptase. *Oncogene* **2014**, *18*, 4643–4652. [CrossRef]
50. Roversi, F.M.; Olalla Saad, S.T.; Machado-Neto, J.A. Serine peptidase inhibitor Kunitz type 2 (SPINT2) in cancer development and progression. *Biomed. Pharmacother.* **2018**, *101*, 278–286. [CrossRef]
51. Yamamoto, K.; Kawaguchi, M.; Shimomura, T.; Izumi, A.; Konari, K.; Honda, A.; Lin, C.Y.; Johnson, M.D.; Yamashita, Y.; Fukushima, T.; et al. Hepatocyte growth factor activator inhibitor-2 (HAI-2)/*SPINT2* contributes to invasive growth of oral squamous cell carcinoma cells. *Oncotarget* **2018**, *8*, 11691–11706. [CrossRef]
52. Van Leenders, G.J.; Schalken, J.A. Epithelial cell differentiation in the human prostate epithelium: implications for the pathogenesis and therapy of prostate cancer. *Crit. Rev. Oncol. Hematol.* **2003**, *46*, 3–10. [CrossRef]
53. Mukai, S.; Yorita, K.; Yamasaki, K.; Nagai, T.; Kamibeppu, T.; Sugie, S.; Kida, K.; Onizuka, C.; Tsukino, H.; Kamimura, T.; et al. Expression of human kallikrein 1-related peptidase 4 (KLK4) and MET phosphorylation in prostate cancer tissue: immunohistochemical analysis. *Hum. Cell.* **2015**, *28*, 133–142. [CrossRef] [PubMed]
54. Mi, J.; Hooker, E.; Balog, S.; Zeng, H.; Johnson, D.T.; He, Y.; Yu, E.J.; Wu, H.; Le, V.; Lee, D.H.; et al. Activation of hepatocyte growth factor/MET signaling initiates oncogenic transformation and enhances tumor aggressiveness in the murine prostate. *J. Biol. Chem.* **2018**, *28*, 20123–20136. [CrossRef] [PubMed]
55. Klezovitch, O.; Chevillet, J.; Mirosevich, J.; Roberts, R.L.; Matusik, R.J.; Vasioukhin, V. Hepsin promotes prostate cancer progression and metastasis. *Cancer Cell* **2004**, *6*, 185–195. [CrossRef]
56. Nandana, S.; Ellwood-Yen, K.; Sawyers, C.; Wills, M.; Weidow, B.; Case, T.; Vasioukhin, V.; Matusik, R. Hepsin cooperates with MYC in the progression of adenocarcinoma in a prostate cancer mouse model. *Prostate* **2010**, *1*, 591–600. [CrossRef]
57. Magee, J.A.; Araki, T.; Patil, S.; Ehrig, T.; True, L.; Humphrey, P.A.; Catalona, W.J.; Watson, M.A.; Milbrandt, J. Expression profiling reveals hepsin overexpression in prostate cancer. *Cancer Res.* **2001**, *61*, 5692–5696.

58. Tang, X.; Mahajan, S.S.; Nguyen, L.T.; Béliveau, F.; Leduc, R.; Simon, J.A.; Vasioukhin, V. Targeted inhibition of cell-surface serine protease Hepsin blocks prostate cancer bone metastasis. *Oncotarget* **2014**, *5*, 1352–1362. [CrossRef]
59. Pal, P.; Xi, H.; Kaushal, R.; Sun, G.; Jin, C.H.; Jin, L.; Suarez, B.K.; Catalona, W.J.; Deka, R. Variants in the HEPSIN gene are associated with prostate cancer in men of European origin. *Hum. Genet.* **2006**, *120*, 187–192. [CrossRef]
60. Knudsen, B.S.; Gmyrek, G.A.; Inra, J.; Scherr, D.S.; Vaughan, E.D.; Nanus, D.M.; Kattan, M.W.; Gerald, W.L.; Vande Woude, G.F. High expression of the Met receptor in prostate cancer metastasis to bone. *Urology* **2002**, *60*, 1113–1117. [CrossRef]
61. Verhoef, E.I.; Kolijn, K.; De Herdt, M.J.; van der Steen, B.; Hoogland, A.M.; Sleddens, H.F.; Looijenga, L.H.; van Leenders, G.J. MET expression during prostate cancer progression. *Oncotarget* **2016**, *24*, 31029–31036. [CrossRef]
62. Nakashiro, K.; Hara, S.; Shinohara, Y.; Oyasu, M.; Kawamata, H.; Shintani, S.; Hamakawa, H.; Oyasu, R. Phenotypic switch from paracrine to autocrine role of hepatocyte growth factor in an androgen-independent human prostatic carcinoma cell line, CWR22R. *Am. J. Pathol.* **2004**, *165*, 533–540. [CrossRef]
63. Maeda, A.; Nakashiro, K.; Hara, S.; Sasaki, T.; Miwa, Y.; Tanji, N.; Yokoyama, M.; Hamakawa, H.; Oyasu, R. Inactivation of AR activates HGF/c-Met system in human prostatic carcinoma cells. *Biochem. Biophys. Res. Commun.* **2006**, *8*, 1158–1165. [CrossRef] [PubMed]
64. Smith, M.; De Bono, J.; Sternberg, C.; Le Moulec, S.; Oudard, S.; De Giorgi, U.; Krainer, M.; Bergman, A.; Hoelzer, W.; De Wit, R.; et al. Phase III Study of Cabozantinib in Previously Treated Metastatic Castration-Resistant Prostate Cancer: COMET-1. *J. Clin. Oncol.* **2016**, *1*, 3005–3013. [CrossRef] [PubMed]
65. Qiao, Y.; Feng, F.Y.; Wang, Y.; Cao, X.; Han, S.; Wilder-Romans, K.; Navone, N.M.; Logothetis, C.; Taichman, R.S.; Keller, E.T.; et al. Mechanistic Support for Combined MET and AR Blockade in Castration-Resistant Prostate Cancer. *Neoplasia* **2016**, *18*, 1–9. [CrossRef]
66. Sanders, A.J.; Parr, C.; Davies, G.; Martin, T.A.; Lane, J.; Mason, M.D.; Jiang, W.G. Genetic reduction of matriptase-1 expression is associated with a reduction in the aggressive phenotype of prostate cancer cells in vitro and in vivo. *J. Exp. Ther. Oncol.* **2006**, *6*, 39–48.
67. Warren, M.; Twohig, M.; Pier, T.; Eickhoff, J.; Lin, C.Y.; Jarrard, D.; Huang, W. Protein expression of matriptase and its cognate inhibitor HAI-1 in human prostate cancer: a tissue microarray and automated quantitative analysis. *Appl. Immunohistochem. Mol. Morphol.* **2009**, *17*, 23–30. [CrossRef]
68. Wu, S.R.; Teng, C.H.; Tu, Y.T.; Ko, C.J.; Cheng, T.S.; Lan, S.W.; Lin, H.Y.; Lin, H.H.; Tu, H.F.; Hsiao, P.W.; et al. The Kunitz Domain I of Hepatocyte Growth Factor Activator Inhibitor-2 Inhibits Matriptase Activity and Invasive Ability of Human Prostate Cancer Cells. *Sci. Rep.* **2017**, *8*, 15101. [CrossRef]
69. Pereira, M.S.; de Almeida, G.C.; Pinto, F.; Viana-Pereira, M.; Reis, R.M. SPINT2 deregulation in prostate carcinoma. *J. Histochem. Cytochem.* **2016**, *64*, 32–41. [CrossRef]
70. Bergum, C.; List, K. Loss of the matriptase inhibitor HAI-2 during prostate cancer progression. *Prostate* **2010**, *15*, 1422–1428. [CrossRef]
71. Wilson, S.; Greer, B.; Hooper, J.; Zijlstra, A.; Walker, B.; Quigley, J.; Hawthorne, S. The membrane-anchored serine protease, TMPRSS2, activates PAR-2 in prostate cancer cells. *Biochem. J.* **2005**, *15 Pt 3*, 967–972. [CrossRef]
72. Matsuyama, S.; Nao, N.; Shirato, K.; Kawase, M.; Saito, S.; Takayama, I.; Nagata, N.; Sekizuka, T.; Katoh, H.; Kato, F.; et al. Enhanced isolation of SARS-CoV-2 by TMPRSS2-expressing cells. *Proc. Natl. Acad. Sci. USA* **2020**, 12. [CrossRef] [PubMed]
73. Uhlén, M.; Fagerberg, L.; Hallström, B.M.; Lindskog, C.; Oksvold, P.; Mardinoglu, A.; Sivertsson, Å.; Kampf, C.; Sjöstedt, E.; Asplund, A.; et al. The Human Protein Atlas, Tissue-based map of the human proteome. *Science* **2015**, *347*, 1260419. [CrossRef] [PubMed]
74. Shen, L.W.; Mao, H.J.; Wu, Y.L.; Tanaka, Y.; Zhang, W. TMPRSS2: A potential target for treatment of influenza virus and coronavirus infections. *Biochimie* **2017**, *142*, 1–10. [CrossRef] [PubMed]

75. St John, J.; Powell, K.; Conley-Lacomb, M.K.; Chinni, S.R. TMPRSS2-ERG Fusion Gene Expression in Prostate Tumor Cells and Its Clinical and Biological Significance in Prostate Cancer Progression. *J. Cancer Sci. Ther.* **2012**, *26*, 94–101. [CrossRef] [PubMed]
76. Krumbholz, M.; Agaimy, A.; Stoehr, R.; Burger, M.; Wach, S.; Taubert, H.; Wullich, B.; Hartmann, A.; Metzler, M. Molecular Composition of Genomic *TMPRSS2-ERG* Rearrangements in Prostate Cancer. *Dis. Markers.* **2019**, 5085373. [CrossRef]
77. Lucas, J.M.; True, L.; Hawley, S.; Matsumura, M.; Morrissey, C.; Vessella, R.; Nelson, P.S. The androgen-regulated type II serine protease TMPRSS2 is differentially expressed and mislocalized in prostate adenocarcinoma. *J. Pathol.* **2008**, *215*, 118–125. [CrossRef]
78. Lucas, J.M.; Heinlein, C.; Kim, T.; Hernandez, S.A.; Malik, M.S.; True, L.D.; Morrissey, C.; Corey, E.; Montgomery, B.; Mostaghel, E.; et al. The androgen-regulated protease TMPRSS2 activates a proteolytic cascade involving components of the tumor microenvironment and promotes prostate cancer metastasis. *Cancer Discov.* **2014**, *4*, 1310–1325. [CrossRef]
79. Ko, C.J.; Huang, C.C.; Lin, H.Y.; Juan, C.P.; Lan, S.W.; Shyu, H.Y.; Wu, S.R.; Hsiao, P.W.; Huang, H.P.; Shun, C.T.; et al. Androgen-Induced TMPRSS2 Activates Matriptase and Promotes Extracellular Matrix Degradation, Prostate Cancer Cell Invasion, Tumor Growth, and Metastasis. *Cancer Res.* **2015**, *15*, 2949–2960. [CrossRef]
80. Chen, S.C.; Kuo, P.L. Bone metastasis from renal cell carcinoma. *Int. J. Mol. Sci.* **2016**, *17*, E987. [CrossRef]
81. Rhoades Smith, K.E.; Bilen, M.A. A Review of Papillary Renal Cell Carcinoma and MET Inhibitors. *Kidney Cancer.* **2019**, *1*, 151–161. [CrossRef]
82. Joffre, C.; Barrow, R.; Ménard, L.; Calleja, V.; Hart, I.R.; Kermorgant, S. A direct role for Met endocytosis in tumorigenesis. *Nat. Cell Biol.* **2011**, *5*, 827–837. [CrossRef] [PubMed]
83. Maher, E.R. Hereditary renal cell carcinoma syndromes: diagnosis, surveillance and management. *World J. Urol.* **2018**, *36*, 1891–1898. [CrossRef] [PubMed]
84. Harshman, L.C.; Choueiri, T.K. Targeting the hepatocyte growth factor/c-Met signaling pathway in renal cell carcinoma. *Cancer J.* **2013**, *19*, 316–323. [CrossRef] [PubMed]
85. Miyata, Y.; Kanetake, H.; Kanda, S. Presence of phosphorylated hepatocyte growth factor receptor/c-Met is associated with tumor progression and survival in patients with conventional renal cell carcinoma. *Clin. Cancer Res.* **2006**, *15*, 4876–4881. [CrossRef]
86. Nandagopal, L.; Sonpavde, G.P.; Agarwal, N. Investigational MET inhibitors to treat Renal cell carcinoma. *Expert Opin. Investig. Drugs* **2019**, *28*, 851–860. [CrossRef]
87. Mukai, S.; Yorita, K.; Kawagoe, Y.; Katayama, Y.; Nakahara, K.; Kamibeppu, T.; Sugie, S.; Tukino, H.; Kamoto, T.; Kataoka, H. Matriptase and MET are prominently expressed at the site of bone metastasis in renal cell carcinoma: immunohistochemical analysis. *Hum. Cell* **2015**, *28*, 44–50. [CrossRef]
88. Yamasaki, K.; Mukai, S.; Sugie, S.; Nagai, T.; Nakahara, K.; Kamibeppu, T.; Sakamoto, H.; Shibasaki, N.; Terada, N.; Toda, Y.; et al. Dysregulated HAI-2 Plays an Important Role in Renal Cell Carcinoma Bone Metastasis through Ligand-Dependent MET Phosphorylation. *Cancers (Basel)* **2018**, *8*, 10. [CrossRef]
89. D'Amico, L.; Belisario, D.; Migliardi, G.; Grange, C.; Bussolati, B.; D'Amelio, P.; Perera, T.; Dalmasso, E.; Dalle Carbonare, L.; Godio, L.; et al. C-met inhibition blocks bone metastasis development induced by renal cancer stem cells. *Oncotarget* **2016**, *19*, 45525–45537. [CrossRef]
90. Choueiri, T.K.; Escudier, B.; Powles, T.; Tannir, N.M.; Mainwaring, P.N.; Rini, B.I.; Hammers, H.J.; Donskov, F.; Roth, B.J.; Peltola, K.; et al. Cabozantinib versus everolimus in advanced renal cell carcinoma (meteor): Final results from a randomised, open-label, phase 3 trial. *Lancet Oncol* **2016**, *17*, 917–927. [CrossRef]
91. Escudier, B.; Powles, T.; Motzer, R.J.; Olencki, T.; Aren Frontera, O.; Oudard, S.; Rolland, F.; Tomczak, P.; Castellano, D.; Appleman, L.J.; et al. Cabozantinib, a new standard of care for patients with advanced renal cell carcinoma and bone metastases? Subgroup analysis of the meteor trial. *J. Clin. Oncol.* **2018**, *36*, 765–772. [CrossRef]
92. Roemer, A.; Schwettmann, L.; Jung, M.; Stephan, C.; Roigas, J.; Kristiansen, G.; Loening, S.A.; Lichtinghagen, R.; Jung, K. The membrane proteases adams and hepsin are differentially expressed in renal cell carcinoma. Are they potential tumor markers? *J. Urol.* **2004**, *172 Pt 6*, 2162–2166. [CrossRef]
93. Yamauchi, M.; Kataoka, H.; Itoh, H.; Seguchi, T.; Hasui, Y.; Osada, Y. Hepatocyte growth factor activator inhibitor types 1 and 2 are expressed by tubular epithelium in kidney and down-regulated in renal cell carcinoma. *J. Urol.* **2004**, *171*, 890–896. [CrossRef] [PubMed]

94. Weber, K.; Doucet, M.; Kominsky, S. Renal cell carcinoma bone metastasis—Elucidating the molecular targets. *Cancer Metastasis Rev.* **2007**, *26*, 691–704. [CrossRef] [PubMed]
95. Abol-Enein, H.; Kava, B.R.; Carmack, A.J. Nonurothelial cancer of the bladder. *Urology* **2007**, *69*, 93–104. [CrossRef] [PubMed]
96. Parr, C.; Jiang, W.G. Expression of hepatocyte growth factor/scatter factor, its activator, inhibitors and the c-Met receptor in human cancer cells. *Int. J. Oncol.* **2001**, *19*, 857–863. [CrossRef] [PubMed]
97. Miyata, Y.; Sagara, Y.; Kanda, S.; Hayashi, T.; Kanetake, H. Phosphorylated hepatocyte growth factor receptor/c-Met is associated with tumor growth and prognosis in patients with bladder cancer: correlation with matrix metalloproteinase-2 and -7 and E-cadherin. *Hum. Pathol.* **2009**, *40*, 496–504. [CrossRef]
98. Yamasaki, K.; Mukai, S.; Nagai, T.; Nakahara, K.; Fujii, M.; Terada, N.; Ohno, A.; Sato, Y.; Toda, Y.; Kataoka, H.; et al. Matriptase-Induced Phosphorylation of MET is Significantly Associated with Poor Prognosis in Invasive Bladder Cancer; an Immunohistochemical Analysis. *Int. J. Mol. Sci.* **2018**, *22*, 19. [CrossRef]
99. Tamatani, T.; Hattori, K.; Iyer, A.; Tamatani, K.; Oyasu, R. Hepatocyte growth factor is an invasion/migration factor of rat urothelial carcinoma cells in vitro. *Carcinogenesis* **1999**, *20*, 957–962. [CrossRef]
100. Nakahara, K.; Yamasaki, K.; Nagai, T.; Fujii, M.; Akioka, T.; Takamori, H.; Terada, N.; Mukai, S.; Sato, Y.; Kamoto, T. Expression of protease activating receptor-2 (PAR-2) is positively correlated with the recurrence of non-muscle invasive bladder cancer: an immunohistochemical analysis. *Res. Rep. Urol.* **2019**, *11*, 97–104. [CrossRef]
101. McNeil, B.K.; Sorbellini, M.; Grubb, R.L., 3rd; Apolo, A.; Cecchi, F.; Athauda, G.; Cohen, B.; Giubellino, A.; Simpson, H.; Agarwal, P.K.; et al. Preliminary evaluation of urinary soluble Met as a biomarker for urothelial carcinoma of the bladder. *J. Transl. Med.* **2014**, *21*, 199. [CrossRef]
102. Matsumoto, K.; Umitsu, M.; De Silva, D.M.; Roy, A.; Bottaro, D.P. Hepatocyte growth factor/MET in cancer progression and biomarker discovery. *Cancer Sci.* **2017**, *108*, 296–307. [CrossRef] [PubMed]
103. Shintani, T.; Kusuhara, Y.; Daizumoto, K.; Dondoo, T.O.; Yamamoto, H.; Mori, H.; Fukawa, T.; Nakatsuji, H.; Fukumori, T.; Takahashi, M.; et al. The Involvement of Hepatocyte Growth Factor-MET-Matrix Metalloproteinase 1 Signaling in Bladder Cancer Invasiveness and Proliferation. Effect of the MET Inhibitor, Cabozantinib (XL184), on Bladder Cancer Cells. *Urology* **2017**, *101*, 169–169.e7. [CrossRef] [PubMed]
104. Sim, W.J.; Iyengar, P.V.; Lama, D.; Lui, S.K.L.; Ng, H.C.; Haviv-Shapira, L.; Domany, E.; Kappei, D.; Tan, T.Z.; Saei, A.; et al. c-Met activation leads to the establishment of a TGFβ-receptor regulatory network in bladder cancer progression. *Nat. Commun.* **2019**, *25*, 4349. [CrossRef] [PubMed]
105. Owusu, B.Y.; Thomas, S.; Venukadasula, P.; Han, Z.; Janetka, J.W.; Galemmo, R.A., Jr.; Klampfer, L. Targeting the tumor-promoting microenvironment in MET-amplified NSCLC cells with a novel inhibitor of pro-HGF activation. *Oncotarget* **2017**, *8*, 63014–63025. [CrossRef] [PubMed]
106. Pennacchietti, S.; Cazzanti, M.; Bertotti, A.; Rideout, W.M., 3rd; Han, M.; Gyuris, J.; Perera, T.; Comoglio, P.M.; Trusolino, L.; Michieli, P. Microenvironment-derived HGF overcomes genetically determined sensitivity to anti-MET drugs. *Cancer Res.* **2014**, *15*, 6598–6609. [CrossRef]
107. Suda, K.; Mizuuchi, H.; Maehara, Y.; Mitsudomi, T. Acquired resistance mechanisms to tyrosine kinase inhibitors in lung cancer with activating epidermal growth factor receptor mutation–diversity, ductility, and destiny. *Cancer Metastasis Rev.* **2012**, *31*, 807–814. [CrossRef]
108. Lee, Y.H.; Apolo, A.B.; Agarwal, P.K.; Bottaro, D.P. Characterization of HGF/Met Signaling in Cell Lines Derived From Urothelial Carcinoma of the Bladder. *Cancers (Basel)* **2014**, *25*, 2313–2329. [CrossRef]
109. Miyata, Y.; Asai, A.; Mitsunari, K.; Matsuo, T.; Ohba, K.; Mochizuki, Y.; Sakai, H. Met in urological cancers. *Cancers (Basel)* **2014**, *16*, 2387–4203. [CrossRef]
110. Han, Z.; Harris, P.K.; Jones, D.E.; Chugani, R.; Kim, T.; Agarwal, M.; Shen, W.; Wildman, S.A.; Janetka, J.W. Inhibitors of HGFA, matriptase, and hepsin serine proteases: A nonkinase strategy to block cell signaling in Cancer. *ACS Med. Chem. Lett.* **2014**, *5*, 1219–2124. [CrossRef]
111. Franco, F.M.; Jones, D.E.; Harris, P.K.; Han, Z.; Wildman, S.A.; Jarvis, C.M.; Janetka, J.W. Structure-based discovery of small molecule hepsin and HGFA protease inhibitors: Evaluation of potency and selectivity derived from distinct binding pockets. *Bioorg. Med. Chem.* **2015**, *23*, 2328–2343. [CrossRef]
112. Han, Z.; Harris, P.K.; Karmakar, P.; Kim, T.; Owusu, B.Y.; Wildman, S.A.; Klampfer, L.; Janetka, J.W. α-Ketobenzothiazole serine protease inhibitors of aberrant HGF/c-MET and MSP/RON kinase pathway signaling in cancer. *ChemMedChem* **2016**, *11*, 585–599. [CrossRef] [PubMed]

113. Forbs, D.; Thiel, S.; Stella, M.C.; Sturzebecher, A.; Schweinitz, A.; Steinmetzer, T.; Stürzebecher, J.; Uhland, K. In vitro inhibition of matriptase prevents invasive growth of cell lines of prostate and colon carcinoma. *Int. J. Oncol.* **2005**, *27*, 1061–1070. [CrossRef] [PubMed]
114. Ustach, C.V.; Huang, W.; Conley-LaComb, M.K.; Lin, C.Y.; Che, M.; Abrams, J.; Kim, H.R. A novel signaling axis of matriptase/PDGF-D/ss-PDGFR in human prostate cancer. *Cancer Res* **2010**, *70*, 9631–9640. [CrossRef] [PubMed]

2

DNA-Methylation-Based Detection of Urological Cancer in Urine: Overview of Biomarkers and Considerations on Biomarker Design, Source of DNA and Detection Technologies

Louise Katrine Larsen [1], Guro Elisabeth Lind [2], Per Guldberg [1] and Christina Dahl [1,*]

[1] Danish Cancer Society Research Center, DK-2100 Copenhagen, Denmark; louisekl@cancer.dk (L.K.L.); perg@cancer.dk (P.G.)

[2] Department of Molecular Oncology, Institute for Cancer Research, Oslo University Hospital, the Norwegian Radium Hospital, NO-0424 Oslo, Norway; Guro.Elisabeth.Lind@rr-research.no

* Correspondence: chd@cancer.dk

Abstract: Changes in DNA methylation have been causally linked with cancer and provide promising biomarkers for detection in biological fluids such as blood, urine, and saliva. The field has been fueled by genome-wide characterization of DNA methylation across cancer types as well as new technologies for sensitive detection of aberrantly methylated DNA molecules. For urological cancers, urine is in many situations the preferred "liquid biopsy" source because it contains exfoliated tumor cells and cell-free tumor DNA and can be obtained easily, noninvasively, and repeatedly. Here, we review recent advances made in the development of DNA-methylation-based biomarkers for detection of bladder, prostate, renal, and upper urinary tract cancers, with an emphasis on the performance characteristics of biomarkers in urine. For most biomarkers evaluated in independent studies, there was great variability in sensitivity and specificity. We discuss issues that impact the outcome of DNA-methylation-based detection of urological cancer and account for the great variability in performance, including genomic location of biomarkers, source of DNA, and technical issues related to the detection of rare aberrantly methylated DNA molecules. Finally, we discuss issues that remain to be addressed to fully exploit the potential of DNA-methylation-based biomarkers in the clinic, including the need for prospective trials and careful selection of control groups.

Keywords: noninvasive detection; DNA methylation biomarkers; bisulfite conversion; urological cancer; bladder cancer; prostate cancer; upper urinary tract cancer; renal cancer

---

1. Introduction

Urological cancers encompass a clinically and molecularly heterogeneous group of neoplasms affecting any region of the urological system. Cancer of the bladder, kidneys, upper urinary tract (ureter and renal pelvis), and prostate are all relatively common and pose specific requirements for diagnosis and follow-up. While kidney and upper urinary tract cancers are detected using imaging techniques, standard work-up for bladder and prostate cancer involves semi-invasive procedures (i.e., cystoscopy and digital rectal examination (DRE), respectively). Cystoscopy is extensively used in clinical practice and poses a significant burden on the healthcare system because it is used as a first-line rule-out test for cancer in patients with relevant symptoms, primarily, hematuria. Other downsides include patient discomfort and anxiety, risk of infectious complications, and high rates of false-positive and false-negative results. Subsequent histopathological assessment of biopsy tissue and surgical resection specimens is the gold standard for cancer diagnosis but also has its limitations, including the subjective evaluation by a pathologist, the need for tissue that is of a certain quality and representative of the tumor, and constraints on sampling frequency. Given these challenges, there is a major unmet need to develop noninvasive methods that could provide clinicians with rapid, objective, and accurate routines for detection of urological cancers.

An important development in cancer care is "liquid biopsy", which involves the analysis of genetic material or tumor cells shed from primary or metastatic tumors into bodily fluids. A rapidly increasing number of studies have demonstrated the potential of liquid biopsies for a wide range of clinical applications, such as initial diagnosis, early detection, and disease monitoring after therapy [1]. Most of this work involves the analysis of cell-free DNA (cfDNA) circulating in the blood; however, for urological cancers, a more convenient liquid biopsy source is voided urine, which is easily and repeatably accessible and contains exfoliated cells and cfDNA from different sites of the urinary system [2]. The advent of high-sensitivity PCR-based technologies has enabled reliable detection of cancer-specific alterations in urine DNA. Because tumor-derived DNA in urine is often present in a large background of DNA derived from normal cells, the most useful DNA biomarkers are those that provide high specificity for malignancy or premalignancy, including mutations, translocations, gene fusions, and aberrant hypermethylation of specific CpG sites. Among these, DNA hypermethylation events represent the most versatile biomarker type because they are common in most cancers and can be easily assessed using well-established techniques. Furthermore, DNA methylation changes are considered early events in tumorigenesis and thus provide potential biomarkers for early diagnosis [3].

Urine-based DNA tests for urological cancer can be divided into two categories depending on the a priori availability of information on the patient's tumor DNA. For detection of recurrence and evaluation of treatment response, DNA from the original tumor can be analyzed to identify specific alterations that may serve as "personalized" biomarkers. For other applications, such as initial examination of patients with symptoms of urological cancer, the genetic and epigenetic makeup of the possible tumor is unknown. In these situations, there is a need for a "universal" or "generic" test that can detect, in principle, any cancer. Because no genetic or epigenetic alteration is present in all cases of a urological cancer type, it is necessary to use a combination of biomarkers. The initial assembly of a biomarker panel is facilitated by information about the performance characteristics of individual biomarkers in terms of sensitivity (the true positive rate), specificity (the true negative rate), and predictive values [4]. If the test is used in individuals with unknown disease status to reduce the use of invasive procedures, the most important performance characteristics are sensitivity and negative predictive value (NPV) to achieve the lowest possible rate of false-negative results. As discussed below, specificity is a less well-defined characteristic that varies based on a number of factors, including control populations and the definition of a false-positive result.

Although the promises of DNA-methylation-based detection of cancer have been recognized since the early 2000s [5], including the potential for detection and management of urological cancers [6], only a few DNA methylation biomarkers have been implemented into routine clinical practice. Navigating towards clinical utility is challenging, requiring optimal study designs (representative and large patient series) as well as robustly designed biomarker assays. Here, we provide an overview of current DNA-methylation-based biomarkers for urological cancer, with an emphasis on their performance characteristics in urine. We discuss potential causes of performance variability across studies and other challenges that must be overcome before clinically useful tests can be developed and implemented. Some of these issues have been discussed in detail elsewhere [7–9] and are only reviewed briefly here.

2. Performance Characteristics of DNA Methylation Biomarkers

To provide an overview of current DNA-methylation-based biomarkers for urine-based detection of urological cancer, we undertook systematic literature searches in PubMed and Embase until February 2019. Details on search strategy, criteria for selection of relevant studies, and data extraction are provided in Supplementary Methods.

2.1. Bladder Cancer

A total of 57 studies met the inclusion criteria (Supplementary Table S1). Fifty-two studies analyzed urine from bladder cancer patients at first diagnosis, using a total of 114 different DNA methylation biomarkers. The sensitivities for 23 biomarkers investigated in more than three studies are shown in Figure 1. Two of these biomarkers each reached a median sensitivity of >80% (*ZNF154* and *POU4F2*) with, however, large variability across studies. The specificities for these biomarkers are shown in Supplementary Figure S1, also demonstrating large interstudy variability. Fifty-two different biomarker combinations, comprising between 2 and 12 individual biomarkers, have been tested for initial diagnosis of bladder cancer. Twenty of these combinations achieved a sensitivity of ≥90% (listed in Table 1).

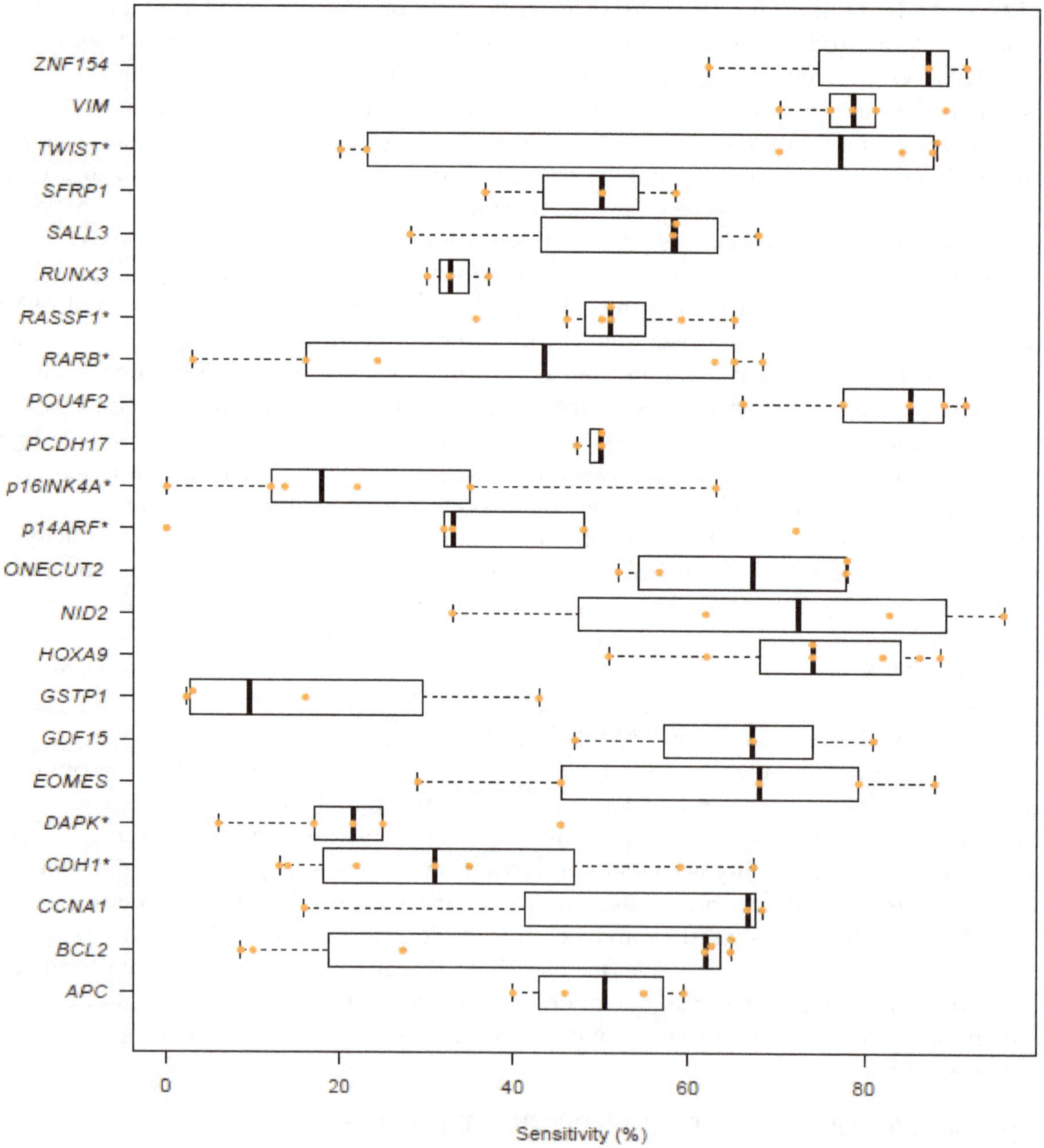

Figure 1. Reported sensitivities of DNA methylation biomarkers for detection of primary bladder cancer. *, Inconsistent nomenclature among studies.

Table 1. DNA-methylation biomarker panels for detection of primary bladder cancer.

Biomarker	Sample Processing	Cases (*n*)	Controls (*n*)	Pathology	Control Population	Method	Sens. (%)	Spec. (%)	Ref.	Year
SOX1, TJP2, MYOD, HOXA9_1, HOXA9_2, VAMP8, CASP8, SPP1, IFNG, CAPG, HLADPA1, RIPK3 (Positive when six or more markers are present)	Sedimentation	73	18	Ta-T4, Grade 1–3	Healthy	Pyrosequencing	100	100	[10]	2013
POU4F2, PCDH17, GDF15	Sedimentation	72	92	Ta-T4, LG, HG	Mixed urologic diseases and healthy	qMSP	97	75	[11]	2016
ZNF671, SFRP1, IRF8	Sedimentation	26	19	Ta-T4, LG, HG	Noncancer, not specified	qMSP	96	84	[12]	2015
POU4F2, EOMES	Sedimentation	72	92	Ta-T4, LG, HG	Mixed urologic diseases and healthy	qMSP	96	88	[11]	2016
TWIST1, NID2	Sedimentation	24	15	Ta-T3, LG, HG	Mixed urologic diseases, and healthy	MSP	96	93	[13]	2013
BCL2, EOMES, VIM, SALL3, CCNA1, HOXA9, POU4F2	Filtration (8 μm)	33	26	Ta-T2, LH, HG, PUNLMP	Mixed urologic diseases, negative findings	qMSP	94		[14]	2015
TWIST1, NID2	Sedimentation	35	57	Ta-T2, LG, HG	Mixed urologic diseases	qMSP	94	91	[15]	2010
VIM, TMEFF2, GDF15	Sedimentation	51	20	Not Specified	Healthy	qMSP	94	100	[16]	2010
VIM, TMEFF2, GDF15, HSPA2	Sedimentation	51	20	Not Specified	Healthy	qMSP	94	100	[16]	2010
SALL3, CFTR, ABCC6, HPR1, RASSF1A, MT1A, ALX4, CDH13, RPRM, MINT1, BRCA1	Sedimentation	132	23	Stage 0a-IV	Mixed urologic diseases	MSP	92	87	[17]	2007
SALL3, CFTR, MT1A, HPP1, ABCC6, RASSF1A, CDH13, RPRM, MINT1, BRCA1, SFRP1	Sedimentation	82	15	Stage pTa-IV	Mixed urologic diseases	MSP	92	73	[18]	2009
POU4F2, PCDH17	Sedimentation	58	90	Ta-T4, LG, HG	Mixed urologic diseases and healthy	qMSP	91	93	[11]	2016
POU4F2, PCDH17, GDF15	Sedimentation	58	90	Ta-T4, LG, HG	Mixed urologic diseases and healthy	qMSP	91	88	[11]	2016
p14ARF, p16INK4A, RASSF1A, DAPK, APC	Sedimentation	113		≥T1, PUNLMP, Grade 1–3	Healthy	MSP	91		[19]	2017
SEPTIN9, SLIT2	Filtration (11 μm)	167	105	Ta-T1 (NMIBC), LG, HG	Patients with negative cystoscopy (hematuria)	qMSP	91	71	[20]	2016
RARβ, DAPK, CDH1, p16	Sedimentation	22	17	NMIBC-MIBC, Grade 1–3	Healthy	MSP	91	76	[21]	2002

Table 1. *Cont.*

Biomarker	Sample Processing	Cases (*n*)	Controls (*n*)	Pathology	Control Population	Method	Sens. (%)	Spec. (%)	Ref.	Year
HOXA9, PCDH17, POU4F2, ONECUT2	Sedimentation	Not specified	Not specified	Ta-T4, LG, HG, PUNLMP	Mixed urologic diseases, hematuria	qMSP	91	73	[22]	2018
HS3ST2, SEPTIN9, SLIT2	Filtration (11 μm)	167	105	Ta-T1 (NMIBC), LG, HG	Patients with negative cystoscopy (hematuria)	qMSP	90	75	[20]	2016
HS3ST2, SLIT2	Filtration (11 μm)	167	105	Ta-T1 (NMIBC), LG, HG	Patients with negative cystoscopy (hematuria)	qMSP	90	34	[20]	2016
HS3ST2, SEPTIN9	Filtration (11 μm)	167	105	Ta-T1 (NMIBC), LG, HG	Patients with negative cystoscopy (hematuria)	qMSP	90	72	[20]	2016
SALL3, CFTR, MT1A, HPP1, ABCC6, RASSF1A, CDH13, RPRM, MINT1, BRCA1	Sedimentation	82	15	Stage Ta-IV	Mixed urologic diseases	MSP	90	80	[18]	2009
ONECUT2, VIM, SALL3, CCNA1, BCL2, EOMES	Filtration (8 μm)	99	376	Ta-T4, LG, HG, PUNLMP	Macroscopic hematuria, no malignancy	qMSP	90	89	[23]	2016

MSP = methylation-specific PCR, qMSP = quantitative MSP, HG = high grade, LG = low grade, PUNLMP = papillary urothelial neoplasm of low malignant potential, NMIBC = nonmuscle invasive bladder cancer, MIBC = muscle invasive bladder cancer.

Table 2. DNA-methylation biomarkers and biomarker panels for detection of recurrent bladder cancer.

Biomarker	Sample Processing	Cases (*n*)	Controls (*n*)	Pathology	Control Population	Method	Sens. (%)	Spec. (%)	Ref.	Year
APC	Sedimentation	15	25	Ta-T1	No recurrence	qMSP	27	80	[24]	2008
BCL2	Sedimentation	15	25	Ta-T1	No recurrence	qMSP	13	96		2008
DAPK	Sedimentation	15	25	Ta-T1	No recurrence	qMSP	0	96		2008
CDH1	Sedimentation	15	25	Ta-T1	No recurrence	qMSP	7	84		2008
EDNRB	Sedimentation	15	25	Ta-T1	No recurrence	qMSP	20	80		2008
EOMES	Sedimentation	139	67	Ta-T1, Grade 1–3	Mixed urologic diseases	qMSP	94	55	[25]	2012
HOXA9	Sedimentation	139	67	Ta-T1, Grade 1–3	Mixed urologic diseases	qMSP	93	55		2012
IGFBP	Sedimentation	15	25	Ta-T1	No recurrence	qMSP	20	84	[24]	2008
MGMT	Sedimentation	15	25	Ta-T1	No recurrence	qMSP	20	92		2008
NID2		48	275	Ta-T3, Grade 1–3	No recurrence	MSP	46	90	[26]	2012
POU4F2	Sedimentation	139	67	Ta-T1, Grade 1–3	Mixed urologic diseases	qMSP	88	64	[25]	2012
RASSF1A	Sedimentation	15	25	Ta-T1	No recurrence	qMSP	50	32	[24]	2008
TERT	Sedimentation	15	25	Ta-T1	No recurrence	qMSP	13	100		2008
TNFRSF25	Sedimentation	15	25	Ta-T1	No recurrence	qMSP	40	56		2008
TWIST1	Sedimentation	139	67	Ta-T1, Grade 1–3	Mixed urologic diseases	qMSP	90	43	[25]	2012
TWIST1		48	275	Ta-T3, Grade 1–3	No recurrence	MSP	75	69	[26]	2012
VIM	Sedimentation	139	67	Ta-T1, Grade 1–3	Mixed urologic diseases	qMSP	90	59	[25]	2012
WIF1	Sedimentation	15	25	Ta-T1	No recurrence	qMSP	20	76	[24]	2008
ZNF154	Sedimentation	139	67	Ta-T1, Grade 1–3	Mixed urologic diseases	qMSP	94	67	[25]	2012
APC_a, TERT_a, TERT_b, EDNRB	Sedimentation	65	29	Ta-T4, Grade 0–3	No recurrence	MS-MLPA	72	55	[27]	2012
APC_a, TERT_a, TERT_b, EDNRB	Sedimentation	49	60	Ta-T1, Grade 1–3	No recurrence	MS-MLPA	63	58		2012
APC_a, TERT_a, TERT_b, EDNRB	Sedimentation	68	91	Ta-T1, Grade 1–3	No BC	MS-MLPA				2012
CFTR, SALL3, TWIST1	Sedimentation	173	285	Ta-T1	Ta-T1	Pyrosequencing	90	31	[28]	2018
HS3ST2, SLIT2, SEPTIN9	Filtration (11 μm)	72	86	Ta-T4, LG, HG	Ta-T4, LG, HG	qMSP			[20]	2016
miR-9-3, miR124-2, miR-124-3, miR-137	Sedimentation	25	107	Ta-T1	No recurrence	Pyrosequencing	62	74	[29]	2018
OTX1, ONECUT2, OSR1	Sedimentation	95	40	NMIBC, Grade 1–3, (recurrence)	No recurrence	SNaPshot	74	Fixed = 90%	[30]	2013
Panel consisting of 41 sequences	Sedimentation	136		≥Ta, LG, HG	Mixed urologic diseases, and healthy	MS-MLPA			[31]	2013
RASSF1A, ECAD, APC, DAPK, MGMT, BCL2, TERT, EDNRB, WIF1, TNFRSF25. IGFBP	Sedimentation	15	25	Ta-T1	No recurrence	qMSP	86	8	[24]	2008
SOX1, IRAK3, L1-MET (*L1-MET* hypomethylated)	Sedimentation	29	54	Ta-T1, LG, HG	Ta-T1, LG, HG	Pyrosequencing	86	89	[32]	2014
SOX1, IRAK3, L1-MET (*L1-MET* hypomethylated)	Sedimentation	134	25	Ta-T1, LG, HG	Ta-T1, LG, HG	Pyrosequencing	80	97		2014

MSP = methylation specific PCR, qMSP = quantitative MSP, HG = high grade, LG = low grade, NMIBC = nonmuscle invasive bladder cancer, BC = bladder cancer, MS-MLPA = methylation-specific multiplex ligation-dependent probe amplification.

Eleven studies investigated recurrent bladder cancer, using 18 individual biomarkers and 8 biomarker panels (Table 2). *ZNF154* and *EOMES* achieved the highest sensitivity (94%), however with a specificity of <70%. The biomarker combination with the highest sensitivity (*CFTR*, *SALL3*, and *TWIST1*; 90%) had a very low specificity (31%). Only one individual biomarker (*TWIST1*) and two panels have been evaluated in more than one study.

2.2. Prostate Cancer

Twenty-seven studies met the inclusion criteria (Supplementary Table S2). Of these, 26 studies contained data on single biomarker performance (48 different biomarkers), with 9 biomarkers tested in 2 or more studies (shown in Figure 2). *GSTP1* was the most extensively studied biomarker (19 studies). The highest median sensitivity was reported for *HOXD3* (76%); most other biomarkers had sensitivities of <50%. The corresponding specificities for these biomarkers are shown in Supplementary Figure S2. Fifteen studies combined two or more biomarkers, with five studies achieving a sensitivity of ≥90% (Table 3).

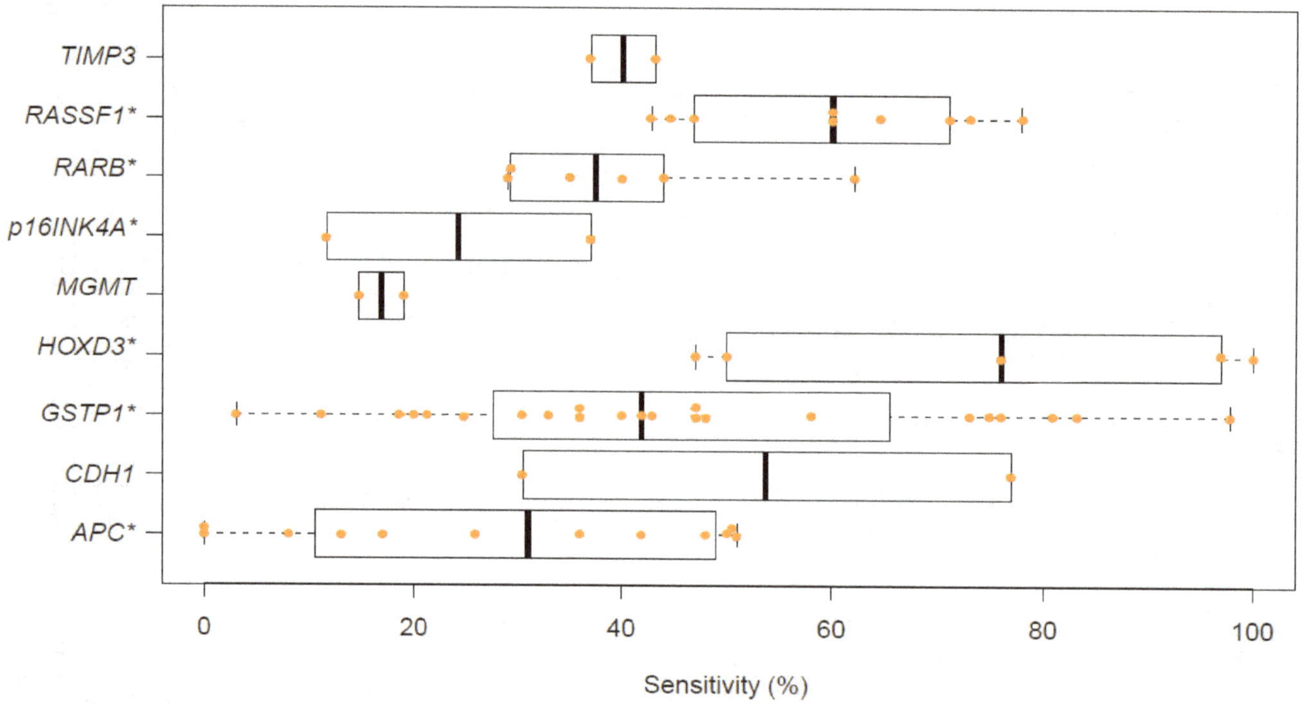

Figure 2. Reported sensitivities of DNA methylation biomarkers for detection of prostate cancer. *, Inconsistent nomenclature among studies.

2.3. Renal Cancer

Five studies met the inclusion criteria (Table 4). Data on single biomarkers were available from four studies for 15 different biomarkers, with sensitivities between 5% and 79% and a generally high specificity (89–100%). *TCF21* was the only biomarker tested in more than one study. Both studies achieved 100% specificity, but the sensitivity varied from 28% to 79%. Three studies evaluated biomarker combinations, with the best performing combination (*VHL*, *p16*, *ARF*, *APC*, *RASSF1A*, and *TIMP3*) achieving a sensitivity of 88% and a specificity of 100%. A similar sensitivity was reported by combining nine biomarkers (*APC*, *ARF*, *CDH1*, *GSTP1*, *MGMT*, *p16*, *RARB2*, *RASSF1A*, and *TIMP3*), with no indication of specificity.

Table 3. DNA-methylation biomarker panels for detection of prostate cancer.

Biomarkers	Urine Collection	Sample Processing	Cancer (*n*)	Controls (*n*)	Pathology	Control Population	Method	Sens. (%)	Spec. (%)	Ref.	Year
GSTP1, RARβ2, APC, miR-34b/c + miR-193b	Morning	Sedimentation	87	32	T2-T3b	Asymptomatic donors	qMSP	100	75	[33]	2018
TGFB2, HOXD3, APC	Post DRE	Sedimentation	10	5	Organ confined	Cancer free (not further specified)	qMSP	100	60	[34]	2014
EDNRB, APC, GSTP1	Post DRE/biopsy	Sedimentation	12	5	GS 6–7	Biopsy Negative	MSP	100	40	[35]	2006
miR-34b/c + miR-193b	Morning	Sedimentation	87	32	T2-T3b	Asymptomatic donors	qMSP	95	84	[33]	2018
GSTP1, RARβ2, APC	Morning	Sedimentation	87	32	T2-T3b	Asymptomatic donors	qMSP	94	84		2018
≥6 positive of 19 markers	First Void	Sedimentation	32	35	GS 6–10	Negative biopsy results	Nested qMSP	94	71	[36]	2018
miR-34b/c + miR-193b	No DRE	Sedimentation	95	46	GS ≥ 6	No urological malignancy, healthy	qMSP	91	98	[37]	2017

MSP = methylation specific PCR, qMSP = quantitative MSP, DRE = digital rectal examination, GS = Gleason score.

Table 4. DNA-methylation biomarkers and biomarker panels for detection of renal cancer.

Biomarker	Sample Processing	Cancer (*n*)	Controls (*n*)	Pathology	Control Population	Method	Sens. (%)	Spec. (%)	Ref.	Year
APC	Sedimentation	26	91	Not specified	Various conditions, malignant and nonmalignant	qMSP	38	96	[38]	2004
ARF	Sedimentation	26	91	Not specified	Various conditions, malignant and nonmalignant	qMSP	31	100		2004
CDH1	Sedimentation	26	91	Not specified	Various conditions, malignant and nonmalignant	qMSP	38	95		2004
GDF15	Sedimentation	19	20	Not specified	Healthy	qMSP	5	100	[16]	2010
GSTP1	Sedimentation	26	91	Not specified	Various conditions, malignant and nonmalignant	qMSP	15	100	[38]	2004
HSPA2	Sedimentation	19	20	Not specified	Healthy	qMSP	11	100	[16]	2010
MGMT	Sedimentation	26	91	Not specified	Various conditions, malignant and nonmalignant	qMSP	8	100	[38]	2004
p16	Sedimentation	26	91	Not specified	Various conditions, malignant and nonmalignant	qMSP	35	100		2004
PCDH17	Sedimentation	50	48	Not specified	Healthy	qMSP	20	100	[39]	2011

Table 4. *Cont.*

Biomarker	Sample Processing	Cancer (*n*)	Controls (*n*)	Pathology	Control Population	Method	Sens. (%)	Spec. (%)	Ref.	Year
RARB2	Sedimentation	26	91	Not specified	Various conditions, malignant and nonmalignant	qMSP	31	91	[38]	2004
RASSF1A	Sedimentation	26	91	Not specified	Various conditions, malignant and nonmalignant	qMSP	65	89		2004
TCF21	Sedimentation	33	15	Grades I–IV	Healthy	Pyrosequencing	79	100	[40]	2016
TCF21	Sedimentation	50	48	Not specified	Healthy	qMSP	28	100	[39]	2011
TIMP3	Sedimentation	26	91	Not specified	Various conditions, malignant and nonmalignant	qMSP	46	91	[38]	2004
TMEFF2	Sedimentation	19	20	Not specified	Healthy	qMSP	11	100	[16]	2010
VIM	Sedimentation	19	20	Not specified	Healthy	qMSP	5	100		2010
PCDH17, TCF21	Sedimentation	50	48	Not specified	Healthy	qMSP	32	100	[39]	2011
APC, ARF, CDH1, GSTP1, MGMT, P16, RAR-β2, RASSF1A, TIMP3	Sedimentation	26	91	Not specified	Various conditions, malignant and nonmalignant	qMSP	88		[38]	2004
VHL, p16/cdkn2a, p14ARF, APC, RASSF1A, Timp-3	Sedimentation	50	24	T1–T3	Healthy, renal stones, benign renal cysts	MSP	88	100	[41]	2004

MSP = methylation specific PCR, qMSP = quantitative MSP.

Table 5. DNA methylation biomarkers and biomarker panels for detection of upper urinary tract tumors.

Biomarkers	Sample Processing	Cancer (*n*)	Controls (*n*)	Pathology	Control Population	Method	Sens. (%)	Spec. (%)	Ref	Year
ABCC6	Sedimentation	98	113	Not specified	Benign urologic conditions	MSP	44	54		2018
BRCA1	Sedimentation	98	113	Not specified	Benign urologic conditions	MSP	26	58		2018
CDH1	Sedimentation	98	113	Not specified	Benign urologic conditions	MSP	28	98		2018
GDF15	Sedimentation	98	113	Not specified	Benign urologic conditions	MSP	30	90		2018
HSPA2	Sedimentation	98	113	Not specified	Benign urologic conditions	MSP	83	36	[42]	2018
RASSF1A	Sedimentation	98	113	Not specified	Benign urologic conditions	MSP	48	73		2018
SALL3	Sedimentation	98	113	Not specified	Benign urologic conditions	MSP	23	80		2018
THBS1	Sedimentation	98	113	Not specified	Benign urologic conditions	MSP	74	25		2018
TMEFF2	Sedimentation	98	113	Not specified	Benign urologic conditions	MSP	67	40		2018
VIM	Sedimentation	98	113	Not specified	Benign urologic conditions	MSP	73	61		2018
VIM	Sedimentation	22	20	Not specified	Healthy	qMSP	82	100	[43]	2014
CDH1, VIM	Sedimentation	98	113	Not specified	Benign urologic conditions	MSP	82	60		2018
CDH1, VIM, RASSF1A	Sedimentation	98	113	Not specified	Benign urologic conditions	MSP	82	60		2018
CDH1, VIM, RASSF1A, HSPA2	Sedimentation	98	113	Not specified	Benign urologic conditions	MSP	85	59		2018
CDH1, VIM, RASSF1A, HSPA2, GDF15	Sedimentation	98	113	Not specified	Benign urologic conditions	MSP	82	65	[42]	2018
CDH1, VIM, RASSF1A, HSPA2, GDF15, TMEFF2	Sedimentation	98	113	Not specified	Benign urologic conditions	MSP	82	68		2018
VIM, GDF15	Sedimentation	22	20	Papillary, invasive, LG, HG	Healthy, renal cell carcinoma, prostate carcinoma	qMSP	91	100	[43]	2014
VIM, GDF15, TMEFF2	Sedimentation	22	20	Papillary, invasive, LG, HG	Healthy, renal cell carcinoma, prostate carcinoma	qMSP	91	100		2014

MSP = methylation specific PCR, qMSP = quantitative MSP, HG = high grade, LG = low grade.

2.4. Upper Urinary Tract Cancer

Only two studies met the inclusion criteria, investigating a total of 10 biomarkers (Table 5). *VIM* was the only biomarker investigated in both studies, achieving a sensitivity of 82% and 73% and a specificity of 100% and 61%. *HSPA2* achieved a sensitivity of 83% but with a specificity of only 36%. Among seven biomarker combinations tested, a combination of *VIM* and *GDF15* reached a sensitivity of 91% and a specificity of 100% in a study with 22 cases and 20 healthy controls, whereas in a study with 98 cases and 113 controls with benign urologic conditions, these two biomarkers in combination with *CDH1*, *RASSF1A*, and *HSPA2* only reached a sensitivity of 82% and a specificity of 65%.

3. Factors Affecting Biomarker Performance

The overall conclusion from our review of DNA-methylation-based biomarkers for detection of urological cancer is that there is great variability in sensitivity and specificity across studies. Below, we discuss clinical and technical factors, which can explain this variability and should be considered when designing studies that eventually should lead to the implementation of urine-based tests in the clinic.

3.1. Urine Collection and Processing

Urine is a complex biological fluid that contains inorganic salts, organic compounds, and multiple cell types, including leukocytes, urothelial cells, renal cells, and prostate cells. Tumor-derived DNA can be present in both the cellular and cell-free fractions of urine, and the procedures used for collection and processing of DNA will greatly impact the outcome of biomarker analysis. Several sources of DNA have been utilized, including (i) whole urine (containing cellular DNA and cfDNA), (ii) urine sediment obtained by centrifugation (containing cellular DNA), (iii) urine supernatant (containing cfDNA), and (iv) cells obtained by immune capture [44] or filtration [14,45,46]. Because cells and DNA in urine are susceptible to degradation upon storage depending on time and temperature, correct storage is important when urine samples are not processed immediately. One study found that DNA in urine stored at room temperature was stable only upon addition of preserving agents but also found that DNA remained stable without the addition of preservatives for up to 28 days when stored at −20 °C or −80 °C [47]. A confounding factor in many studies is that samples containing DNA of insufficient quantity or quality were excluded from analysis. Such sample selection bias may lead to an overestimation of performance characteristics.

The vast majority of studies included in this review utilized sedimented urine as the source of DNA. The procedure for collection of urine sediments is simple and inexpensive but has several limitations in addition to storage challenges and processing time, including the co-sedimentation of normal cells and the presence of crystals and substances that may inhibit downstream PCR analyses [48]. A recent study showed that the sensitivity for detection of bladder cancer using *TERT* promoter mutations as a biomarker was higher in sedimented samples compared with cfDNA [2]. However, in leukocyte-rich urine, the sensitivity was higher in cfDNA using next-generation sequencing (NGS), probably because of a higher ratio of tumor-to-wildtype DNA compared with urine sediments. An alternative approach to enriching for tumor DNA is size-based cell selection, utilizing a filter with a pore size that enables capture of tumor cells with the passage of smaller-sized normal cells, at the same time removing inhibitory substances. One study comparing sedimentation and filtration of urine samples from patients with bladder cancer showed a higher sensitivity for filtration, particularly for low-grade tumors [46].

Another factor that should be considered when designing urine-based assays for urological cancer is that the concentrations of cells and DNA in urine are not constant. Shedding of cells and release of DNA through apoptosis or necrosis are stochastic and depend on several factors, including the size and location of the tumor. In prostate cancer, higher sensitivities have been achieved after physical manipulation of the prostate, such as massage and DRE. Another approach to increase the sensitivity is repeated urine sampling. In a study of men with high-grade prostate cancer, analysis of urine cells collected by filtration on different days without prior DRE showed a great interday variation in the presence of DNA methylation biomarkers, with some samples giving a false-negative result [49]. A study of patients with small low-grade bladder tumors showed that analysis of pooled urine samples collected over 24 h resulted in a sensitivity of 100%, whereas it was only 75% when a single urine sample was analyzed [50].

3.2. Bisulfite Treatment, Detection Technologies, and Sample Scoring

With few exceptions, the studies included in this review used treatment of DNA with sodium bisulfite to selectively convert unmethylated cytosines to uracil (leaving methylated cytosines as cytosine). These methylation-dependent C-to-U changes can subsequently be analyzed using PCR-based technologies to ascertain the methylation status [50]. Although the basic protocol for bisulfite conversion is simple and well described, it has a number of limitations that can introduce biases. Treatment of DNA with bisulfite introduces DNA strand breaks and results in highly fragmented single-stranded DNA, leading to degradation of up to 90% of the input DNA [51] and severely reducing the number of molecules effectively available for PCR amplification. The loss of DNA may be further aggravated by incomplete DNA recovery after bisulfite conversion. Recovery depends on the length of input DNA, with higher recovery for high-molecular-weight DNA. In urine, cfDNA has a large component of mononucleosomal (178 bp) DNA, posing specific requirements for extraction procedures [52]. Another limitation inherent to bisulfite treatment is incomplete conversion, which may lead to false-positive results because unconverted unmethylated CpG sites are falsely interpreted as methylated. A comparison of 12 commercially available bisulfite conversion kits showed a large variability in recovery and conversion efficiency [53]. Furthermore, several factors have been shown to affect the technical variability of PCR-based analysis of bisulfite-treated DNA, including the amount of bisulfite-converted template in the PCR, the amount of DNA input in the bisulfite conversion, and storage (bisulfite-converted DNA is less stable than genomic DNA) [54].

A wide range of PCR methods have been used for downstream biomarker evaluation. The most frequently used methods are methylation-specific PCR (MSP) and quantitative MSP (qMSP). Conventional MSP [55] was the method of choice in earlier studies but has also been used in more recent studies. This method is easy to perform and requires no specialized equipment but has several limitations, including the qualitative readout. The most frequently used method in more recent studies is qMSP based on the MethyLight technology [56], which provides a semiquantitative readout. Other methods include pyrosequencing [55], methylation-sensitive single nucleotide primer extension (MS-SnuPE) [57], methylation-sensitive high-resolution melting (MS-HRM) [58], and methylation-specific multiplex ligation-dependent probe amplification (MS-MLPA). [59] A systematic evaluation and comparison of assays for measuring DNA methylation at specific CpG sites was recently conducted by the BLUEPRINT Consortium [60]. Most methods performed well in distinguishing methylated from unmethylated DNA but all had limitations in detecting low-abundant molecules. It is likely that the field will be markedly advanced with the introduction of newer technologies such as NGS and digital PCR, which enable DNA quantification with superior sensitivity and accuracy.

A general limitation in most studies reviewed here was the lack of information about assay performance in terms of limit of blank (LoB), limit of detection (LoD), and limit of quantitation (LoQ), which are critical parameters describing the smallest concentration of a biomarker that can be reliably measured [61]. In most cases, there were no predefined thresholds for interpreting assay signals, and several studies did not indicate the number of positive biomarkers required for scoring a sample positive.

3.3. Genomic Location of Biomarker Assays

The most commonly used strategy to identify and develop new DNA methylation biomarkers is targeting functionally relevant locations, such as CpG islands where methylation affects gene expression.

The three biomarkers *TWIST1*, *OTX1*, and *ONECUT2* included in the commercial AssureMDx test, evaluating the risk for bladder cancer in patients with hematuria, are examples of this [11]. Whereas the biomarker for *TWIST1* is located in the gene promoter and associated with loss of gene expression, the assays for *OTX1* and *ONECUT2* are located in regions associated with increased gene expression [8].

Detailed promoter methylation studies have demonstrated that some CpG sites may influence gene expression more than others. This was first shown in 2002, when Deng et al. reported that methylation of CpG sites in a proximal region of *MHL1* was associated with lack of expression, whereas CpG sites in the distal part of the promoter tended to be methylated independently of MLH1 expression [62]. Designing biomarker assays close to the transcription start site generally increases the likelihood of hitting a location where the DNA methylation status will have a functional effect.

Independent of whether DNA methylation is functionally important or not, detailed knowledge of the methylation pattern of the individual CpG sites (e.g., through TCGA data) in a genomic region of interest is useful prior to biomarker assay design. Methylation density may vary considerably within a genomic region, potentially affecting the sensitivity and specificity of a biomarker assay. From a biomarker perspective, CpG sites that most robustly separate cases from controls and reach the highest sensitivity and specificity (independent of functional effect) would be highly attractive.

3.4. Sensitivity, Specificity, and Control Populations

Most DNA methylation biomarkers reviewed here were originally discovered by analysis of DNA from tumor biopsies, using adjacent tumor-free tissue or normal tissue as control. The sensitivity of a biomarker may here be defined as the proportion of tumors positive for this biomarker. However, a biomarker with high sensitivity in tumor tissue may not necessarily provide the same sensitivity in urine because this will depend on the shedding of tumor cells or cfDNA. Only a few studies have compared urine and tumor tissue from the same patients, suggesting that the sensitivity is generally lower in urine. As larger tumors will shed more material than smaller tumors, sensitivity is highly dependent on the cohort composition, with studies having a higher proportion of advanced cancers achieving higher sensitivity. Only a few studies have evaluated the sensitivity of biomarkers in large prospective studies enrolling patients consecutively and in an unbiased manner.

The specificity of a urinary DNA methylation biomarker is the probability of a negative test result in individuals without cancer. Based on the data compiled in this review, the specificity of DNA methylation biomarkers was relatively high in renal carcinoma (>90%) but generally lower in prostate cancer and recurrent bladder cancer. Although these figures may reflect a true difference in the ability of biomarkers to discriminate between cancer and no cancer, it is important to consider that specificity is affected by choice of control group. In the ideal situation, cases and controls should be age and sex matched. Notably, because epigenetic modifications (including DNA methylation) increase with age, the use of a non-age-matched control group could introduce significant bias. Another important factor is the clinical status of the control group. In many studies, including those on renal carcinoma, the control population consisted of healthy individuals. To evaluate the specificity of a test in a more realistic setting, the control population should consist of individuals with symptoms relevant for the specific cancer. Examples of such control groups include individuals with hematuria (in the case of bladder cancer) and increased prostate-specific antigen (PSA) levels (in the case of prostate cancer). One caveat here is that some patients with a positive urine test may have early cancers or precursor lesions that are molecularly detectable but still undetectable using current scanning or endoscopic procedures.

None of the biomarkers or biomarker panels for bladder cancer detected recurrence with a sensitivity or specificity of more than 90%, despite better performance of the same biomarkers for detection of primary bladder tumors [13]. The lower sensitivity may be explained by the fact that recurrent tumors are usually smaller than primary tumors and therefore are less prone to shed material into urine [13]. The lower specificity may at least in part be ascribed to challenges in the study design. While control groups for evaluating specificity at first diagnosis of bladder cancer are usually individuals with no prior history of bladder cancer, controls for recurrence are groups of patients showing negative follow-up cystoscopy. It is possible that these patients have residual DNA biomarkers in the urine due to incomplete tumor resection or the emergence of an as-yet undetectable recurrent tumor, thereby resulting in a lower specificity. Longitudinal studies where the patient is his/her own control may be more accurate, at least when it comes to the sensitivity.

4. Conclusions

Studies over more than a decade have demonstrated the great potential of DNA methylation biomarkers for urine-based detection of urological cancer. However, the bewildering number of biomarkers currently under evaluation and the great variability in biomarker performance across studies hamper successful translation into clinically useful tests. We have highlighted a number of factors, which directly impact the performance of urinary DNA methylation biomarkers, including technical issues related to the design and implementation of biomarker assays. Guidelines for these procedural issues should be clearly defined to ensure reproducibility and eventually facilitate the development of clinically useful urinary tests for urological cancer.

Author Contributions: Conceptualization, L.K.L, G.E.L., P.G., and C.D.; Methodology, L.K.L.; Formal Analysis, L.K.L. and C.D.; Writing–Original Draft Preparation, L.K.L., G.E.L., P.G., and C.D.; Writing—Review and Editing, L.K.L., G.E.L., P.G., and C.D.; Supervision, P.G.; Funding Acquisition, P.G.

References

1. Heitzer, E.; Haque, I.S.; Roberts, C.E.S.; Speicher, M.R. Current and future perspectives of liquid biopsies in genomics-driven oncology. *Nat. Rev. Genet.* **2019**, *20*, 71–88. [CrossRef]
2. Stasik, S.; Salomo, K.; Heberling, U.; Froehner, M.; Sommer, U.; Baretton, G.B.; Ehninger, G.; Wirth, M.P.; Thiede, C.; Fuessel, S. Evaluation of tert promoter mutations in urinary cell-free DNA and sediment DNA for detection of bladder cancer. *Clin. Biochem.* **2019**, *64*, 60–63. [CrossRef]
3. Baylin, S.B.; Jones, P.A. A decade of exploring the cancer epigenome—Biological and translational implications. *Nat. Rev. Cancer.* **2011**, *11*, 726–734. [CrossRef]
4. Trevethan, R. Sensitivity, specificity, and predictive values: Foundations, pliabilities, and pitfalls in research and practice. *Front Public Health* **2017**, *5*, 307. [CrossRef] [PubMed]
5. Laird, P.W. The power and the promise of DNA methylation markers. *Nat. Rev. Cancer* **2003**, *3*, 253–266. [CrossRef]
6. Cairns, P. Gene methylation and early detection of genitourinary cancer: The road ahead. *Nat. Rev. Cancer* **2007**, *7*, 531–543. [CrossRef] [PubMed]
7. Kandimalla, R.; van Tilborg, A.A.; Zwarthoff, E.C. DNA methylation-based biomarkers in bladder cancer. *Nat. Rev. Urol.* **2013**, *10*, 327–335. [CrossRef] [PubMed]
8. Koch, A.; Joosten, S.C.; Feng, Z.; de Ruijter, T.C.; Draht, M.X.; Melotte, V.; Smits, K.M.; Veeck, J.; Herman, J.G.; Van Neste, L.; et al. Analysis of DNA methylation in cancer: Location revisited. *Nat. Rev. Clin. Oncol.* **2018**, *15*, 459–466. [CrossRef] [PubMed]
9. Bosschieter, J.; Lutz, C.; Segerink, L.I.; Vis, A.N.; Zwarthoff, E.C.; van Moorselaar, R.J.A.; van Rhijn, B.W.; Heymans, M.W.; Jansma, E.P.; Steenbergen, R.D.; et al. The diagnostic accuracy of methylation markers in urine for the detection of bladder cancer: A systematic review. *Epigenomics* **2018**, *10*, 673–687. [CrossRef] [PubMed]
10. Chihara, Y.; Kanai, Y.; Fujimoto, H.; Sugano, K.; Kawashima, K.; Liang, G.; Jones, P.A.; Fujimoto, K.; Kuniyasu, H.; Hirao, Y. Diagnostic markers of urothelial cancer based on DNA methylation analysis. *BMC Cancer* **2013**, *13*, 275. [CrossRef]
11. Wang, Y.; Yu, Y.; Ye, R.; Zhang, D.; Li, Q.; An, D.; Fang, L.; Lin, Y.; Hou, Y.; Xu, A.; et al. An epigenetic biomarker combination of pcdh17 and pou4f2 detects bladder cancer accurately by methylation analyses of urine sediment DNA in han chinese. *Oncotarget* **2016**, *7*, 2754–2764. [CrossRef]

12. Yeh, C.M.; Chen, P.C.; Hsieh, H.Y.; Jou, Y.C.; Lin, C.T.; Tsai, M.H.; Huang, W.Y.; Wang, Y.T.; Lin, R.I.; Chen, S.S.; et al. Methylomics analysis identifies znf671 as an epigenetically repressed novel tumor suppressor and a potential non-invasive biomarker for the detection of urothelial carcinoma. *Oncotarget* **2015**, *6*, 29555–29572. [CrossRef]
13. Yegin, Z.; Gunes, S.; Buyukalpelli, R. Hypermethylation of twist1 and nid2 in tumor tissues and voided urine in urinary bladder cancer patients. *DNA Cell Biol.* **2013**, *32*, 386–392. [CrossRef]
14. Andersson, E.; Dahmcke, C.M.; Steven, K.; Larsen, L.K.; Guldberg, P. Filtration device for on-site collection, storage and shipment of cells from urine and its application to DNA-based detection of bladder cancer. *PLoS ONE* **2015**, *10*, e0131889. [CrossRef]
15. Renard, I.; Joniau, S.; van Cleynenbreugel, B.; Collette, C.; Naome, C.; Vlassenbroeck, I.; Nicolas, H.; de Leval, J.; Straub, J.; Van Criekinge, W.; et al. Identification and validation of the methylated twist1 and nid2 genes through real-time methylation-specific polymerase chain reaction assays for the noninvasive detection of primary bladder cancer in urine samples. *Eur. Urol.* **2010**, *58*, 96–104. [CrossRef]
16. Costa, V.L.; Henrique, R.; Danielsen, S.A.; Duarte-Pereira, S.; Eknaes, M.; Skotheim, R.I.; Rodrigues, A.; Magalhaes, J.S.; Oliveira, J.; Lothe, R.A.; et al. Three epigenetic biomarkers, gdf15, tmeff2, and vim, accurately predict bladder cancer from DNA-based analyses of urine samples. *Clin. Cancer Res.* **2010**, *16*, 5842–5851. [CrossRef]
17. Yu, J.; Zhu, T.; Wang, Z.; Zhang, H.; Qian, Z.; Xu, H.; Gao, B.; Wang, W.; Gu, L.; Meng, J.; et al. A novel set of DNA methylation markers in urine sediments for sensitive/specific detection of bladder cancer. *Clin. Cancer Res.* **2007**, *13*, 7296–7304. [CrossRef]
18. Sun, J.; Chen, Z.; Zhu, T.; Yu, J.; Ma, K.; Zhang, H.; He, Y.; Luo, X.; Zhu, J. Hypermethylated sfrp1, but none of other nine genes "informative" for western countries, is valuable for bladder cancer detection in mainland china. *J. Cancer Res. Clin. Oncol.* **2009**, *135*, 1717–1727. [CrossRef]
19. Pietrusinski, M.; Kepczynski, L.; Jedrzejczyk, A.; Borkowska, E.; Traczyk-Borszynska, M.; Constantinou, M.; Kauzewski, B.; Borowiec, M. Detection of bladder cancer in urine sediments by a hypermethylation panel of selected tumor suppressor genes. *Cancer Biomark.* **2017**, *18*, 47–59. [CrossRef]
20. Roperch, J.P.; Grandchamp, B.; Desgrandchamps, F.; Mongiat-Artus, P.; Ravery, V.; Ouzaid, I.; Roupret, M.; Phe, V.; Ciofu, C.; Tubach, F.; et al. Promoter hypermethylation of hs3st2, septin9 and slit2 combined with fgfr3 mutations as a sensitive/specific urinary assay for diagnosis and surveillance in patients with low or high-risk non-muscle-invasive bladder cancer. *BMC Cancer* **2016**, *16*, 704. [CrossRef]
21. Chan, M.W.; Chan, L.W.; Tang, N.L.; Tong, J.H.; Lo, K.W.; Lee, T.L.; Cheung, H.Y.; Wong, W.S.; Chan, P.S.; Lai, F.M.; et al. Hypermethylation of multiple genes in tumor tissues and voided urine in urinary bladder cancer patients. *Clin. Cancer Res.* **2002**, *8*, 464–470. [PubMed]
22. Wu, Y.; Jiang, G.; Zhang, N.; Liu, S.; Lin, X.; Perschon, C.; Zheng, S.L.; Ding, Q.; Wang, X.; Na, R.; et al. Hoxa9, pcdh17, pou4f2, and onecut2 as a urinary biomarker combination for the detection of bladder cancer in chinese patients with hematuria. *Eur. Urol. Focus* **2018**. [CrossRef] [PubMed]
23. Dahmcke, C.M.; Steven, K.E.; Larsen, L.K.; Poulsen, A.L.; Abdul-Al, A.; Dahl, C.; Guldberg, P. A prospective blinded evaluation of urine-DNA testing for detection of urothelial bladder carcinoma in patients with gross hematuria. *Eur. Urol.* **2016**, *70*, 916–919. [CrossRef] [PubMed]
24. Roupret, M.; Hupertan, V.; Yates, D.R.; Comperat, E.; Catto, J.W.; Meuth, M.; Lackmichi, A.; Ricci, S.; Lacave, R.; Gattegno, B.; et al. A comparison of the performance of microsatellite and methylation urine analysis for predicting the recurrence of urothelial cell carcinoma, and definition of a set of markers by bayesian network analysis. *BJU Int.* **2008**, *101*, 1448–1453. [CrossRef]
25. Reinert, T.; Borre, M.; Christiansen, A.; Hermann, G.G.; Orntoft, T.F.; Dyrskjot, L. Diagnosis of bladder cancer recurrence based on urinary levels of eomes, hoxa9, pou4f2, twist1, vim, and znf154 hypermethylation. *PLoS ONE* **2012**, *7*, e46297. [CrossRef] [PubMed]
26. Fernandez, C.A.; Millholland, J.M.; Zwarthoff, E.C.; Feldman, A.S.; Karnes, R.J.; Shuber, A.P. A noninvasive multi-analyte diagnostic assay: Combining protein and DNA markers to stratify bladder cancer patients. *Res. Rep. Urol.* **2012**, *4*, 17–26. [CrossRef]

27. Zuiverloon, T.C.; Beukers, W.; van der Keur, K.A.; Munoz, J.R.; Bangma, C.H.; Lingsma, H.F.; Eijkemans, M.J.; Schouten, J.P.; Zwarthoff, E.C. A methylation assay for the detection of non-muscle-invasive bladder cancer (nmibc) recurrences in voided urine. *BJU Int.* **2012**, *109*, 941–948. [CrossRef]
28. van der Heijden, A.G.; Mengual, L.; Ingelmo-Torres, M.; Lozano, J.J.; van Rijt-van de Westerlo, C.C.M.; Baixauli, M.; Geavlete, B.; Moldoveanud, C.; Ene, C.; Dinney, C.P.; et al. Urine cell-based DNA methylation classifier for monitoring bladder cancer. *Clin. Epigenetics* **2018**, *10*, 71. [CrossRef]
29. Shindo, T.; Shimizu, T.; Nojima, M.; Niinuma, T.; Maruyama, R.; Kitajima, H.; Kai, M.; Itoh, N.; Suzuki, H.; Masumori, N. Evaluation of urinary DNA methylation as a marker for recurrent bladder cancer: A 2-center prospective study. *Urology* **2018**, *113*, 71–78. [CrossRef]
30. Kandimalla, R.; Masius, R.; Beukers, W.; Bangma, C.H.; Orntoft, T.F.; Dyrskjot, L.; van Leeuwen, N.; Lingsma, H.; van Tilborg, A.A.; Zwarthoff, E.C. A 3-plex methylation assay combined with the fgfr3 mutation assay sensitively detects recurrent bladder cancer in voided urine. *Clin. Cancer Res.* **2013**, *19*, 4760–4769. [CrossRef]
31. Zuiverloon, T.C.; Beukers, W.; van der Keur, K.A.; Nieuweboer, A.J.; Reinert, T.; Dyrskjot, L.; Orntoft, T.F.; Zwarthoff, E.C. Combinations of urinary biomarkers for surveillance of patients with incident nonmuscle invasive bladder cancer: The european fp7 uromol project. *J. Urol.* **2013**, *189*, 1945–1951. [CrossRef] [PubMed]
32. Su, S.F.; de Castro Abreu, A.L.; Chihara, Y.; Tsai, Y.; Andreu-Vieyra, C.; Daneshmand, S.; Skinner, E.C.; Jones, P.A.; Siegmund, K.D.; Liang, G. A panel of three markers hyper- and hypomethylated in urine sediments accurately predicts bladder cancer recurrence. *Clin. Cancer Res.* **2014**, *20*, 1978–1989. [CrossRef] [PubMed]
33. Moreira-Barbosa, C.; Barros-Silva, D.; Costa-Pinheiro, P.; Torres-Ferreira, J.; Constancio, V.; Freitas, R.; Oliveira, J.; Antunes, L.; Henrique, R.; Jeronimo, C. Comparing diagnostic and prognostic performance of two-gene promoter methylation panels in tissue biopsies and urines of prostate cancer patients. *Clin. Epigenetics* **2018**, *10*, 132. [CrossRef] [PubMed]
34. Olkhov-Mitsel, E.; Zdravic, D.; Kron, K.; van der Kwast, T.; Fleshner, N.; Bapat, B. Novel multiplex methylight protocol for detection of DNA methylation in patient tissues and bodily fluids. *Sci. Rep.* **2014**, *4*, 4432. [CrossRef]
35. Rogers, C.G.; Gonzalgo, M.L.; Yan, G.; Bastian, P.J.; Chan, D.Y.; Nelson, W.G.; Pavlovich, C.P. High concordance of gene methylation in post-digital rectal examination and post-biopsy urine samples for prostate cancer detection. *J. Urol.* **2006**, *176*, 2280–2284. [CrossRef] [PubMed]
36. Brikun, I.; Nusskern, D.; Decatus, A.; Harvey, E.; Li, L.; Freije, D. A panel of DNA methylation markers for the detection of prostate cancer from fv and dre urine DNA. *Clin. Epigenetics* **2018**, *10*, 91. [CrossRef] [PubMed]
37. Torres-Ferreira, J.; Ramalho-Carvalho, J.; Gomez, A.; Menezes, F.D.; Freitas, R.; Oliveira, J.; Antunes, L.; Bento, M.J.; Esteller, M.; Henrique, R.; et al. Mir-193b promoter methylation accurately detects prostate cancer in urine sediments and mir-34b/c or mir-129-2 promoter methylation define subsets of clinically aggressive tumors. *Mol. Cancer* **2017**, *16*, 26. [CrossRef] [PubMed]
38. Hoque, M.O.; Begum, S.; Topaloglu, O.; Jeronimo, C.; Mambo, E.; Westra, W.H.; Califano, J.A.; Sidransky, D. Quantitative detection of promoter hypermethylation of multiple genes in the tumor, urine, and serum DNA of patients with renal cancer. *Cancer Res.* **2004**, *64*, 5511–5517. [CrossRef] [PubMed]
39. Costa, V.L.; Henrique, R.; Danielsen, S.A.; Eknaes, M.; Patricio, P.; Morais, A.; Oliveira, J.; Lothe, R.A.; Teixeira, M.R.; Lind, G.E.; et al. Tcf21 and pcdh17 methylation: An innovative panel of biomarkers for a simultaneous detection of urological cancers. *Epigenetics* **2011**, *6*, 1120–1130. [CrossRef]
40. Xin, J.; Xu, R.; Lin, S.; Xin, M.; Cai, W.; Zhou, J.; Fu, C.; Zhen, G.; Lai, J.; Li, Y.; et al. Clinical potential of tcf21 methylation in the diagnosis of renal cell carcinoma. *Oncol. Lett.* **2016**, *12*, 1265–1270. [CrossRef]
41. Battagli, C.; Uzzo, R.G.; Dulaimi, E.; De Caceres, I.I.; Krassenstein, R.; Al-Saleem, T.; Greenberg, R.E.; Cairns, P. Promoter hypermethylation of tumor suppressor genes in urine from kidney cancer patients. *Cancer Res.* **2003**, *63*, 8695–8699. [PubMed]
42. Dulaimi, E.; Uzzo, R.G.; Greenberg, R.E.; Al-Saleem, T.; Cairns, P. Detection of bladder cancer in urine by a tumor suppressor gene hypermethylation panel. *Clin. Cancer Res.* **2004**, *10*, 1887–1893. [CrossRef] [PubMed]

43. Friedrich, M.G.; Weisenberger, D.J.; Cheng, J.C.; Chandrasoma, S.; Siegmund, K.D.; Gonzalgo, M.L.; Toma, M.I.; Huland, H.; Yoo, C.; Tsai, Y.C.; et al. Detection of methylated apoptosis-associated genes in urine sediments of bladder cancer patients. *Clin. Cancer Res.* **2004**, *10*, 7457–7465. [CrossRef] [PubMed]
44. Macgregor-Ramiasa, M.; McNicholas, K.; Ostrikov, K.; Li, J.; Michael, M.; Gleadle, J.M.; Vasilev, K. A platform for selective immuno-capture of cancer cells from urine. *Biosens. Bioelectron.* **2017**, *96*, 373–380. [CrossRef] [PubMed]
45. Birkhahn, M.; Mitra, A.P.; Williams, A.J.; Barr, N.J.; Skinner, E.C.; Stein, J.P.; Skinner, D.G.; Tai, Y.C.; Datar, R.H.; Cote, R.J. A novel precision-engineered microfiltration device for capture and characterisation of bladder cancer cells in urine. *Eur. J. Cancer* **2013**, *49*, 3159–3168. [CrossRef]
46. Andersson, E.; Steven, K.; Guldberg, P. Size-based enrichment of exfoliated tumor cells in urine increases the sensitivity for DNA-based detection of bladder cancer. *PLoS ONE* **2014**, *9*, e94023. [CrossRef]
47. Bosschieter, J.; Bach, S.; Bijnsdorp, I.V.; Segerink, L.I.; Rurup, W.F.; van Splunter, A.P.; Bahce, I.; Novianti, P.W.; Kazemier, G.; van Moorselaar, R.J.A.; et al. A protocol for urine collection and storage prior to DNA methylation analysis. *PLoS ONE* **2018**, *13*, e0200906. [CrossRef]
48. Lin, S.Y.; Linehan, J.A.; Wilson, T.G.; Hoon, D.S.B. Emerging utility of urinary cell-free nucleic acid biomarkers for prostate, bladder, and renal cancers. *Eur. Urol. Focus* **2017**, *3*, 265–272. [CrossRef]
49. Larsen, L.K.; Jakobsen, J.S.; Abdul-Al, A.; Guldberg, P. Noninvasive detection of high grade prostate cancer by DNA methylation analysis of urine cells captured by microfiltration. *J. Urol.* **2018**, *200*, 749–757. [CrossRef]
50. Dahl, C.; Guldberg, P. DNA methylation analysis techniques. *Biogerontology* **2003**, *4*, 233–250. [CrossRef]
51. Grunau, C.; Clark, S.J.; Rosenthal, A. Bisulfite genomic sequencing: Systematic investigation of critical experimental parameters. *Nucleic Acids Res.* **2001**, *29*, E65. [CrossRef]
52. Russo, I.J.; Ju, Y.; Gordon, N.S.; Zeegers, M.P.; Cheng, K.K.; James, N.D.; Bryan, R.T.; Ward, D.G. Toward personalised liquid biopsies for urothelial carcinoma: Characterisation of ddpcr and urinary cfdna for the detection of the tert 228 g>a/t mutation. *Bladder Cancer* **2018**, *4*, 41–48. [CrossRef]
53. Worm Orntoft, M.B.; Jensen, S.O.; Hansen, T.B.; Bramsen, J.B.; Andersen, C.L. Comparative analysis of 12 different kits for bisulfite conversion of circulating cell-free DNA. *Epigenetics* **2017**, *12*, 626–636. [CrossRef]
54. Pharo, H.D.; Honne, H.; Vedeld, H.M.; Dahl, C.; Andresen, K.; Liestol, K.; Jeanmougin, M.; Guldberg, P.; Lind, G.E. Experimental factors affecting the robustness of DNA methylation analysis. *Sci. Rep.* **2016**, *6*, 33936. [CrossRef]
55. Tost, J.; Gut, I.G. DNA methylation analysis by pyrosequencing. *Nat. Protoc.* **2007**, *2*, 2265–2275. [CrossRef]
56. Eads, C.A.; Danenberg, K.D.; Kawakami, K.; Saltz, L.B.; Blake, C.; Shibata, D.; Danenberg, P.V.; Laird, P.W. Methylight: A high-throughput assay to measure DNA methylation. *Nucleic Acids Res.* **2000**, *28*, E32. [CrossRef]
57. Gonzalgo, M.L.; Jones, P.A. Rapid quantitation of methylation differences at specific sites using methylation-sensitive single nucleotide primer extension (ms-snupe). *Nucleic Acids Res.* **1997**, *25*, 2529–2531. [CrossRef]
58. Wojdacz, T.K.; Dobrovic, A. Methylation-sensitive high resolution melting (ms-hrm): A new approach for sensitive and high-throughput assessment of methylation. *Nucleic Acids Res.* **2007**, *35*, e41. [CrossRef]
59. Nygren, A.O.; Ameziane, N.; Duarte, H.M.; Vijzelaar, R.N.; Waisfisz, Q.; Hess, C.J.; Schouten, J.P.; Errami, A. Methylation-specific mlpa (ms-mlpa): Simultaneous detection of cpg methylation and copy number changes of up to 40 sequences. *Nucleic Acids Res.* **2005**, *33*, e128. [CrossRef]
60. consortium, B. Quantitative comparison of DNA methylation assays for biomarker development and clinical applications. *Nat. Biotechnol.* **2016**, *34*, 726–737. [CrossRef]
61. Armbruster, D.A.; Pry, T. Limit of blank, limit of detection and limit of quantitation. *Clin. Biochem. Rev.* **2008**, *29* (Suppl. 1), S49–S52.
62. Deng, G.; Peng, E.; Gum, J.; Terdiman, J.; Sleisenger, M.; Kim, Y.S. Methylation of hmlh1 promoter correlates with the gene silencing with a region-specific manner in colorectal cancer. *Br. J. Cancer* **2002**, *86*, 574–579. [CrossRef]
63. Fantony, J.J.; Longo, T.A.; Gopalakrishna, A.; Owusu, R.; Lance, R.S.; Foo, W.C.; Inman, B.A.; Abern, M.R. Urinary nid2 and twist1 methylation to augment conventional urine cytology for the detection of bladder cancer. *Cancer Biomark.* **2017**, *18*, 381–387. [CrossRef]

64. Sathyanarayana, U.G.; Maruyama, R.; Padar, A.; Suzuki, M.; Bondaruk, J.; Sagalowsky, A.; Minna, J.D.; Frenkel, E.P.; Grossman, H.B.; Czerniak, B.; et al. Molecular detection of noninvasive and invasive bladder tumor tissues and exfoliated cells by aberrant promoter methylation of laminin-5 encoding genes. *Cancer Res.* **2004**, *64*, 1425–1430. [CrossRef]
65. Urakami, S.; Shiina, H.; Enokida, H.; Kawakami, T.; Kawamoto, K.; Hirata, H.; Tanaka, Y.; Kikuno, N.; Nakagawa, M.; Igawa, M.; et al. Combination analysis of hypermethylated wnt-antagonist family genes as a novel epigenetic biomarker panel for bladder cancer detection. *Clin. Cancer Res.* **2006**, *12*, 2109–2116. [CrossRef]
66. Hoque, M.O.; Begum, S.; Topaloglu, O.; Chatterjee, A.; Rosenbaum, E.; Van Criekinge, W.; Westra, W.H.; Schoenberg, M.; Zahurak, M.; Goodman, S.N.; et al. Quantitation of promoter methylation of multiple genes in urine DNA and bladder cancer detection. *J. Natl. Cancer Inst.* **2006**, *98*, 996–1004. [CrossRef]
67. Yates, D.R.; Rehman, I.; Meuth, M.; Cross, S.S.; Hamdy, F.C.; Catto, J.W. Methylational urinalysis: A prospective study of bladder cancer patients and age stratified benign controls. *Oncogene* **2006**, *25*, 1984–1988. [CrossRef]
68. Bayramov, B.; Gunes, S.; Buyukalpelli, R.; Aydin, O.; Henkel, R. Promoter methylation analysis of cdh1 and p14arf genes in patients with urothelial bladder cancer. *Oncol. Targets* **2018**, *11*, 4189–4196. [CrossRef]
69. Guo, R.Q.; Xiong, G.Y.; Yang, K.W.; Zhang, L.; He, S.M.; Gong, Y.Q.; He, Q.; Li, X.Y.; Wang, Z.C.; Bao, Z.Q.; et al. Detection of urothelial carcinoma, upper tract urothelial carcinoma, bladder carcinoma, and urothelial carcinoma with gross hematuria using selected urine-DNA methylation biomarkers: A prospective, single-center study. *Urol. Oncol.* **2018**, *36*, 342.e315–342.e323. [CrossRef]
70. Mijnes, J.; Veeck, J.; Gaisa, N.T.; Burghardt, E.; de Ruijter, T.C.; Gostek, S.; Dahl, E.; Pfister, D.; Schmid, S.C.; Knuchel, R.; et al. Promoter methylation of DNA damage repair (ddr) genes in human tumor entities: Rbbp8/ctip is almost exclusively methylated in bladder cancer. *Clin. Epigenetics* **2018**, *10*, 15. [CrossRef]
71. Fantony, J.J.; Abern, M.R.; Gopalakrishna, A.; Owusu, R.; Jack Tay, K.; Lance, R.S.; Inman, B.A. Multi-institutional external validation of urinary twist1 and nid2 methylation as a diagnostic test for bladder cancer. *Urol. Oncol.* **2015**, *33*, 387.e381–387.e386. [CrossRef]
72. Maldonado, L.; Brait, M.; Michailidi, C.; Munari, E.; Driscoll, T.; Schultz, L.; Bivalacqua, T.; Schoenberg, M.; Sidransky, D.; Netto, G.J.; et al. An epigenetic marker panel for recurrence risk prediction of low grade papillary urothelial cell carcinoma (lgpucc) and its potential use for surveillance after transurethral resection using urine. *Oncotarget* **2014**, *5*, 5218–5233. [CrossRef]
73. Hayashi, M.; Bernert, H.; Kagohara, L.T.; Maldonado, L.; Brait, M.; Schoenberg, M.; Bivalacqua, T.; Netto, G.J.; Koch, W.; Sidransky, D.; et al. Epigenetic inactivation of vgf associated with urothelial cell carcinoma and its potential as a non-invasive biomarker using urine. *Oncotarget* **2014**, *5*, 3350–3361. [CrossRef]
74. Abern, M.R.; Owusu, R.; Inman, B.A. Clinical performance and utility of a DNA methylation urine test for bladder cancer. *Urol. Oncol.* **2014**, *32*, 51.e21–51.e26. [CrossRef]
75. Beukers, W.; Kandimalla, R.; van Houwelingen, D.; Kovacic, H.; Chin, J.F.; Lingsma, H.F.; Dyrskjot, L.; Zwarthoff, E.C. The use of molecular analyses in voided urine for the assessment of patients with hematuria. *PLoS ONE* **2013**, *8*, e77657. [CrossRef]
76. Garcia-Baquero, R.; Puerta, P.; Beltran, M.; Alvarez, M.; Sacristan, R.; Alvarez-Ossorio, J.L.; Sanchez-Carbayo, M. Methylation of a novel panel of tumor suppressor genes in urine moves forward noninvasive diagnosis and prognosis of bladder cancer: A 2-center prospective study. *J. Urol.* **2013**, *190*, 723–730. [CrossRef]
77. Scher, M.B.; Elbaum, M.B.; Mogilevkin, Y.; Hilbert, D.W.; Mydlo, J.H.; Sidi, A.A.; Adelson, M.E.; Mordechai, E.; Trama, J.P. Detecting DNA methylation of the bcl2, cdkn2a and nid2 genes in urine using a nested methylation specific polymerase chain reaction assay to predict bladder cancer. *J. Urol.* **2012**, *188*, 2101–2107. [CrossRef]
78. Karnes, R.J.; Fernandez, C.A.; Shuber, A.P. A noninvasive multianalyte urine-based diagnostic assay for urothelial cancer of the bladder in the evaluation of hematuria. *Mayo Clin. Proc.* **2012**, *87*, 835–842. [CrossRef]
79. Zhao, Y.; Guo, S.; Sun, J.; Huang, Z.; Zhu, T.; Zhang, H.; Gu, J.; He, Y.; Wang, W.; Ma, K.; et al. Methylcap-seq reveals novel DNA methylation markers for the diagnosis and recurrence prediction of bladder cancer in a chinese population. *PLoS ONE* **2012**, *7*, e35175. [CrossRef]
80. Eissa, S.; Zohny, S.F.; Shehata, H.H.; Hegazy, M.G.; Salem, A.M.; Esmat, M. Urinary retinoic acid receptor-beta2 gene promoter methylation and hyaluronidase activity as noninvasive tests for diagnosis of bladder cancer. *Clin. Biochem.* **2012**, *45*, 402–407. [CrossRef]

81. Reinert, T.; Modin, C.; Castano, F.M.; Lamy, P.; Wojdacz, T.K.; Hansen, L.L.; Wiuf, C.; Borre, M.; Dyrskjot, L.; Orntoft, T.F. Comprehensive genome methylation analysis in bladder cancer: Identification and validation of novel methylated genes and application of these as urinary tumor markers. *Clin. Cancer Res.* **2011**, *17*, 5582–5592. [CrossRef]
82. Eissa, S.; Swellam, M.; El-Khouly, I.M.; Kassim, S.K.; Shehata, H.; Mansour, A.; Esmat, M.; Nossier, A.I.; Hamdy, M.A.; Awad, N.M.; et al. Aberrant methylation of rarbeta2 and apc genes in voided urine as molecular markers for early detection of bilharzial and nonbilharzial bladder cancer. *Cancer Epidemiol. Biomark. Prev.* **2011**, *20*, 1657–1664. [CrossRef] [PubMed]
83. Chen, P.C.; Tsai, M.H.; Yip, S.K.; Jou, Y.C.; Ng, C.F.; Chen, Y.; Wang, X.; Huang, W.; Tung, C.L.; Chen, G.C.; et al. Distinct DNA methylation epigenotypes in bladder cancer from different chinese sub-populations and its implication in cancer detection using voided urine. *BMC Med. Genom.* **2011**, *4*, 45. [CrossRef] [PubMed]
84. Chung, W.; Bondaruk, J.; Jelinek, J.; Lotan, Y.; Liang, S.; Czerniak, B.; Issa, J.P. Detection of bladder cancer using novel DNA methylation biomarkers in urine sediments. *Cancer Epidemiol. Biomark. Prev.* **2011**, *20*, 1483–1491. [CrossRef]
85. Serizawa, R.R.; Ralfkiaer, U.; Steven, K.; Lam, G.W.; Schmiedel, S.; Schuz, J.; Hansen, A.B.; Horn, T.; Guldberg, P. Integrated genetic and epigenetic analysis of bladder cancer reveals an additive diagnostic value of fgfr3 mutations and hypermethylation events. *Int. J. Cancer* **2011**, *129*, 78–87. [CrossRef] [PubMed]
86. Vinci, S.; Giannarini, G.; Selli, C.; Kuncova, J.; Villari, D.; Valent, F.; Orlando, C. Quantitative methylation analysis of bcl2, htert, and dapk promoters in urine sediment for the detection of non-muscle-invasive urothelial carcinoma of the bladder: A prospective, two-center validation study. *Urol. Oncol.* **2011**, *29*, 150–156. [CrossRef]
87. Lin, H.H.; Ke, H.L.; Huang, S.P.; Wu, W.J.; Chen, Y.K.; Chang, L.L. Increase sensitivity in detecting superficial, low grade bladder cancer by combination analysis of hypermethylation of e-cadherin, p16, p14, rassf1a genes in urine. *Urol. Oncol.* **2010**, *28*, 597–602. [CrossRef]
88. Pu, R.T.; Laitala, L.E.; Clark, D.P. Methylation profiling of urothelial carcinoma in bladder biopsy and urine. *Acta Cytol.* **2006**, *50*, 499–506. [CrossRef]
89. Padrao, N.A.; Monteiro-Reis, S.; Torres-Ferreira, J.; Antunes, L.; Leca, L.; Montezuma, D.; Ramalho-Carvalho, J.; Dias, P.C.; Monteiro, P.; Oliveira, J.; et al. Microrna promoter methylation: A new tool for accurate detection of urothelial carcinoma. *Br. J. Cancer* **2017**, *116*, 634–639. [CrossRef]
90. Shimizu, T.; Suzuki, H.; Nojima, M.; Kitamura, H.; Yamamoto, E.; Maruyama, R.; Ashida, M.; Hatahira, T.; Kai, M.; Masumori, N.; et al. Methylation of a panel of microrna genes is a novel biomarker for detection of bladder cancer. *Eur. Urol.* **2013**, *63*, 1091–1100. [CrossRef]
91. van Kessel, K.E.; Van Neste, L.; Lurkin, I.; Zwarthoff, E.C.; Van Criekinge, W. Evaluation of an epigenetic profile for the detection of bladder cancer in patients with hematuria. *J. Urol.* **2016**, *195*, 601–607. [CrossRef]
92. Chan, M.W.; Chan, L.W.; Tang, N.L.; Lo, K.W.; Tong, J.H.; Chan, A.W.; Cheung, H.Y.; Wong, W.S.; Chan, P.S.; Lai, F.M.; et al. Frequent hypermethylation of promoter region of rassf1a in tumor tissues and voided urine of urinary bladder cancer patients. *Int. J. Cancer* **2003**, *104*, 611–616. [CrossRef]
93. Zhao, F.; Olkhov-Mitsel, E.; Kamdar, S.; Jeyapala, R.; Garcia, J.; Hurst, R.; Hanna, M.Y.; Mills, R.; Tuzova, A.V.; O'Reilly, E.; et al. A urine-based DNA methylation assay, procure, to identify clinically significant prostate cancer. *Clin. Epigenetics* **2018**, *10*, 147. [CrossRef]
94. Yao, L.; Ren, S.; Zhang, M.; Du, F.; Zhu, Y.; Yu, H.; Zhang, C.; Li, X.; Yang, C.; Liu, H.; et al. Identification of specific DNA methylation sites on the y-chromosome as biomarker in prostate cancer. *Oncotarget* **2015**, *6*, 40611–40621. [CrossRef]
95. Haluskova, J.; Lachvac, L.; Nagy, V. The investigation of gstp1, apc and rassf1 gene promoter hypermethylation in urine DNA of prostate-diseased patients. *Bratislava Lek Listy* **2015**, *116*, 79–82. [CrossRef]
96. Zhang, L.; Zhang, Q.; Li, L.; Wang, Z.; Ying, J.; Fan, Y.; He, Q.; Lv, T.; Han, W.; Li, J.; et al. Dlec1, a 3p tumor suppressor, represses nf-kappab signaling and is methylated in prostate cancer. *J. Mol. Med. (Berl.)* **2015**, *93*, 691–701. [CrossRef]
97. Daniunaite, K.; Jarmalaite, S.; Kalinauskaite, N.; Petroska, D.; Laurinavicius, A.; Lazutka, J.R.; Jankevicius, F. Prognostic value of rassf1 promoter methylation in prostate cancer. *J. Urol.* **2014**, *192*, 1849–1855. [CrossRef]
98. Dimitriadis, E.; Kalogeropoulos, T.; Velaeti, S.; Sotiriou, S.; Vassiliou, E.; Fasoulis, L.; Klapsas, V.; Synesiou, M.; Apostolaki, A.; Trangas, T.; et al. Study of genetic and epigenetic alterations in urine samples as diagnostic markers for prostate cancer. *Anticancer Res.* **2013**, *33*, 191–197.

99. Daniunaite, K.; Berezniakovas, A.; Jankevicius, F.; Laurinavicius, A.; Lazutka, J.R.; Jarmalaite, S. Frequent methylation of rassf1 and rarb in urine sediments from patients with early stage prostate cancer. *Medicina (Kaunas)* **2011**, *47*, 147–153.
100. Prior, C.; Guillen-Grima, F.; Robles, J.E.; Rosell, D.; Fernandez-Montero, J.M.; Agirre, X.; Catena, R.; Calvo, A. Use of a combination of biomarkers in serum and urine to improve detection of prostate cancer. *World J. Urol.* **2010**, *28*, 681–686. [CrossRef]
101. Payne, S.R.; Serth, J.; Schostak, M.; Kamradt, J.; Strauss, A.; Thelen, P.; Model, F.; Day, J.K.; Liebenberg, V.; Morotti, A.; et al. DNA methylation biomarkers of prostate cancer: Confirmation of candidates and evidence urine is the most sensitive body fluid for non-invasive detection. *Prostate* **2009**, *69*, 1257–1269. [CrossRef] [PubMed]
102. Woodson, K.; O'Reilly, K.J.; Hanson, J.C.; Nelson, D.; Walk, E.L.; Tangrea, J.A. The usefulness of the detection of gstp1 methylation in urine as a biomarker in the diagnosis of prostate cancer. *J. Urol.* **2008**, *179*, 508–511. [CrossRef]
103. Roupret, M.; Hupertan, V.; Yates, D.R.; Catto, J.W.; Rehman, I.; Meuth, M.; Ricci, S.; Lacave, R.; Cancel-Tassin, G.; de la Taille, A.; et al. Molecular detection of localized prostate cancer using quantitative methylation-specific pcr on urinary cells obtained following prostate massage. *Clin. Cancer Res.* **2007**, *13*, 1720–1725. [CrossRef] [PubMed]
104. Hoque, M.O.; Topaloglu, O.; Begum, S.; Henrique, R.; Rosenbaum, E.; Van Criekinge, W.; Westra, W.H.; Sidransky, D. Quantitative methylation-specific polymerase chain reaction gene patterns in urine sediment distinguish prostate cancer patients from control subjects. *J. Clin. Oncol.* **2005**, *23*, 6569–6575. [CrossRef] [PubMed]
105. Goessl, C.; Muller, M.; Heicappell, R.; Krause, H.; Straub, B.; Schrader, M.; Miller, K. DNA-based detection of prostate cancer in urine after prostatic massage. *Urology* **2001**, *58*, 335–338. [CrossRef]
106. Baden, J.; Green, G.; Painter, J.; Curtin, K.; Markiewicz, J.; Jones, J.; Astacio, T.; Canning, S.; Quijano, J.; Guinto, W.; et al. Multicenter evaluation of an investigational prostate cancer methylation assay. *J. Urol.* **2009**, *182*, 1186–1193. [CrossRef] [PubMed]
107. Vener, T.; Derecho, C.; Baden, J.; Wang, H.; Rajpurohit, Y.; Skelton, J.; Mehrotra, J.; Varde, S.; Chowdary, D.; Stallings, W.; et al. Development of a multiplexed urine assay for prostate cancer diagnosis. *Clin. Chem.* **2008**, *54*, 874–882. [CrossRef]
108. Gonzalgo, M.L.; Pavlovich, C.P.; Lee, S.M.; Nelson, W.G. Prostate cancer detection by gstp1 methylation analysis of postbiopsy urine specimens. *Clin. Cancer Res.* **2003**, *9*, 2673–2677.
109. Jeronimo, C.; Usadel, H.; Henrique, R.; Silva, C.; Oliveira, J.; Lopes, C.; Sidransky, D. Quantitative gstp1 hypermethylation in bodily fluids of patients with prostate cancer. *Urology* **2002**, *60*, 1131–1135. [CrossRef]
110. Goessl, C.; Muller, M.; Heicappell, R.; Krause, H.; Miller, K. DNA-based detection of prostate cancer in blood, urine, and ejaculates. *Ann. N. Y. Acad. Sci.* **2001**, *945*, 51–58. [CrossRef]
111. Dumache, R.; Popescu, S.; Minciu, R.; Negru, S.; Puiu, M. Molecular detection of prostate cancer by methylation-specific polymerase chain reaction from urine specimens. *J. Med. Biochem.* **2013**, *32*, 233–237. [CrossRef]

3

Angiogenesis Inhibition in Prostate Cancer

Chandrani Sarkar [1,2], Sandeep Goswami [1], Sujit Basu [1,2,3] and Debanjan Chakroborty [1,*]

1 Department of Pathology, Ohio State University, Columbus, OH 43210, USA; Chandrani.Sarkar@osumc.edu (C.S.); Sandeep.Goswami@osumc.edu (S.G.); Sujit.Basu@osumc.edu (S.B.)
2 Comprehensive Cancer Center, Ohio State University, Columbus, OH 43210, USA
3 Department of Medical Oncology, Ohio State University, Columbus, OH 43210, USA
* Correspondence: Debanjan.Chakroborty@osumc.edu

Abstract: Prostate cancer (PCa), like all other solid tumors, relies on angiogenesis for growth, progression, and the dissemination of tumor cells to other parts of the body. Despite data from in vitro and in vivo preclinical studies, as well as human specimen studies indicating the crucial role played by angiogenesis in PCa, angiogenesis inhibition in clinical settings has not shown significant benefits to patients, thus challenging the inclusion and usefulness of antiangiogenic agents for the treatment of PCa. However, one of the apparent reasons why these antiangiogenic agents failed to meet expectations in PCa can be due to the choice of the antiangiogenic agents, because the majority of these drugs target vascular endothelial growth factor-A (VEGFA) and its receptors. The other relevant causes might be inappropriate drug combinations, the duration of treatment, and the method of endpoint determination. In this review, we will first discuss the role of angiogenesis in PCa growth and progression. We will then summarize the different angiogenic growth factors that influence PCa growth dynamics and review the outcomes of clinical trials conducted with antiangiogenic agents in PCa patients and, finally, critically assess the current status and fate of antiangiogenic therapy in this disease.

Keywords: prostate cancer; angiogenesis; angiogenic growth factors; antiangiogenic therapy

1. Introduction

Prostate cancer (PCa) is the most commonly diagnosed non-skin cancer in the United States and the second major cause of cancer-related death in men [1]. Although nearly 80% of cases are diagnosed as localized diseases that can be cured by radiotherapy or surgery, there is relapse of the disease in 30–60% of patients [2,3]. Androgen deprivation therapy (ADT) is commonly used in PCa treatment to block the androgens required for cancer growth [4–6]. However, aggressive disease relapse frequently occurs following ADT, and the disease becomes castration-resistant prostate cancer (CRPC) [4–8]. Treatment and management thus pose a real challenge at this stage of the disease [7,8]. Advancement of clinical research over the last two decades, along with the approval of several targeted and immunomodulatory agents, together with chemotherapeutic agents such as docetaxel, prednisone, and mitoxantrone, have substantially changed the treatment landscape of metastatic CRPC (mCRPC). Although these agents have shown significant benefits to a percentage of patients, these benefits are short-lived [9–13]. Accordingly, there is a constant need to identify newer and better treatments that can be used alone or in combination with currently available therapies for better disease management and outcomes.

Angiogenesis, the sprouting of new blood vessels from pre-existing vessels, is essential for tumor growth and metastasis [14–17]. Inhibiting angiogenesis has emerged as an effective strategy for the treatment of many solid tumors [18–20]. Unlike other angiogenic solid tumors, the inhibition of angiogenesis in PCa did not meet the clinical expectations, thereby igniting concerns about its relevance in PCa progression [21–25]. However, several preclinical observations as well as studies involving patient samples and cell lines support and reinforce the importance of angiogenesis in PCa [21,23–25]. Based on our current knowledge and relevant reports in literature, we will here discuss the importance of angiogenesis in PCa and the relevance of antiangiogenic strategies for the management of this disease.

2. Angiogenesis and Tumor Progression

Angiogenesis, a multistep process tightly regulated by several stimulatory and inhibitory growth factors, is essential not only for normal physiological processes but also for abnormal conditions, such as tumor growth [14,15,22,26]. Tumor growth often depends on its ability to sustain adequate blood supply by newly formed blood vessels (neovessels), thus making angiogenesis a rate-limiting step [14–16,26,27]. Vascular endothelial growth factors (VEGFs) are the most prominent and well-studied proangiogenic factors associated with tumor growth, including PCa [15,22,25]. Other angiogenic factors, such as fibroblast growth factors (FGFs), angiopoietins (Ang), hepatocyte growth factor (HGF), epidermal growth factor (EGF), platelet-derived growth factor (PDGF), placental growth factor (PlGF), insulin-like growth factors (IGFs), tumor necrosis factor (TNF), interleukin-6 (IL-6), and lysophosphatidic acid (LPA), have also been mentioned in the literature [22,28]. The antiangiogenic factors include angiostatin, endostatin, platelet factor-4 (PF4), tissue inhibitors of metalloproteinases (TIMPs), interleukins (ILs), and interferons (IFs) [22,25]. The neovessels formed during tumorigenesis differ from normal vasculature both in structure and in function, as they lack hierarchy, are chaotic in their arrangement, and the blood flow in them is sluggish [25,27,29,30].

Dr. Folkman, in his pioneer study, first described the essential role of angiogenesis in tumor growth in 1971, which led to the idea that targeting this process might be a promising therapeutic strategy to combat the growth and metastatic spread of cancer. Accordingly, antiangiogenic agents have been developed and tested in clinics, and many have been approved for the treatment of different cancer types [31].

3. Angiogenesis and Prostate Cancer

Preclinical animal experiments and studies with clinical samples have indicated significant angiogenic activity within malignant prostate tumor tissues often measured as microvessel density (MVD), a well-established marker of angiogenesis, which correlated well with the tumor growth, Gleason score, and metastasis in PCa [23,25,32]. Thus, MVD in PCa has been designated as a valuable prognostic indicator that may predict the clinical and biochemical recurrence of the disease [23,25,32–35]. In addition, several reports have demonstrated the importance of angiogenic factors such as VEGFs, FGFs, ILs, transforming growth factor β (TGFβ), and different metalloproteinases which support the role of angiogenesis in PCa progression. However, the presently approved antiangiogenic agents could not meet acceptable outcomes in PCa patients, as was expected from the results of preclinical studies [23–25,36]. Although, in some cases, the response rate and progression-free survival were significantly improved, the overall survival (OS) did not increase following treatment [25]. Because there are discrepancies between these results and the reports from the preclinical animal studies and histopathology studies using PCa samples, it would be therefore prudent to discuss and analyze the possible reasons for these apparent differences.

3.1. Angiogenic Growth Factors in Prostate Cancer

Vascular Endothelial Growth factors (VEGFs): VEGFs are part of the platelet-derived growth factor family and have been most extensively studied and described among all the angiogenic growth factors. VEGFs (VEGFA, VEGFB, VEGFC, and VEGFD) along with their cognate cell surface receptors (VEGFR1, VEGFR2, VEGFR3) play critical roles in PCa starting from cell growth to motility and cellular dissemination to other parts of the body [14,21,22]. Vascular endothelial growth factor

–A (VEGFA), which is a 45 KDa heparin-binding protein, is the most predominant growth factor among all the VEGFs [14,22,37]. VEGFA has long been identified to influence every aspect of endothelial cell (EC) behavior and the maintenance of vascular integrity, and therefore plays a crucial role during tumor growth [14,17,22,37] and is overexpressed in PCa [37,38]. Both human PCa and PCa tissues of animal origin, including prostate tumors isolated from TRansgenic Adenocarcinoma Mouse Prostate (TRAMP)models, show an increased expression of VEGFA in comparison to normal prostate tissues [21,22,37–41]. Along with prostatic glandular epithelial cells, non-vascular cells of the tumor microenvironment, such as macrophages, fibroblasts, and mast cells, also secrete VEGFA [42,43]. The role of VEGFA in PCa progression is further evident from studies that correlate the increased VEGFA expression in PCa tissues to angiogenesis, advanced disease stages, increased recurrence, and decreased survival among patients [41,44,45]. Increased amounts of VEGFA are also present in the urine samples of PCa patients, which has been reported to serve as a prognostic indicator of hormone-refractory PCa progression and survivability of these patients [46,47]. In addition, the results from several preclinical studies indicate that VEGFA inhibition or treatment with anti-VEGFA antibodies blocks the growth of human prostate tumors through suppression of angiogenesis [21,22,48], further supporting the role of VEGFA-mediated angiogenesis in PCa growth and progression. Reports also show the efficacy of anti-VEGFA treatment in combination with other therapeutic agents in preclinical mouse PCa models [49,50]. Interestingly, a dose-dependent regulation in the expression of VEGFA and its receptor FLT1 (FMS-like tyrosine kinase receptor domain 1) or VEGFR1 by androgen during PCa progression has been reported [51]. The expression of VEGFR1 has been further correlated with higher MVD, advanced pathologic state, and poor outcome in PCa [51]. Moreover, patients with advanced PCa receiving ADT show genetic polymorphisms in the androgen receptor (AR) binding site of FLT1 [52,53]. These reports, therefore, indicate that the expression of VEGFA and its receptors in PCa are subjected to androgen regulation, which together regulates the process of angiogenesis.

Fibroblast growth factors (FGFs): In addition to the VEGF family, the FGF family of growth factors is another major cytokine family that plays diverse roles during PCa progression [54,55]. FGFs are potent mitogens to many cell types, including ECs, and are expressed in many tissues, where they play significant roles in both physiological and pathological processes [54,55]. FGFs, particularly FGF2, FGF7, and FGF10, play vital roles in normal prostatic development, such as organogenesis, tissue homeostasis, and the acquisition of androgen dependency [54–56]. Both PCa cells and stromal cells in the PCa microenvironment secrete FGFs and express FGF receptors (FGFRs) [54,56,57]. FGF1 and FGF2 were among the first identified angiogenic factors which promote angiogenesis during tumor growth [57]. FGF/FGFR signaling regulates PCa angiogenesis both in a VEGFA-dependent and -independent manner [54–59]. Enhanced FGF levels and FGFR expressions such as type 1 FGFR (FGFR1), together with aberrant FGFR signaling and the loss of the intrinsic FGF7/FGF10-type 2 FGFR (FGFR2), are associated with enhanced PCa growth and angiogenesis [54,57,58]. The serum basic FGF (bFGF) level has also been shown to increase in PCa patients [59]. Furthermore, the correlation between FGF8 expression and VEGFA has been reported to be associated with advanced disease stage, higher serum PSA values, and poor survival [60]. These studies on the FGF/FGFR signaling cascade form the basis of FGF/VEGFR dual inhibition as a therapeutic strategy in PCa [61]. The prognostic implication of FGF, however, is controversial, as some studies have failed to find any relation between the FGF expression and PCa disease stage [62,63]. The specific role of FGF thus needs to be studied in more details.

Matrix metalloproteinases (MMPs): MMPs, together with TIMPs, form a classic regulatory unit that drives angiogenic processes both positively and negatively [64,65]. Metalloproteinases are zinc-containing calcium-dependent endopeptidases belonging to the metzincin superfamily [64,65]. Although MMPs are better known for their roles in tumor invasion and metastasis, as they help in breaking down the connective tissue barrier and thus help cancer cells to metastasize, they also play a crucial role in regulating angiogenesis by controlling EC attachment /detachment to the extracellular matrix, therefore helping in EC migration and invasion [64–66]. The expression of TIMPs controls the

MMP activities in the tissue environment, and an imbalance in the expression of MMPs and TIMPs has been shown in PCa angiogenesis [64]. Studies reveal a higher MMPs to TIMPs ratio in advanced PCa tumors (Gleason score of 8 and above) compared to tumors with a favorable prognosis (Gleason score of less than 6) [67]. Knowledge about the involvement of MMPs in PCa progression is mostly derived from knockdown and overexpression studies using animal models of PCa due to the lack of availability of specific MMP inhibitors [68]. Among different members of the metalloproteinase family, the roles of MMP-2, -7, -9, and MT1-MMP are well documented in PCa. MMP-2, MMP-7, and MMP-9 have been shown to stimulate PCa angiogenesis, as conditional knockouts of these MMPs in mice resulted in PCa that showed reduced vascularity and angiogenesis [68]. While MMP-2 deficiency is associated with a reduction in the number of immature blood vessels along with reduced tumor burden, MMP-9 primarily plays a role in vascular remodeling [68]. Studies have further shown that knocking down of MMP-9 in PCa cells has a negative effect on the expression of proangiogenic molecules, such as VEGFA and intercellular adhesion molecule1 (ICAM-1). It helps in the upregulation of the expression of angiostatin and other endogenous inhibitors of angiogenesis in PCa [64,69–71]. Furthermore, not only in primary tumors, MMPs, specifically MMP-9, derived from osteoclasts directly affect angiogenesis in the prostate tumor-bone microenvironment [72]. However, controversies exist regarding the roles of MMPs in PCa progression, particularly that of MMP-9, as some studies correlate the increased expression of MMP-9 with a high Gleason score, disease progression, and poorer clinical outcomes [68,73]. On the contrary, others fail to demonstrate MMP-9 expression in PCa and describe the increased perivascular invasion of PCa cells in mice lacking MMP9 [68,73].

Transforming growth factor (TGF) β: TGFβ, a pleiotropic molecule comprised of three isoforms, exhibits potent tumor suppressor properties in the early stages of tumor development [74,75], while harboring a tumor-promoting effect during the later stages of tumor progression [75,76]. This paradoxical nature of TGFβ in PCa is mostly due to its capability to differentially activate the ERK/MAP kinase pathway in benign and malignant PCa cells [76]. Although no unanimous opinion exists regarding the time point when TGFβ switches from being a tumor suppressor to a tumor promoter, studies mostly report that it acts in the interphase of stromal -epithelial interaction and exerts its effect through three different TGFβ receptors—TGFβ1, TGFβ2, and TGFβ3on tumor cells, as well as on nonmalignant stromal cells such as fibroblasts and ECs [76]. Increased TGFβ1 in PCa tissues and high levels of TGFβ1 in the urinary and serum samples of PCa patients have been reported to be associated with enhanced angiogenesis, metastasis, and poor clinical outcomes [76,77]. TGFβ indirectly affects PCa angiogenesis via the upregulation of VEGFA through the activation of SMAD-mediated transcriptional regulation and activation of the Src/Focal Adhesion Kinase (FAK)/Protein kinase B (PKB or AKT) signaling pathways [78]. TGFβ also regulates PCa angiogenesis by promoting the differentiation of cancer-associated fibroblasts (CAFs), which in turn promote tumor angiogenesis through increased VEGFA production [79]. Besides this, VEGFA also influences TGFβ expression through a positive feedback mechanism [78]. However, some studies also report the negative association between TGFβ and VEGFA expression, especially in ECs [79]. Among the TGFβ receptors, TGFβ1 expression is associated with higher clinical tumor stages and a lower 5-year survival rate. Furthermore, apigenin, a natural flavone compound, and an inhibitor for TGFβ have been shown to inhibit angiogenesis in PCa through the suppression of VEGFA, which further proves the role of TGFβ in PCa angiogenesis [78].

Cyclooxygenases: Cyclooxygenases are enzymes that form prostaglandins and thromboxanes from arachidonic acids and are mainly associated with inflammatory responses [80,81]. Fatty acids and inflammation and their role in genitourinary cancer is an actively growing area of research [80,81]. Although clinical data at this point does not strongly support the effect of nonsteroidal anti-inflammatory drugs (NSAIDs) in inhibiting or preventing PCa progression in patients, the results from several preclinical studies are encouraging [80–82]. Cyclooxygenases and their eicosanoids products, prostaglandins and thromboxanes, play multiple roles in the regulation of EC biology [82]. There are two different forms of cyclooxygenase: cyclooxygenase 1 (COX1), which is expressed constitutively, and cyclooxygenase 2 (COX2), which expresses under the influence of various growth factors and cytokines [80,81]. The increased expression of COX2 has been reported in different cell types of the tumor microenvironment, and it promotes angiogenesis through enhanced VEGFA production, EC mobilization, vascular sprouting, and increased EC survival [82]. COX2 has been reported to overexpress in PCa tissues compared to the normal prostate, which shows low to no expression [83–85]. Increased COX2 expression is associated with increased MVDs in PCa tissues [84,85]. The inhibition of COX2 with its specific inhibitor, NS398, inhibits the growth of PC3 human prostate tumors in athymic mice through the suppression of neovessel formation in these tumors [85]. The inhibition of COX2 induces apoptosis in ECs via the suppression of AKT phosphorylation in PCa [86]. Importantly, epidemiologic studies show a lower risk of PCa in men taking aspirin and other NSAIDs, which has been attributed to COX2 inhibition that leads to the inhibition of subsequent angiogenesis [80,81]. However, specific patient data showing the grade-specific upregulation of COX2 in PCa is still lacking and is needed in order to ascertain the role of COX2 in PCa in a more definitive way.

Interleukins (ILs): ILs, which are cytokines primarily secreted by leukocytes, play a major role in shaping the tumor microenvironment during tumor progression primarily through their immune regulatory properties [87,88]. In addition to lymphocytes, monocytes, and macrophages, ECs in the tumor microenvironment are regarded as major contributors of ILs [88]. To date, 50 different ILs have been identified [89]. ILs play diverse roles in PCa, such as being molecular determinants of progression from androgen-dependent to androgen-independent stages, or acting as tumor suppressors [90]. They regulate EC properties and angiogenesis in PCa either positively or negatively [91,92]. While some ILs, such as IL8, have been linked to increased PCa angiogenesis, others such as IL27 and IL10 have been linked to angiogenesis suppression in PCa [93–95]. IL8 expression in PCa has been shown to correlate with intra-tumoral MVD [93]. In addition, PCa cells transfected with IL8 have been shown to grow faster in mice with increased tumor vascularity compared to non-transfected cells [93]. As a result, targeting IL8 in PCa has emerged as a novel strategy for PCa treatment [93]. Other ILs such as IL27 and IL10, however, negatively regulate the process of angiogenesis during PCa progression. Rather than directly affecting ECs, the antiangiogenic properties of IL27 are mediated through the downregulation of proangiogenic-related genes such as FLT1, prostaglandin G/H synthase 1/cyclooxygenase-1 (PTGS1/COX-1), and FGFR3s and the upregulation of antiangiogenic genes such as CXCL10 and TIMP3 [94]. In addition to IL27, IL10 also negatively affects proangiogenic cells in the tumor microenvironment, such as activated macrophages, by inhibiting proangiogenic MMP2 and upregulating TIMP 1 and thereby suppressing the process of angiogenesis during PCa progression [95].

Other factors: In addition to the above factors, in recent years, there have been reports that other novel factors. such as microRNAs (miRNAs), which are short segments (21- to 25-nucleotides) of non-coding RNAs; long noncoding RNAs (lncRNAs), which are RNA transcripts longer than 200 nucleotides that do not encode proteins; and extracellular vesicles (EVs), which are small cell-derived membranous structures containing proteins, lipids, and genetic material, either directly or indirectly affect the angiogenic response in PCa [96–102]. In the past decades, these factors have attracted attention, as they play important roles in the progression of the disease. Increasing evidence indicates that cancer cells communicate among themselves as well as with cells of the surrounding microenvironment via the secretion and transfer of these factors. We will discuss some of these recent findings.

miRNAs can modulate the functions of ECs via non-cell-autonomous as well as cell-autonomous mechanisms, and thus regulate angiogenesis [103]. They regulate the expressions of both pro- or anti-angiogenic growth factors, and target the growth factor receptors and signaling molecules required in the process. Both the upregulation and downregulation of miRNAs have impact on PCa progression and angiogenesis. While miRNAs such as miR-296, miR-30d, miR-323, miR-21, and miR-182 are upregulated in PCa [104–109], the decreased expressions of miR-195, miR-218, and miR-146a are also shown to be associated with increased angiogenesis in PCa [97,110 112]. The upregulation of miR-30d [104] and miR-323 [105] were reported to enhance VEGF synthesis and secretion by PCa cells and therefore promote VEGF-mediated angiogenesis in PCa. miR-296, which is frequently upregulated in PCa, regulates the levels of VEGF and PDGF receptors in angiogenic ECs [108,109]. miR-21 and miR-182 regulate the expression of HIF1α and thereby HIF 1α-mediated angiogenesis [106,107]. The decreased expression of miR-146a was reported in CRPC, where it regulates the expression of epidermal growth factor receptor (EGFR) and MMP2 in PCa tissues [112]. On the other hand, the decreased expression of miR-195 in PCa results in the upregulation of ribosomal protein S6 kinase B1 (RPS6KB1), which leads to increased expressions of MMP-9 and VEGF proteins, which regulate angiogenesis [110]. miR-218, which inhibits angiogenesis through targeting the rapamycin-insensitive companion of mTOR (RICTOR)/VEGFA axis, is also downregulated during PCa progression [97]. In addition, the reduced expression of miR-130b in PCa tissues correlates with poor prognosis and increased angiogenesis, as the miR-130b/TNF-α/NF-κB/VEGFA loop inhibits PCa angiogenesis [113].

Among the lncRNAs, prostate cancer antigens (PCAs) and prostate cancer-associated transcripts (PCAT) are of immense interest, as they regulate several aspects of PCa progression. PCA3, a prostate-specific RNA which is overexpressed in more than 95% of PCa patients' urine samples, has been reported to regulate the expression of genes involved in angiogenesis, in addition to genes controlling signal transduction and apoptosis [114,115]. The knockdown of lncRNas, PCAT3, and PCAT9 in PCa cells leads to the suppression of VEGF synthesis and angiogenesis via the modulation of the miR-203/SNAI2 axis [116]. RBMS3-AS3, which poorly expresses in PCa, can suppress PCa angiogenesis and cell proliferation by upregulating the expression of an intrinsic angiogenesis inhibitor, vasohibin1 (VASH1), through the RBMS3-AS3/miR-4534/VASH1 axis [117].

EVs, including apoptotic bodies, microvesicles, and exosomes, play vital roles in vascular development, growth, and maturation [118]. EVs can act both in a positive and negative way to modulate the process of tumor growth and angiogenesis, therefore they are considered as promising targets for therapeutic intervention [102,119,120]. While exosomes secreted from PCa cells, cells in the PCa microenvironment, and also from PCa stem cells mostly promote angiogenesis, exosomes derived from other cell types and tissues have been reported to negatively affect the process and thereby PCa growth, suggesting a crucial role of EVs in tumor angiogenesis, which largely depends on their origin [102,120,121]. Cancer-derived EVs bestow aggressive phenotypes to cancer cells by affecting ECs within the tumor microenvironment and promoting angiogenesis. The exosomes in bodily fluids, secreted during hypoxia or acidocis, cause increased angiogenesis [122]. EVs contain miRNAs, mRNAs, and proteins that mediate the communication between various cell types and ECs and induce either pro- or antiangiogenic signaling. Sphingomyelin transferred into ECs by EVs secreted by PCa cells promotes the migration and proangiogenic activity of these cells [123]. Exosomes from PCa cell lines contain TGFβ1, which stimulates the differentiation of fibroblasts to highly aggressive myofibroblasts [124,125], an important source of matrix-remodeling proteins within the tumor microenvironment, via the activation of TGFβ/SMAD3 signaling, and thereby support PCa angiogenesis [124,125]. PCa cell-derived exosomes promote the differentiation of mesenchymal stem cells (MSCs) to proangiogenic myofibroblasts that support angiogenesis during PCa progression [126]. Furthermore, PCa-associated exosomes contain c-Src, IGF-1R, and FAK proteins that promote angiogenesis and PCa development [127]. Prostate-specific membrane antigen (PSMA), which is an important tumor marker for PCa progression, including angiogenesis and metastasis, is enriched in exosomes derived from PCa cells [128].

A schematic diagram representing the role of angiogenic growth factors in PCa is presented in Figure 1.

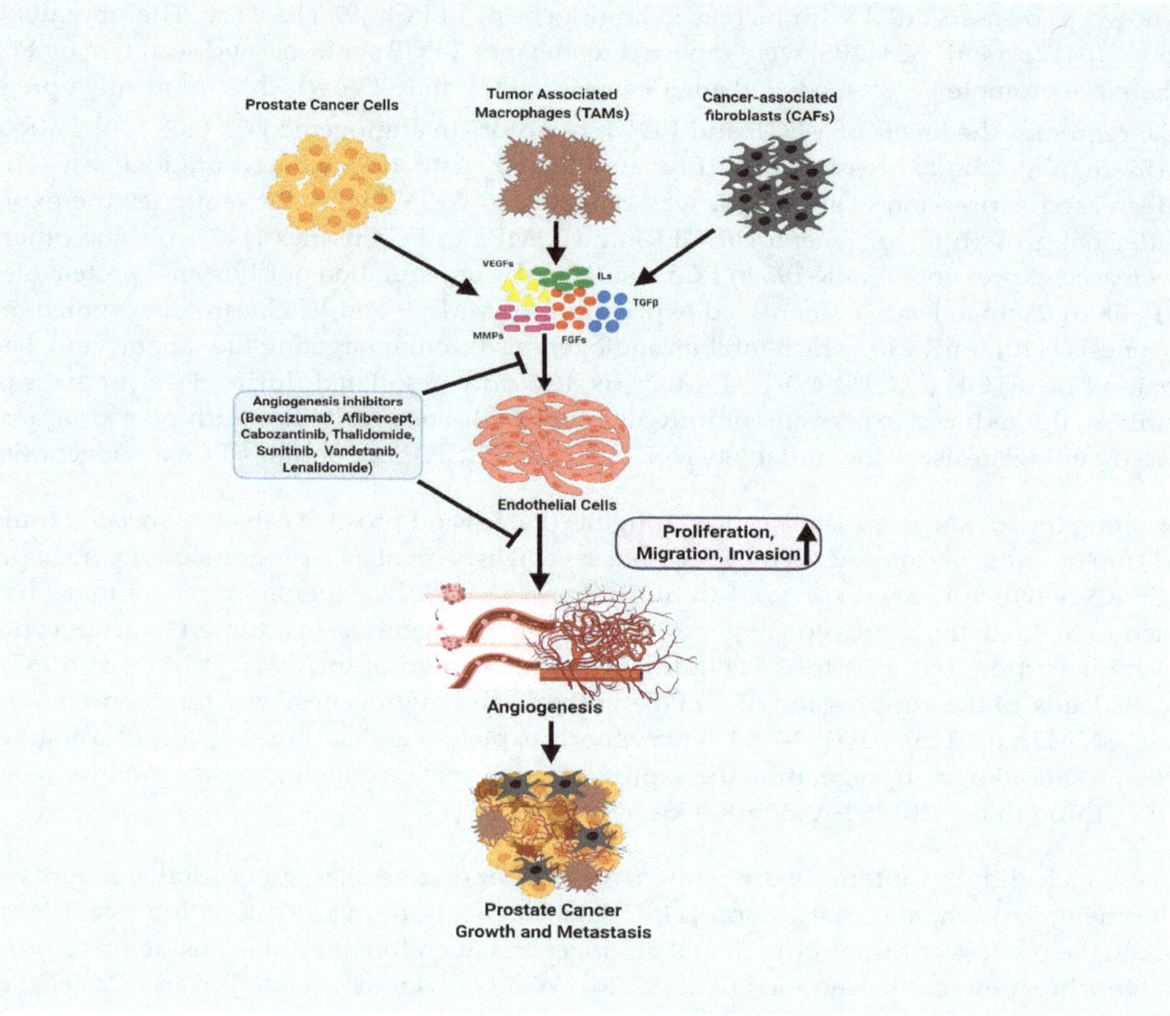

Figure 1. Schematic diagram of the role of angiogenic growth factors in prostate cancer (created with BioRender.com https://biorender.com/). VEGFs = Vascular endothelial growth factors; ILs = Interleukins, MMPs = Matrix metalloproteinases; FGFs = Fibroblast growth factors; TGFβ = Transforming growth factor beta.

3.2. *Current Antiangiogenic Treatment Strategies for Prostate Cancer*

Several mechanisms, such as inhibiting the activity of the proangiogenic factors directly, blocking the receptors of these proangiogenic factors, or elevating the levels of endogenous antiangiogenic factors, can be employed to inhibit angiogenesis [24,25]. In PCa, strategies were mainly designed to inhibit the proangiogenic factors or target downstream signaling effector pathways using monoclonal antibodies or small molecule inhibitors or using agents that are capable of immune modulation. Due to the multitude of factors regulating the process of angiogenesis, monotherapy, as well as combination therapy with different chemotherapeutic agents or antiangiogenic agents, have been tested for optimal therapeutic effects. Since VEGFA is a critical growth factor associated with PCa, it has been extensively studied [25,41,44,45]. As the overexpression of VEGFA correlates with poor prognosis and metastasis, the main antiangiogenic strategies in PCa at present were designed to mainly inhibit the VEGF pathway by targeting VEGFA or its receptors [25,41,44,45]. In this section, we will discuss some of these prominent antiangiogenic strategies that were developed for the treatment of PCa.

Bevacizumab is a humanized anti-VEGF monoclonal IgG1 antibody (molecular weight, 149 kDa) that selectively binds to and neutralizes VEGF, thereby preventing it from binding to its cell surface VEGFRs, leading to reduced MVD in tumors, thus limiting the blood supply to tumor tissues and lowering interstitial tissue pressure and vascular permeability [25]. A Phase II trial with bevacizumab in combination with ADT consisting of 102 recurrent hormone-sensitive PCa patients reported a significant improvement in relapse-free survival (RFS). Hypertension was the most commonly observed adverse effect in these patients [129]. Other Phase II studies with CRPC patients where bevacizumab was combined with docetaxel, thalidomide, and prednisone [130] or where bevacizumab was combined with estramustine and docetaxel for the treatment of HRPC or CRPC patients [131,132] have all demonstrated that the combination with bevacizumab was tolerated and led to encouraging antitumor activity, median survival and OS. On the contrary, the Phase III Cancer and Leukemia Group B (CALGB)trial that followed with 1050 metastatic PCa patients demonstrated some improvement in progression-free survival (PFS) with the combination therapy; there was no significant increase in OS. Bevacizumab also showed other adverse events (AE), which included cardiovascular and neutropenic complications [133]. Furthermore, in a very recent Phase I/II trial in patients with mCRPC, bevacizumab when used in combination with temsirolimus showed limited clinical activity, and only a transient decrease in the circulating tumor cells (CTC) level was observed, which was associated with significant AE [134]. These studies thus indicate that the addition of bevacizumab to standard therapy does not result in any significant clinical benefit in CRPC.

Sunitinib is a novel oral small-molecule tyrosine kinase inhibitor that targets VEGFR1 and VEGFR2. [135]. Not many clinical studies have been conducted using sunitinib in PCa. In a randomized, placebo-controlled, Phase III trial conducted with 873 progressive mCRPC patients who either received prednisone in combination with sunitinib or prednisone alone, sunitinib did not improve OS and severe AE was reported, which led to the discontinuation of the study [136].

Vandetanib is an oral multi-tyrosine kinase inhibitor that targets VEGFR2, epidermal growth factor receptor (EGFR), and RET (rearranged during transfection) pathways in cancer [25]. In a randomized, double-blinded, placebo-controlled Phase II trial of vandetanib in combination with docetaxel/prednisolone in 86 hormone-refractory PCa patients, the combination with vandetanib did not demonstrate any benefit [137]. Additionally, in another randomized Phase II trial with mCRPC patients, a combination of vandetanib with bicalutamide did not exhibit superior efficacy compared to the treatment with bicalutamide alone. These approaches were also associated with considerable toxicity [138].

Aflibercept (VEGF Trap) is a recombinant human fusion protein comprised of extracellular domains of human VEGFR1 and 2 fused to the constant region (Fc) of human immunoglobulin G1 (IgG1), which has a very high VEGF binding affinity and binds to all isomers of the VEGFA and B family and PlGF [25]. In a Phase III double-blinded randomized trial, where men with mCRPC received aflibercept with docetaxel and prednisone as first-line chemotherapy, no improvement in OS was reported. Furthermore, a high incidence of severe AE and treatment-related fatal events were reported in the aflibercept group compared to the placebo group [139].

Thalidomide is an oral agent that inhibits the activity of angiogenic factors such as VEGF, bFGF, and IL-6. In CRPC patients who have failed multiple therapies, thalidomide monotherapy showed some clinical activity [140]. Results from an open-label Phase II trial of thalidomide in patients with androgen-independent PCa [141] indicated thalidomide to be an option for patients who do not respond to other forms of therapy. Upon combination with docetaxel in a randomized Phase II trial, more than half (53%) of the CRPC patients had a PSA decrease of at least 50%, as compared to 35% of the patients in the docetaxel-alone treatment arm [142].

Lenalidomide is a thalidomide derivative that inhibits VEGF-mediated phosphatidylinositol-3,4,5-trisphosphate (PI3K)-Akt signaling pathway. The results of an open-label, Phase II clinical trial with 63 CRPC patients where lenalidomide was combined with docetaxel, bevacizumab, and prednisone showed that combining different angiogenesis inhibitors was safe with appropriate supportive measures and could potentially provide clinical benefit to patients [143]. In a Phase I/II double-blinded, randomized study with 60 non-metastatic PCa patients, treatment with lenalidomide showed an acceptable toxicity, with disease stabilization and reduction in PSA [144]. However, in a randomized, double-blind, placebo-controlled, Phase III study with 1059 chemotherapy-naive mCRPC patients, a combination of lenalidomide with docetaxel and prednisone resulted in a significantly worse OS with increased AE such as hematological side effects, diarrhea, pulmonary embolism, and asthenia [145].

Cabozantinib is an orally available small-molecule inhibitor of kinases, including VEGFR2. Preclinical studies show that cabozantinib can effectively inhibit PCa growth and metastasis by suppressing angiogenesis [146]. Clinical studies conducted so far with cabozantinib have demonstrated positive effects mostly in context to bone metastasis inhibition, bone lesion resolution, and improvement in patient CTC counts [25]. In a Phase II randomized trial of cabozantinib with patients with advanced solid tumors, randomization was halted, and the patients were unblinded because the drug showed efficacy and the largest PFS improvement in CRPC patients [147]. Furthermore, cabozantinib treatment also reduced soft tissue and bone lesions, bone turnover markers, pain, and narcotic use [148]. However, in a Phase III study with previously treated mCRPC patients, cabozantinib did not improve the OS, disease progression, or PSA response [149].

From the results of the clinical studies that have been summarized in Table 1, it can be concluded that the antiangiogenic approach in PCa has only been moderately successful. Treatment-related toxicities, often grade 3 or greater, were observed with these agents, which also resulted in treatment-related deaths. The main AE reported were hypertension, gastrointestinal perforation, proteinuria, hemorrhage, thrombosis, fistula formation, cardiac toxicity, endocrine dysfunction, and reversible posterior leukoencephalopathy [25,150].

Table 1. Summary of clinical studies of antiangiogenic drugs in the treatment of prostate cancer.

Drug	Mechanism of Action	Phase	Drugs in Combination Treatment	Outcomes	Adverse Events	Reference
Bevacizumab (Avastin®; Genentech, Inc.)	Recombinant humanized monoclonal antibody against VEGF-A	I/II	Temsirolimus	Transient decrease in circulating tumor cell levels in metastatic CRPC patients	• Anorexia • Fatigue • Mucositis • Lymphopenia • Thrombocytopenia	[134]
		II	ADT	Significant improvement in relapse-free survival in recurrent hormone-sensitive PCa patients	• Hypertension • Musculoskeletal pain • Infection • Headache	[129]
			Docetaxel, Thalidomide, and Prednisone	Improved median survival in CRPC patients	• Neutropenia • Anemia • Thrombocytopenia • Constipation	[130]
			Estramustine and Docetaxel	Improved overall survival in CRPC patients	• Leukopenia • Neutropenia • Fatigue • Pulmonary embolism • Deep venous thrombosis • Epistaxis • Hypertension	[132]
		III	Docetaxel and Prednisone	No improvement in overall survival in metastatic CRPC patients	• Neutropenia • Fatigue • Leucopenia • Hypertension • GI hemorrhage and perforation • Mucositis	[133]

Table 1. *Cont.*

Drug	Mechanism of Action	Phase	Drugs in Combination Treatment	Outcomes	Adverse Events	Reference
Sunitinib malate (Sutent®, Pfizer)	Novel oral small-molecule tyrosine kinase inhibitor that targets VEGFR1 and VEGFR2	III	Prednisone	No improvement in overall survival in metastatic CRPC patients	• Diarrhea • Nausea • Vomiting • Fatigue • Hand/Foot Syndrome • Hypertension • Mucosal inflammation • Asthenia	[136]
Vandetanib (Caprelsa, AstraZeneca & Sanofi)	Oral multi-tyrosine kinase inhibitor that targets VEGFR2, epidermal growth factor receptor (EGFR), and RET pathways in cancer	II	Docetaxel and Prednisolone	No efficacy benefit in HRPC patients	• Fatigue • Diarrhea • Nausea • Erythematous and exfoliative rash	[137]
			Bicalutamide	No efficacy benefit in metastatic CRPC patients	• Hypertension • Fatigue • Diarrhea • Dyspnea • Skin rash • Hand/Foot syndrome • Anorexia • Prolonged QTc interval	[138]
Aflibercept/VEGF Trap (Eylea and Zaltrap, Regeneron Pharmaceuticals)	Recombinant human fusion protein that has high VEGF binding affinity and binds to all isomers of the VEGFA and B family and placental growth factor (PGF)	III	Docetaxel and Prednisone	No improvement in overall survival in metastatic CRPC patients	• Hypertension • Vascular Disorder • GI hemorrhage • Epistaxis • Perforation • Stomatitis • Ulceration	[139]
Thalidomide (Thalomid, Celgene)	Oral agent that inhibits VEGF, bFGF, and IL-6	II	Docetaxel	PSA decrease in CRPC patients	• Thrombocytopenia • Anemia • Venous thromboembolism	[142]

Table 1. *Cont.*

Drug	Mechanism of Action	Phase	Drugs in Combination Treatment	Outcomes	Adverse Events	Reference
Lenalidomide (Revlimid, Celgene)	Thalidomide derivative that inhibits VEGF-mediated phosphatidylinositol-3,4,5-trisphosphate (PI3K)-Akt signaling pathway	I/II		Disease stabilization and reduction of PSA in non-metastatic PCa patients	• Neutropenia • Venous thromboembolism • Fatigue • Hyperglycemia • Constipation • Anemia	[144]
		II	Docetaxel, Bevacizumab, and Prednisone	PSA decline and partial responses in CRPC patients	• Neutropenia • Anemia • Thrombocytopenia • Diarrhea • Fatigue	[143]
		III	Docetaxel and Prednisone	Significantly worse overall survival in chemotherapy-naive metastatic CRPC patients	• Hematological side effects • Diarrhea • Pulmonary embolism • Asthenia • Pneumonia	[145]
Cabozantinib (Cometriq™ and Cabometyx™, Exelixis Inc.)	Orally available small-molecule inhibitor of kinases, including VEGFR2	II		Proliferation-free survival improvement in CRPC patients	• Fatigue • Diarrhea • Hypertension • Muscle spasms • Asthenia	[147]
		III		No improvement in overall survival, disease progression, or PSA response in previously treated metastatic CRPC patients. Some improvement in bone scan response, radiographic progression-free survival, symptomatic skeletal events, circulating tumor cell conversion, and bone biomarkers	• Nausea • Diarrhea • Fatigue • Asthenia • Weight loss • Constipation • Anemia • Hypertension • Bone pain	[149]

4. Conclusions and Future Direction

In summary, there is substantial evidence regarding the critical role of angiogenesis in the progression of PCa, with studies reporting correlations between expressions of angiogenic markers, Gleason scores, metastatic disease progression, and clinical outcomes [23,25,32–35]. Several studies have also demonstrated the efficacies of antiangiogenic agents in preclinical PCa models [23,25]. However, despite these promising results, antiangiogenic treatment has only been moderately successful in some hormone-sensitive PCa patients [96]. On the contrary, in mCRPC, which to date has limited treatment options, antiangiogenic treatment has failed to show any significant effects in terms of improvement in OS or improvement in the quality of life of patients in the clinics [21,25].

Reviews on PCa and angiogenesis have discussed many factors that may be responsible for the moderate effectiveness of antiangiogenic agents in PCa [22,151,152]. Importantly, the failure of these agents may be attributed to several factors, such as differences in the design of clinical trials from preclinical studies, choosing appropriate angiogenic agents or combination of agents, the determination of treatment response and endpoints, and lastly the side effects encountered by the patients [23,25].

Treatment response measured as a decrease in the PSA level, improvement in PFS, or OS may not also be sufficient and appropriate for antiangiogenic agents, as the PSA level may not always accurately indicate the clinical status and disease progression, and these drugs often increase the PSA level despite a positive disease response [22,23,25]. The measurement of alternative biomarkers such as CTCcounts in the peripheral blood samples isolated from patients can be an indicator of drug efficacy as CTC counts can predict OS better than PSA levels at all time points [153,154]. OS as an endpoint may not be the best evaluator of survival benefit from an antiangiogenic agent, considering the long survival rate of PCa patients normally, and PFS is not an ideal endpoint to determine the efficacy of a drug, as it may or may not necessarily translate into an OS improvement [23]. Therefore, new biomarkers of disease progression and the establishment of clinical endpoints following the administration of antiangiogenic agents may help in the determination of the efficacy of these drugs. Furthermore, at present there are no established markers to assess the angiogenic activity in PCa. MVD, which is considered as a potent surrogate marker, may not be an independent prognostic factor in untreated tumors, and studies have not yet established a strong correlation between MVD and the effectiveness of antiangiogenic agents in PCa [155]. The determination of vascularization in two-dimensional histological slides may not also be the most appropriate method for evaluating the efficacy of antiangiogenic agents [155–157]. With improved imaging techniques and other noninvasive techniques such as Doppler, it will be prudent to assess the whole vascular architecture within the tumors. Moreover, the study of the functional aspects of angiogenesis, such as the detection of vascular permeability and blood flow in tumors, will help to provide previously unavailable information and also help in decision-making [29,156,157].

Finally, although several growth factors regulate angiogenesis in PCa, most of the preclinical studies and clinical trials have been undertaken with anti-VEGFA or anti-VEGFR agents, which demonstrated modest clinical response and severe AE in patients. Therefore, it will be necessary to investigate the roles of other novel proangiogenic growth factors in PCa, which will identify newer, effective, and safe antiangiogenic agents for the treatment of PCa. Resistance, both intrinsic and acquired, to the currently used antiangiogenic agents is another possible reason for the suboptimal performance of these agents in the clinics. A number of growth factors can activate different signaling pathways during the process of angiogenesis in PCa. Recent findings indicate the probable regulatory roles of miRNAs, lncRNAs, and EVs in PCa angiogenesis. Therefore, targeting the angiogenic process using agents that are capable of inhibiting multiple pathways or by combining agents that can target different pathways may help to overcome drug resistance and result in better clinical outcomes. Combination therapy with antiangiogenic agents have actually shown promising results in clinics [143,151]. Furthermore, to find out more effective drug combinations and minimize toxicity, detailed studies determining the effective dose of each drug in a combination and monitoring the pharmacodynamic endpoints is required. Importantly, a deeper understanding of the process of angiogenesis and signaling pathways regulating the process is needed in order to design novel targeted antiangiogenic therapies in PCa.

Author Contributions: Conceptualization, C.S. and D.C.; Writing—original draft preparation, C.S., S.G., and D.C.; Writing—review and editing, C.S., S.B., and D.C. All authors have read and agreed to the published version of the manuscript.

References

1. Siegel, R.L.; Miller, K.D.; Jemal, A. Cancer statistics, 2020. *CA Cancer J. Clin.* **2020**, *70*, 7–30. [CrossRef] [PubMed]
2. Merino, M.; Pinto, A.; González, R.; Espinosa, E. Antiangiogenic agents and endothelin antagonists in advanced castration resistant prostate cancer. *Eur. J. Cancer* **2011**, *47*, 1846–1851. [CrossRef]
3. Shipley, W.U.; Seiferheld, W.; Lukka, H.R.; Major, P.P.; Heney, N.M.; Grignon, D.J.; Sartor, O.; Patel, M.P.; Bahary, J.P.; Zietman, A.L.; et al. NRG Oncology RTOG Radiation with or without Antiandrogen Therapy in Recurrent Prostate Cancer. *N. Engl. J. Med.* **2017**, *376*, 417–428. [CrossRef] [PubMed]
4. Cannata, D.H.; Kirschenbaum, A.; Levine, A.C. Androgen deprivation therapy as primary treatment for prostate cancer. *J. Clin. Endocrinol. Metab.* **2012**, *97*, 360–365. [CrossRef] [PubMed]
5. Schmidt, L.J.; Tindall, D.J. Androgen receptor: Past, present and future. *Curr. Drug Targets.* **2013**, *14*, 401–407. [CrossRef]
6. Yap, T.A.; Smith, A.D.; Ferraldeschi, R.; Al-Lazikani, B.; Workman, P.; de Bono, J.S. Drug discovery in advanced prostate cancer: Translating biology into therapy. *Nat. Rev. Drug Discov.* **2016**, *15*, 699–718. [CrossRef]
7. Katsogiannou, M.; Ziouziou, H.; Karaki, S.; Andrieu, C.; Henry de Villeneuve, M.; Rocchi, P. The hallmarks of castration-resistant prostate cancers. *Cancer Treat. Rev.* **2015**, *41*, 588–597. [CrossRef]
8. Craft, N.; Chhor, C.; Tran, C.; Belldegrun, A.; DeKernion, J.; Witte, O.N.; Said, J.; Reiter, R.E.; Sawyers, C.L. Evidence for clonal outgrowth of androgen-independent prostate cancer cells from androgen-dependent tumors through a two-step process. *Cancer Res.* **1999**, *59*, 5030–5036.
9. Pham, T.; Sadowski, M.C.; Li, H.; Richard, D.J.; d'Emden, M.C.; Richard, K. Advances in hormonal therapies for hormone naïve and castration-resistant prostate cancers with or without previous chemotherapy. *Exp. Hematol. Oncol.* **2016**, *22*, 5. [CrossRef]
10. Donkena, K.V.; Yuan, H.; Young, C.Y. Recent advances in understanding hormonal therapy resistant prostate cancer. *Curr. Cancer Drug Targets* **2010**, *10*, 402–410. [CrossRef]
11. Janiczek, M.; Szylberg, Ł.; Kasperska, A.; Kowalewski, A.; Parol, M.; Antosik, P.; Radecka, B.; Marszałek, A. Immunotherapy as a Promising Treatment for Prostate Cancer: A Systematic Review. *J. Immunol. Res.* **2017**, *2017*, 4861570. [CrossRef]
12. Nevedomskaya, E.; Baumgart, S.J.; Haendler, B. Recent Advances in Prostate Cancer Treatment and Drug Discovery. *Int. J. Mol. Sci.* **2018**, *19*, 1359. [CrossRef] [PubMed]
13. Sumanasuriya, S.; De Bono, J. Treatment of Advanced Prostate Cancer-A Review of Current Therapies and Future Promise. *Cold Spring Harb. Perspect. Med.* **2018**, *8*, a030635. [CrossRef] [PubMed]
14. Carmeliet, P.; Jain, R.K. Angiogenesis in cancer and other diseases. *Nature* **2000**, *407*, 249–257. [CrossRef]
15. Basu, S.; Nagy, J.A.; Pal, S.; Vasile, E.; Eckelhoefer, I.A.; Bliss, V.S.; Manseau, E.J.; Dasgupta, P.S.; Dvorak, H.F.; Mukhopadhyay, D. The neurotransmitter dopamine inhibits angiogenesis induced by vascular permeability factor/vascular endothelial growth factor. *Nat. Med.* **2001**, *5*, 569–574. [CrossRef]
16. Bielenberg, D.R.; Zetter, B.R. The Contribution of Angiogenesis to the Process of Metastasis. *Cancer J.* **2015**, *21*, 267–273. [CrossRef] [PubMed]
17. Chakroborty, D.; Sarkar, C.; Basu, B.; Dasgupta, P.S.; Basu, S. Catecholamines regulate tumor angiogenesis. *Cancer Res.* **2009**, *69*, 3727–3730. [CrossRef]
18. Chakroborty, D.; Sarkar, C.; Mitra, R.B.; Banerjee, S.; Dasgupta, P.S.; Basu, S. Depleted dopamine in gastric cancer tissues: Dopamine treatment retards growth of gastric cancer by inhibiting angiogenesis. *Clin. Cancer Res.* **2004**, *10*, 4349–4356. [CrossRef]

19. Sarkar, C.; Chakroborty, D.; Dasgupta, P.S.; Basu, S. Dopamine is a safe antiangiogenic drug which can also prevent 5-fluorouracil induced neutropenia. *Int. J. Cancer* **2015**, *137*, 744–749. [CrossRef]
20. Schmidt, T.; Carmeliet, P. Angiogenesis: A target in solid tumors, also in leukemia? *Hematol. Am. Soc. Hematol. Educ. Program* **2011**, *2011*, 1–8. [CrossRef]
21. Guo, Y.; Wang, S.; Hoot, D.R.; Clinton, S.K. Suppression of VEGF-mediated autocrine and paracrine interactions between prostate cancer cells and vascular endothelial cells by soy isoflavones. *J. Nutr. Biochem.* **2007**, *18*, 408–417. [CrossRef] [PubMed]
22. Hwang, C.; Heath, E.I. Angiogenesis inhibitors in the treatment of prostate cancer. *J. Hematol. Oncol.* **2010**, *3*, 26. [CrossRef] [PubMed]
23. Bilusic, M.; Wong, Y.N. Anti-angiogenesis in prostate cancer: Knocked down but not out. *Asian J. Androl.* **2014**, *16*, 372–377. [CrossRef]
24. Aragon-Ching, J.B.; Jain, L.; Gulley, J.L.; Arlen, P.M.; Wright, J.J.; Steinberg, S.M.; Draper, D.; Venitz, J.; Jones, E.; Chen, C.C.; et al. Final analysis of a phase II trial using sorafenib for metastatic castration-resistant prostate cancer. *BJU Int.* **2009**, *103*, 1636–1640. [CrossRef]
25. Mukherji, D.; Temraz, S.; Wehbe, D.; Shamseddine, A. Angiogenesis and antiangiogenic therapy in prostate cancer. *Crit. Rev. Oncol. Hematol.* **2013**, *87*, 122–131. [CrossRef]
26. Carmeliet, P. Angiogenesis in health and disease. *Nat. Med.* **2003**, *9*, 653–660. [CrossRef]
27. Hanahan, D.; Folkman, J. Patterns and emerging mechanisms of the angiogenic switch during tumorigenesis. *Cell* **1996**, *86*, 353–364. [CrossRef]
28. Rivera-Lopez, C.M.; Tucker, A.L.; Lynch, K.R. Lysophosphatidic acid (LPA) and angiogenesis. *Angiogenesis* **2008**, *11*, 301–310. [CrossRef]
29. Chakroborty, D.; Sarkar, C.; Yu, H.; Wang, J.; Liu, Z.; Dasgupta, P.S.; Basu, S. Dopamine stabilizes tumor blood vessels by upregulating angiopoietin 1 expression in pericytes and Kruppel-like factor-2 expression in tumor endothelial cells. *Proc. Natl. Acad. Sci. USA* **2011**, *108*, 20730–20735. [CrossRef]
30. Winkler, F.; Kozin, S.V.; Tong, R.T.; Chae, S.S.; Booth, M.F.; Garkavtsev, I.; Xu, L.; Hicklin, D.J.; Fukumura, D.; di Tomaso, E.; et al. Kinetics of vascular normalization by VEGFR2 blockade governs brain tumor response to radiation: Role of oxygenation, angiopoietin-1, and matrix metalloproteinases. *Cancer Cell.* **2004**, *6*, 553–563. [CrossRef]
31. Folkman, J. Tumor angiogenesis: Therapeutic implications. *N. Engl. J. Med.* **1971**, *21*, 1182–1186. [CrossRef]
32. Gettman, M.T.; Pacelli, A.; Slezak, J.; Bergstralh, E.J.; Zincke, H.; Bostwick, D.G. Role of microvessel density inpredicting recurrence in pathologic Stage T3 prostatic adenocarcinoma. *Urology* **1999**, *54*, 479–485. [CrossRef]
33. Weidner, N.; Carroll, P.R.; Flax, J.; Blumenfeld, W.; Folkman, J. Tumor angiogenesis correlates with metastasis in invasive prostate carcinoma. *Am. J. Pathol.* **1993**, *143*, 401–409. [PubMed]
34. Siegal, J.A.; Yu, E.; Brawer, M.K. Topography of neovascularity in human prostate carcinoma. *Cancer* **1995**, *75*, 2545–2551. [CrossRef]
35. Brawer, M.K.; Deering, R.E.; Brown, M.; Preston, S.D.; Bigler, S.A. Predictors of pathologic stage in prostatic carcinoma. The role of neovascularity. *Cancer* **1994**, *73*, 678–687. [CrossRef]
36. Chi, K.N.; Ellard, S.L.; Hotte, S.J.; Czaykowski, P.; Moore, M.; Ruether, J.D.; Schell, A.J.; Taylor, S.; Hansen, C.; Gauthier, I.; et al. A phase II study of sorafenib in patients with chemo-naive castration-resistant prostate cancer. *Ann. Oncol.* **2008**, *19*, 746–751. [CrossRef]
37. Dvorak, H.F. Vascular permeability factor/vascular endothelial growth factor: A critical cytokine in tumor angiogenesis and a potential target for diagnosis and therapy. *J. Clin. Oncol.* **2002**, *20*, 4368–4380. [CrossRef]
38. Roberts, E.; Cossigny, D.A.; Quan, G.M. The role of vascular endothelial growth factor in metastatic prostate cancer to the skeleton. *Prostate Cancer* **2013**, 418340. [CrossRef]
39. Jackson, M.W.; Roberts, J.S.; Heckford, S.E.; Ricciardelli, C.; Stahl, J.; Choong, C.; Horsfall, D.J.; Tilley, W.D. A potential autocrine role for vascular endothelial growth factor in prostate cancer. *Cancer Res.* **2002**, *62*, 854–859.
40. Huss, W.J.; Hanrahan, C.F.; Barrios, R.J.; Simons, J.W.; Greenberg, N.M. Angiogenesis and prostate cancer: Identification of a molecular progression switch. *Cancer Res.* **2001**, *61*, 2736–2743.
41. Strohmeyer, D.; Rössing, C.; Bauerfeind, A.; Kaufmann, O.; Schlechte, H.; Bartsch, G.; Loening, S. Vascular endothelial growth factor and its Fargoncorrelation with angiogenesis and p53 expression in prostate cancer. *Prostate* **2000**, *45*, 216–224. [CrossRef]

42. Chen, P.C.; Cheng, H.C.; Wang, J.; Wang, J.; Wang, S.W.; Tai, H.C.; Lin, C.W.; Tang, C.H. Prostate cancer-derived CCN3 induces M2 macrophage infiltration and contributes to angiogenesis in prostate cancer microenvironment. *Oncotarget* **2014**, *5*, 1595–1608. [CrossRef] [PubMed]
43. Taverna, G.; Giusti, G.; Seveso, M.; Hurle, R.; Colombo, P.; Stifter, S.; Grizzi, F. Mast cells as a potential prognostic marker in prostate cancer. *Dis. Markers* **2013**, *35*, 711–720. [CrossRef] [PubMed]
44. Aragon-Ching, J.B.; Dahut, W.L. VEGF inhibitors and prostate cancer therapy. *Curr. Mol. Pharmacol.* **2009**, *2*, 161–168. [CrossRef] [PubMed]
45. Borre, M.; Nerstrøm, B.; Overgaard, J. Association between immunohistochemical expression of vascular endothelial growth factor (VEGF), VEGF-expressing neuroendocrine-differentiated tumor cells, and outcome in prostate cancer patients subjected to watchful waiting. *Clin. Cancer Res.* **2000**, *6*, 1882–1890.
46. Jamaspishvili, T.; Kral, M.; Khomeriki, I.; Student, V.; Kolar, Z.; Bouchal, J. Urine markers in monitoring for prostate cancer. *Prostate Cancer Prostatic Dis.* **2010**, *13*, 12–19. [CrossRef]
47. George, D.J.; Halabi, S.; Shepard, T.F.; Vogelzang, N.J.; Hayes, D.F.; Small, E.J.; Kantoff, P.W. Prognostic significance of plasma vascular endothelial growth factor levels in patients with hormone-refractory prostate cancer treated on Cancer and Leukemia Group B 9480. *Clin. Cancer Res.* **2001**, *7*, 1932–1936.
48. Mateus, P.A.M.; Kido, L.A.; Silva, R.S.; Cagnon, V.H.A.; Montico, F. Association of anti-inflammatory and antiangiogenic therapies negatively influences prostate cancer progression in TRAMP mice. *Prostate* **2019**, *79*, 515–535. [CrossRef]
49. Zurita, A.J.; George, D.J.; Shore, N.D.; Liu., G.; Wilding, G.; Hutson, T.E.; Kozloff, M.; Mathew, P.; Harmon, C.S.; Wang, S.L.; et al. Sunitinib in combination with docetaxel and prednisone in chemotherapy-naive patients with metastatic, castration-resistant prostate cancer: A phase 1/2 clinical trial. *Ann. Oncol.* **2012**, *23*, 688–694. [CrossRef]
50. Antonarakis, E.S.; Armstrong, A.J. Emerging therapeutic approaches in the management of metastatic castration-resistant prostate cancer. *Prostate Cancer Prostatic Dis.* **2011**, *14*, 206–218. [CrossRef]
51. Sieveking, D.P.; Lim, P.; Chow, R.W.; Dunn, L.L.; Bao, S.; McGrath, K.C.; Heather, A.K.; Handels, D.J.; Celermajer, D.S.; Ng, M.K. A sex-specific role for androgens in angiogenesis. *J. Exp. Med.* **2010**, *207*, 345–352. [CrossRef] [PubMed]
52. Pallares, J.; Rojo, F.; Iriarte, J.; Morote, J.; Armadans, L.I.; de Torres, I. Study of microvessel density and the expression of the angiogenic factors VEGF, bFGF and the receptors Flt-1 and FLK-1 in benign, premalignant and malignant prostate tissues. *Histol. Histopathol.* **2006**, *21*, 857–865. [CrossRef] [PubMed]
53. Huang, C.N.; Huang, S.P.; Pao, J.B.; Hour, T.C.; Chang, T.Y.; Lan, Y.H.; Lu, T.-L.; Lee, H.-Z.; Juang, S.-H.; Huang, C.Y.; et al. Genetic polymorphisms in androgen receptor-binding sites predict survival in prostate cancer patients receiving androgen-deprivation therapy. *Ann. Oncol.* **2012**, *23*, 707–713. [CrossRef] [PubMed]
54. Huss, W.J.; Barrios, R.J.; Foster, B.A.; Greenberg, N.M. Differential expression of specific FGF ligand and receptor isoforms during angiogenesis associated with prostate cancer progression. *Prostate* **2003**, *54*, 8–16. [CrossRef] [PubMed]
55. Doll, J.A.; Reiher, F.K.; Crawford, S.E.; Pins, M.R.; Campbell, S.C.; Bouck, N.P. Thrombospondin-1, vascular endothelial growth factor and fibroblast growth factor-2 are key functional regulators of angiogenesis in the prostate. *Prostate* **2001**, *49*, 293–305. [CrossRef] [PubMed]
56. Thomson, A.A. Role of androgens and fibroblast growth factors in prostatic development. *Reproduction* **2001**, *121*, 187–195. [CrossRef]
57. Kwabi-Addo, B.; Ozen, M.; Ittmann, M. The role of fibroblast growth factors and their receptors in prostate cancer. *Endocr. Relat. Cancer* **2004**, *11*, 709–724. [CrossRef]
58. Wang, C.; Liu, Z.; Ke, Y.; Wang, F. Intrinsic FGFR2 and Ectopic FGFR1 Signaling in the Prostate and Prostate Cancer. *Front. Genet.* **2019**, *10*, 12. [CrossRef]
59. Meyer, G.E.; Yu, E.; Siegal, J.A.; Petteway, J.C.; Blumenstein, B.A.; Brawer, M.K. Serum basic fibroblast growth factor in men with and without prostate carcinoma. *Cancer* **1995**, *76*, 2304–2311. [CrossRef]
60. West, A.F.; O'Donnell, M.; Charlton, R.G.; Neal, D.E.; Leung, H.Y. Correlation of vascular endothelial growth factor expression with fibroblast growth factor-8 expression and clinico-pathologic parameters in human prostate cancer. *Br. J. Cancer* **2001**, *85*, 576–583. [CrossRef]

61. Bok, R.A.; Halabi, S.; Fei, D.T.; Rodriquez, C.R.; Hayes, D.F.; Vogelzang, N.J.; Kantoff, P.; Shuman, M.A.; Small, E.J. Vascular endothelial growth factor and basic fibroblast growth factor urine levels as predictors of outcome in hormone-refractory prostate cancer patients: A cancer and leukemia group B study. *Cancer Res.* **2001**, *61*, 2533–2536. [PubMed]
62. Dorkin, T.J.; Robinson, M.C.; Marsh, C.; Bjartell, A.; Neal, D.E.; Leung, H.Y. FGF8 over-expression in prostate cancer is associated with decreased patient survival and persists in androgen independent disease. *Oncogene* **1999**, *18*, 2755–2761. [CrossRef] [PubMed]
63. Casanovas, O.; Hicklin, D.J.; Bergers, G.; Hanahan, D. Drug resistance by evasion of antiangiogenic targeting of VEGF signaling in late-stage pancreatic islet tumors. *Cancer Cell.* **2005**, *8*, 299–309. [CrossRef]
64. Gong, Y.; Chippada-Venkata, U.D.; Oh, W.K. Roles of matrix metalloproteinases and their natural inhibitors in prostate cancer progression. *Cancers* **2014**, *6*, 1298–1327. [CrossRef] [PubMed]
65. Kessenbrock, K.; Plaks, V.; Werb, Z. Matrix metalloproteinases: Regulators of the tumor microenvironment. *Cell* **2010**, *141*, 52–67. [CrossRef] [PubMed]
66. Gialeli, C.; Theocharis, A.D.; Karamanos, N.K. Roles of matrix metalloproteinases in cancer progression and their pharmacological targeting. *FEBS J.* **2011**, *278*, 16–27. [CrossRef] [PubMed]
67. Wood, M.; Fudge, K.; Mohler, J.L.; Frost, A.R.; Garcia, F.; Wang, M.; Stearns, M.E. In situ hybridization studies of metallo-proteinases 2 and 9 and TIMP-1 and TIMP-2 expression in human prostate cancer. *Clin. Exp. Metastasis* **1997**, *15*, 246–258. [CrossRef]
68. Littlepage, L.E.; Sternlicht, M.D.; Rougier, N.; Phillips, J.; Gallo, E.; Yu, Y.; Williams, K.; Brenot, A.; Gordon, J.I.; Werb, Z. Matrix metalloproteinases contribute distinct roles in neuroendocrine prostate carcinogenesis, metastasis, and angiogenesis progression. *Cancer Res.* **2010**, *70*, 2224–2234. [CrossRef]
69. Aalinkeel, R.; Nair, M.P.; Sufrin, G.; Mahajan, S.D.; Chadha, K.C.; Chawda, R.P.; Schwartz, S.A. Gene expression of angiogenic factors correlates with metastatic potential of prostate cancer cells. *Cancer Res.* **2004**, *64*, 5311–5321. [CrossRef]
70. Aalinkeel, R.; Nair, B.B.; Reynolds, J.L.; Sykes, D.E.; Mahajan, S.D.; Chadha, K.C.; Schwartz, S.A. Overexpression of MMP-9 contributes to invasiveness of prostate cancer cell line LNCaP. *Immunol. Investig.* **2011**, *40*, 447–464. [CrossRef]
71. Gupta, A.; Zhou, C.Q.; Chellaiah, M.A. Osteopontin and MMP9: Associations with VEGF Expression/Secretion and Angiogenesis in PC3 Prostate Cancer Cells. *Cancers* **2013**, *5*, 617–638. [CrossRef] [PubMed]
72. Bruni-Cardoso, A.; Johnson, L.C.; Vessella, R.L.; Peterson, T.E.; Lynch, C.C. Osteoclast-derived matrix metalloproteinase-9 directly affects angiogenesis in the prostate tumor-bone microenvironment. *Mol. Cancer Res.* **2010**, *8*, 459–470. [CrossRef] [PubMed]
73. Trudel, D.; Fradet, Y.; Meyer, F.; Têtu, B. Matrix metalloproteinase 9 is associated with Gleason score in prostate cancer but not with prognosis. *Hum. Pathol.* **2010**, *41*, 1694–1701. [CrossRef] [PubMed]
74. Akhurst, R.J.; Derynck, R. TGF-beta signaling in cancer–a double-edged sword. *Trends Cell Biol.* **2001**, *11*, S44–S51. [CrossRef] [PubMed]
75. Inman, G.J. Switching TGFβ from a tumor suppressor to a tumor promoter. *Curr. Opin. Genet. Dev.* **2011**, *21*, 93–99. [CrossRef] [PubMed]
76. Principe, D.R.; Doll, J.A.; Bauer, J.; Jung, B.; Munshi, H.G.; Bartholin, L.; Pasche, B.; Lee, C.; Grippo, P.J. TGF-β: Duality of function between tumor prevention and carcinogenesis. *J. Natl. Cancer Inst.* **2014**, *106*, djt369. [CrossRef]
77. Lu, S.; Lee, J.; Revelo, M.; Wang, X.; Lu, S.; Dong, Z. Smad3 is overexpressed in advanced human prostate cancer and necessary for progressive growth of prostate cancer cells in nude mice. *Clin. Cancer Res.* **2007**, *13*, 5692–5702. [CrossRef]
78. Mirzoeva, S.; Franzen, C.A.; Pelling, J.C. Apigenin inhibits TGF-β-induced VEGF expression in human prostate carcinoma cells via a Smad2/3- and Src-dependent mechanism. *Mol. Carcinog.* **2014**, *53*, 598–609. [CrossRef]
79. Ji, H.; Li, Y.; Jiang, F.; Wang, X.; Zhang, J.; Shen, J.; Yanget, X. Inhibition of transforming growth factor beta/SMAD signal by MiR-155 is involved in arsenic trioxide-induced anti-angiogenesis in prostate cancer. *Cancer Sci.* **2014**, *105*, 1541–1549. [CrossRef]
80. Mahmud, S.; Franco, E.; Aprikian, A. Prostate cancer and use of nonsteroidal anti-inflammatory drugs: Systematic review and meta-analysis. *Br. J. Cancer* **2004**, *90*, 93–99. [CrossRef]

81. Cai, T.; Santi, R.; Tamanini, I.; Galli, I.C.; Perletti, G.; Bjerklund Johansen, T.E.; Nesi, G. Current Knowledge of the Potential Links between Inflammation and Prostate Cancer. *Int. J. Mol. Sci.* **2019**, *20*, 3833. [CrossRef] [PubMed]
82. Masferrer, J.L.; Leahy, K.M.; Koki, A.T.; Zweifel, B.S.; Settle, S.L.; Woerner, B.M.; Edwaeds, D.A.; Flickinger, A.G.; More, R.J.; Seibert, K. Antiangiogenic and antitumor activities of cyclooxygenase-2 inhibitors. *Cancer Res.* **2000**, *60*, 1306–1311. [PubMed]
83. Khor, L.Y.; Bae, K.; Pollack, A.; Hammond, M.E.; Grignon, D.J.; Venkatesan, V.M.; Rosenthal, S.A.; Ritter, M.A.; Sandler, H.M.; Hanks, G.E.; et al. COX-2 expression predicts prostate-cancer outcome: Analysis of data from the RTOG 92-02 trial. *Lancet Oncol.* **2007**, *8*, 912–920. [CrossRef]
84. Dandekar, D.S.; Lokeshwar, B.L. Inhibition of cyclooxygenase (COX)-2 expression by Tet-inducible COX-2 antisense cDNA in hormone-refractory prostate cancer significantly slows tumor growth and improves efficacy of chemotherapeutic drugs. *Clin. Cancer Res.* **2004**, *10*, 8037–8047. [CrossRef]
85. Liu, X.H.; Kirschenbaum, A.; Yao, S.; Lee, R.; Holland, J.F.; Levine, A.C. Inhibition of cyclooxygenase-2 suppresses angiogenesis and the growth of prostate cancer in vivo. *J. Urol.* **2000**, *164*, 820–825. [CrossRef]
86. Gately, S. The contributions of cyclooxygenase-2 to tumor angiogenesis. *Cancer Metastasis Rev.* **2000**, *19*, 19–27. [CrossRef]
87. Setrerrahmane, S.; Xu, H. Tumor-related interleukins: Old validated targets for new anti-cancer drug development. *Mol. Cancer* **2017**, *16*, 153. [CrossRef]
88. Anestakis, D.; Petanidis, S.; Kalyvas, S.; Nday, C.M.; Tsave, O.; Kioseoglou, E.; Salifoglou, A. Mechanisms and applications of interleukins in cancer immunotherapy. *Int. J. Mol. Sci.* **2015**, *16*, 1691–1710. [CrossRef]
89. Jiang, X.; Wang, J.; Deng, X.; Xiong, F.; Ge, J.; Xiang, B.; Wu, X.; Ma, J.; Zhou, M.; Li, X.; et al. Role of the tumor microenvironment in PD-L1/PD-1-mediated tumor immune escape. *Mol. Cancer* **2019**, *18*, 10. [CrossRef]
90. Araki, S.; Omori, Y.; Lyn, D.; Lyn, D.; Singh, R.K.; Meinbach, D.M.; Sandman, Y.; Lokeshwar, V.B.; Lokeshwar, B.L. Interleukin-8 is a molecular determinant of androgen independence and progression in prostate cancer. *Cancer Res.* **2007**, *67*, 6854–6862. [CrossRef]
91. Inoue, K.; Slaton, J.W.; Eve, B.Y.; Kim, S.J.; Perrotte, P.; Balbay, M.D.; Yano, S.; Bar-Eli, M.; Radinsky, R.; Pettaway, C.A.; et al. Interleukin 8 expression regulates tumorigenicity and metastases in androgen-independent prostate cancer. *Clin. Cancer Res.* **2000**, *6*, 2104–2119. [PubMed]
92. Middleton, K.; Jones, J.; Lwin, Z.; Coward, J.I. Interleukin-6: An angiogenic target in solid tumours. *Crit. Rev. Oncol. Hematol.* **2014**, *89*, 129–139. [CrossRef] [PubMed]
93. Roumeguère, T.; Legrand, F.; Rassy, E.E.; Kaitouni, M.; Albisinni, S.; Rousseau, A.; Vanhaeverbeek, M.; Rorive, S.; Decaestecker, C.; Debeir, O.; et al. A prospective clinical study of the implications of IL-8 in the diagnosis, aggressiveness and prognosis of prostate cancer. *Future Sci. OA* **2017**, *4*, FSO266. [CrossRef] [PubMed]
94. Di Carlo, E.; Sorrentino, C.; Zorzoli, A.; Di Meo, S.; Tupone, M.G.; Ognio, E.; Mincione, G.; Airoldi, I. The antitumor potential of Interleukin-27 in prostate cancer. *Oncotarget* **2014**, *5*, 10332–10341. [CrossRef]
95. Stearns, M.E.; Wang, M.; Hu, Y.; Garcia, F.U.; Rhim, J. Interleukin 10 blocks matrix metalloproteinase-2 and membrane type 1-matrix metalloproteinase synthesis in primary human prostate tumor lines. *Clin. Cancer Res.* **2003**, *3*, 1191–1199.
96. Vanacore, D.; Boccellino, M.; Rossetti, S.; Cavaliere, C.; D'Aniello, C.; Di Franco, R.; Romano, F.J.; Montanari, M.; Mantia, E.L.; Piscitelli, R.; et al. Micrornas in prostate cancer: An overview. *Oncotarget* **2017**, *8*, 50240–50251. [CrossRef]
97. Guan, B.; Wu, K.; Zeng, J.; Xu, S.; Mu, L.; Gao, Y.; Wang, K.; Ma, Z.; Tian, J.; Shi, Q.; et al. Tumor-suppressive microRNA-218 inhibits tumor angiogenesis via targeting the mTOR component RICTOR in prostate cancer. *Oncotarget* **2017**, *8*, 8162–8172. [CrossRef]
98. Misawa, A.; Takayama, K.I.; Inoue, S. Long non-coding RNAs and prostate cancer. *Cancer Sci.* **2017**, *108*, 2107–2114. [CrossRef]
99. Takayama, K.I.; Misawa, A.; Inoue, S. Significance of microRNAs in Androgen Signaling and Prostate Cancer Progression. *Cancers* **2017**, *9*, 102. [CrossRef]
100. Saber, S.H.; Ali, H.E.A.; Gaballa, R.; Gaballah, M.; Ali, H.I.; Zerfaoui, M.; Elmageed, Z.Y.A. Exosomes are the Driving Force in Preparing the Soil for the Metastatic Seeds: Lessons from the Prostate Cancer. *Cells* **2020**, *9*, 564. [CrossRef]

101. Liu, C.M.; Hsieh, C.L.; Shen, C.N.; Lin, C.C.; Shigemura, K.; Sung, S.Y. Exosomes from the tumor microenvironment as reciprocal regulators that enhance prostate cancer progression. *Int. J. Urol.* **2016**, *23*, 734–744. [CrossRef] [PubMed]
102. Vlaeminck-Guillem, V. Extracellular Vesicles in Prostate Cancer Carcinogenesis, Diagnosis, and Management. *Front. Oncol.* **2018**, *8*, 222. [CrossRef] [PubMed]
103. Wang, Y.; Wang, L.; Chen, C.; Chu, X. New insights into the regulatory role of microRNA in tumor angiogenesis and clinical implications. *Mol. Cancer* **2018**, *17*, 22. [CrossRef] [PubMed]
104. Lin, Z.Y.; Chen, G.; Zhang, Y.Q.; He, H.C.; Liang, Y.X.; Ye, J.H.; Liang, Y.K.; Mo, R.J.; Lu, J.M.; Zhou, Y.J.; et al. MicroRNA-30d promotes angiogenesis and tumor growth via MYPT1/c-JUN/VEGFA pathway and predicts aggressive outcome in prostate cancer [published correction appears in prostate cancer. *Mol. Cancer* **2019**, 18, 122]. *Mol. Cancer* **2017**, *16*, 48. [CrossRef] [PubMed]
105. Gao, Q.; Yao, X.; Zheng, J. MiR-323 Inhibits Prostate Cancer Vascularization Through Adiponectin Receptor. *Cell Physiol. Biochem.* **2015**, *36*, 1491–1498. [CrossRef]
106. Li, Y.; Zhang, D.; Wang, X.; Yao, X.; Ye, C.; Zhang, S.; Wang, H.; Chang, C.; Xia, H.; Wang, Y.; et al. Hypoxia-inducible miR-182 enhances HIF1α signaling via targeting PHD2 and FIH1 in prostate cancer. *Sci. Rep.* **2015**, *5*, 12495. [CrossRef]
107. Liu, L.Z.; Li, C.; Chen, Q.; Jing, Y.; Carpenter, R.; Jiang, Y.; Kung, H.F.; Lai, L.; Jiang, B.H. MiR-21 induced angiogenesis through AKT and ERK activation and HIF-1α expression. *PLoS ONE.* **2011**, *6*, e19139. [CrossRef]
108. Würdinger, T.; Tannous, B.A.; Saydam, O.; Skog, J.; Grau, S.; Soutschek, J.; Weissleder, R.; Breakefield, X.O.; Krichevsky, A.M. miR-296 regulates growth factor receptor overexpression in angiogenic endothelial cells. *Cancer Cell.* **2008**, *14*, 382–393. [CrossRef]
109. Lou, W.; Liu, J.; Gao, Y.; Lou, W.; Liu, J.; Gao, Y.; Zhong, G.; Chen, D.; Shen, J.; Ding, B.; et al. MicroRNAs in cancer metastasis and angiogenesis. *Oncotarget* **2017**, *8*, 115787–115802. [CrossRef]
110. Cai, C.; Chen, Q.B.; Han, Z.D.; Zhang, Y.Q.; He, H.C.; Chen, J.H.; Chen, Y.R.; Yang, S.B.; Wu, Y.D.; Qin, G.Q.; et al. miR-195 Inhibits Tumor Progression by Targeting RPS6KB1 in Human Prostate Cancer. *Clin. Cancer Res.* **2015**, *21*, 4922–4934. [CrossRef]
111. Cai, C.; He, H.; Duan, X.; Wu, W.; Mai, Z.; Zhang, T.; Fan, J.; Deng, T.; Zhong, W.; Liu, Y.; et al. miR-195 inhibits cell proliferation and angiogenesis in human prostate cancer by downregulating PRR11 expression. *Oncol. Rep.* **2018**, *39*, 1658–1670. [CrossRef]
112. Xu, B.; Wang, N.; Wang, X.; Tong, N.; Shao, N.; Tao, J.; Li, P.; Niu, X.; Feng, N.; Zhang, L.; et al. MiR-146a suppresses tumor growth and progression by targeting EGFR pathway and in a p-ERK-dependent manner in castration-resistant prostate cancer. *Prostate* **2012**, *72*, 1171–1178. [CrossRef]
113. Mu, H.Q.; He, Y.H.; Wang, S.B.; Yang, S.; Wang, Y.J.; Nan, C.J.; Bao, Y.F.; Xie, Q.P.; Chen, Y.H. MiR-130b/TNF-α/NF-κB/VEGFA loop inhibits prostate cancer angiogenesis. *Clin. Transl. Oncol.* **2020**, *22*, 111–121. [CrossRef] [PubMed]
114. De Oliveira, J.C.; Oliveira, L.C.; Mathias, C.; Pedroso, G.A.; Lemos, D.S.; Salviano-Silva, A.; Gradia, D.F.; Jucoski, T.S.; Lobo-Alves, S.C.; Zamalde, E.P.; et al. Long non-coding RNAs in cancer: Another layer of complexity. *J. Gene Med.* **2019**, *21*, e3065. [CrossRef]
115. Salameh, A.; Lee, A.K.; Cardó-Vila, M.; Nunes, D.; Efstathiou, E.; Staquicini, F.; Dobroff, A.S.; Machio, S.; Navone, N.; Hpsoya, H.; et al. PRUNE2 is a human prostate cancer suppressor regulated by the intronic long noncoding RNA PCA3. *Proc. Natl. Acad. Sci. USA* **2015**, *112*, 8403–8408. [CrossRef] [PubMed]
116. Tao, F.; Tian, X.; Zhang, Z. The PCAT3/PCAT9-miR-203-SNAI2 axis functions as a key mediator for prostate tumor growth and progression. *Oncotarget* **2018**, *9*, 12212–12225. [CrossRef] [PubMed]
117. Jiang, Z.; Zhang, Y.; Chen, X.; Wu, P.; Chen, D. Long noncoding RNA RBMS3-AS3 acts as a microRNA-4534 sponge to inhibit the progression of prostate cancer by upregulating VASH1. *Gene Ther.* **2020**, *27*, 143–156. [CrossRef]
118. Naito, Y.; Yoshioka, Y.; Yamamoto, Y.; Ochiya, T. How cancer cells dictate their microenvironment: Present roles of extracellular vesicles. *Cell Mol. Life Sci.* **2017**, *74*, 697–713. [CrossRef] [PubMed]
119. Ciardiello, C.; Leone, A.; Budillon, A. The Crosstalk between Cancer Stem Cells and Microenvironment Is Critical for Solid Tumor Progression: The Significant Contribution of Extracellular Vesicles. *Stem Cells Int.* **2018**, 6392198. [CrossRef]

120. Alcayaga-Miranda, F.; González, P.L.; Lopez-Verrilli, A.; Varas-Godoy, M.; Aguila-Díaz, C.; Contreras, L.; Khoury, M. Prostate tumor-induced angiogenesis is blocked by exosomes derived from menstrual stem cells through the inhibition of reactive oxygen species. *Oncotarget* **2016**, *7*, 44462–44477. [CrossRef]
121. Lorenc, T.; Klimczyk, K.; Michalczewska, I.; Słomka, M.; Kubiak-Tomasze wska, G.; Olejarz, W. Exosomes in Prostate Cancer Diagnosis, Prognosis and Therapy. *Int. J. Mol. Sci.* **2020**, *21*, 2118. [CrossRef] [PubMed]
122. Mashouri, L.; Yousefi, H.; Aref, A.R.; Ahadi, A.M.; Molaei, F.; Alahari, S.K. Exosomes: Composition, biogenesis, and mechanisms in cancer metastasis and drug resistance. *Mol. Cancer* **2019**, *18*, 75. [CrossRef] [PubMed]
123. Kim, C.W.; Lee, H.M.; Lee, T.H.; Kang, C.; Kleinman, H.K.; Gho, Y.S. Extracellular membrane vesicles from tumor cells promote angiogenesis via sphingomyelin. *Cancer Res.* **2002**, *62*, 6312–6317.
124. Webber, J.; Steadman, R.; Mason, M.D.; Tabi, Z.; Clayton, A. Cancer exosomes trigger fibroblast to myofibroblast differentiation. *Cancer Res.* **2010**, *70*, 9621–9630. [CrossRef]
125. Webber, J.P.; Spary, L.K.; Sanders, A.J.; Chowdhury, R.; Jiang, W.G.; Steadman, R.; Wymant, J.; Jones, A.T.; Kynastion, H.; Tabi, Z.; et al. Differentiation of tumour-promoting stromal myofibroblasts by cancer exosomes. *Oncogene* **2015**, *34*, 290–302. [CrossRef]
126. Chowdhury, R.; Webber, J.P.; Gurney, M.; Mason, M.D.; Tabi, Z.; Clayton, A. Cancer exosomes trigger mesenchymal stem cell differentiation into pro-angiogenic and pro-invasive myofibroblasts. *Oncotarget* **2015**, *6*, 715–731. [CrossRef]
127. DeRita, R.M.; Zerlanko, B.; Singh, A.; Lu, H.; Iozzo, R.V.; Benovic, J.L.; Languino, L.R. c-Src, Insulin-Like Growth Factor I Receptor, G-Protein-Coupled Receptor Kinases and Focal Adhesion Kinase are Enriched Into Prostate Cancer Cell Exosomes. *J. Cell. Biochem.* **2017**, *118*, 66–73. [CrossRef]
128. Liu, T.; Mendes, D.E.; Berkman, C.E. Functional prostate-specific membrane antigen is enriched in exosomes from prostate cancer cells. *Int. J. Oncol.* **2014**, *44*, 918–922. [CrossRef]
129. McKay, R.R.; Zurita, A.J.; Werner, L.; Bruce, J.Y.; Carducci, M.A.; Stein, M.N.; Heath, E.I.; Hussain, A.; Tran, T.H.; Sweeney, C.J.; et al. A Randomized Phase II Trial of Short-Course Androgen Deprivation Therapy With or Without Bevacizumab for Patients With Recurrent Prostate Cancer After Definitive Local Therapy. *J. Clin. Oncol.* **2016**, *34*, 1913–1920. [CrossRef]
130. Ning, Y.M.; Gulley, J.L.; Arlen., P.M.; Woo, S.; Steinberg, S.M.; Wright, J.J.; Parnes, H.L.; Trepel, J.B.; Lee, M.; Kim, Y.S.; et al. Phase II trial of bevacizumab, thalidomide, docetaxel, and prednisone in patients with metastatic castration-resistant prostate cancer. *J. Clin. Oncol.* **2010**, *28*, 2070–2076. [CrossRef]
131. Picus, J.; Halabi, S.; Rini, B.; Vogelzang, N.; Whang, Y.; Kaplan, E.; Kelly, W.; Small, E. The use of bevacizumab (B) with docetaxel (D) and estramustine (E) in hormone refractory prostate cancer (HRPC): Initial results of CALGB 90006 (abstract 1578). *Proc. Am. Soc. Oncol.* **2003**, *22*, 393.
132. Picus, J.; Halabi, S.; Kelly, W.K.; Vogelzang, N.J.; Whang, Y.E.; Kaplan, E.B.; Stadler, W.M.; Small, E.J.; The Cancer and Leukemia Group B. A phase 2 study of estramustine, docetaxel, and bevacizumab in men with castrate-resistant prostate cancer: Results from Cancer and Leukemia Group B Study 90006. *Cancer* **2011**, *117*, 526–533. [CrossRef] [PubMed]
133. Kelly, W.K.; Halabi, S.; Carducci, M.; George, D.; Mahoney, J.F.; Stadler, W.M.; Morris, M.; Kantoff, P.; Monk, J.P.; Kaplan, E.; et al. Randomized, double-blind, placebo-controlled phase III trial comparing docetaxel and prednisone with or without bevacizumab in men with metastatic castration-resistant prostate cancer: CALGB 90401. *J. Clin. Oncol.* **2012**, *30*, 1534–1540. [CrossRef] [PubMed]
134. Barata, P.C.; Cooney, M.; Mendiratta, P.; Gupta, R.; Dreicer, R.; Garcia, J.A. Phase I/II study evaluating the safety and clinical efficacy of temsirolimus and bevacizumab in patients with chemotherapy refractory metastatic castration-resistant prostate cancer. *Investig. New Drugs* **2019**, *37*, 331–337. [CrossRef] [PubMed]
135. Mendel, D.B.; Laird, A.D.; Xin, X.; Louie, S.G.; Christensen, J.G.; Li, G.; Schreck, R.E.; Abrams, T.J.; Ngai, T.J.; Lee, L.B.; et al. In vivo antitumor activity of SU11248, a novel tyrosine kinase inhibitor targeting vascular endothelial growth factor and platelet-derived growth factor receptors: Determination of a pharmacokinetic/pharmacodynamic relationship. *Clin. Cancer Res.* **2003**, *9*, 327–337. [PubMed]
136. Michaelson, M.D.; Oudard, S.; Ou, Y.C.; Sengeløv, L.; Saad, F.; Houede, N.; Ostler, P.; Stenzl, A.; Daugaard, G.; Jones, R.; et al. Randomized, placebo-controlled, phase III trial of sunitinib plus prednisone versus prednisone alone in progressive, metastatic, castration-resistant prostate cancer. *J. Clin. Oncol.* **2014**, *32*, 76–82. [CrossRef] [PubMed]

137. Horti, J.; Widmark, A.; Stenzl, A.; Federico, M.H.; Abratt, R.P.; Sanders, N.; Pover, G.M.; Bodrogi, I. A randomized, double-blind, placebo-controlled phase II study of vandetanib plus docetaxel/prednisolone in patients with hormone-refractory prostate cancer. *Cancer Biother. Radiopharm.* **2009**, *24*, 175–180. [CrossRef]
138. Azad, A.A.; Beardsley, E.K.; Hotte, S.J.; Ellard, S.L.; Klotz, L.; Chin, J.; Kollmannsberger, C.; Mukherjee, S.D.; Chi, K.N. A randomized phase II efficacy and safety study of vandetanib (ZD6474) in combination with bicalutamide versus bicalutamide alone in patients with chemotherapy naïve castration-resistant prostate cancer. *Investig. New Drugs* **2014**, *32*, 746–752. [CrossRef]
139. Tannock, I.F.; Fizazi, K.; Ivanov, S.; Karlsson, C.T.; Fléchon, A.; Skoneczna, I.; Orlandi, F.; Gravis, G.; Matveev, V.; Bavbek, S.; et al. Aflibercept versus placebo in combination with docetaxel and prednisone for treatment of men with metastatic castration-resistant prostate cancer (VENICE): A phase 3, double-blind randomised trial. *Lancet Oncol.* **2013**, *14*, 760–768. [CrossRef]
140. Figg, W.D.; Dahut, W.; Duray, P.; Hamilton, M.; Tompkins, A.; Steinberg, S.M.; Jones, E.; Premkumar, A.; MarstonLinehan, W.; KayFloeter, M.; et al. A randomized phase II trial of thalidomide, an angiogenesis inhibitor, in patients with androgen-independent prostate cancer. *Clin. Cancer Res.* **2001**, *7*, 1888–1893.
141. Drake, M.J.; Robson, W.; Mehta, P.; Schofield, I.; Neal, D.E.; Leung, H.Y. An open-label phase II study of low-dose thalidomide in androgen-independent prostate cancer. *Br. J. Cancer* **2003**, *88*, 822–827. [CrossRef] [PubMed]
142. Figg, W.D.; Arlen, P.; Gulley, J.; Fernandez, P.; Noone, M.; Fedenko, K.; Hamilton, M.; Parker, C.; Kruger, E.A.; Pluda, J.; et al. A randomized phase II trial of docetaxel (taxotere) plus thalidomide in androgen-independent prostate cancer. *Semin. Oncol.* **2001**, *28*, 62–66. [CrossRef]
143. Madan, R.A.; Karzai, F.H.; Ning, Y.M.; Adesunloye, B.A.; Huang, X.; Harold, N.; Couvillon, A.; Chun, G.; Cordes, L.; Sissung, T.; et al. Phase II trial of docetaxel, bevacizumab, lenalidomide and prednisone in patients with metastatic castration-resistant prostate cancer. *BJU Int.* **2016**, *11*, 590–597. [CrossRef] [PubMed]
144. Keizman, D.; Zahurak, M.; Sinibaldi, V.; Carducci, M.; Denmeade, S.; Drake, C.; Pili, R.; Antonarakis, E.S.; Hudock, S.; Eisenberger, M. Lenalidomide in non-metastatic biochemically relapsed prostate cancer: Results of a phase I/II double-blinded, randomized study. *Clin. Cancer Res.* **2010**, *16*, 5269–5276. [CrossRef]
145. Petrylak, D.P.; Vogelzang, N.J.; Budnik, N.; Jan Wiechno, P.; Sternberg, C.N.; Doner, K.; Bellmunt, J.; Burke, J.M.; de Olza, M.O.; Choudhury, A.; et al. Docetaxel and prednisone with or without lenalidomide in chemotherapy-naive patients with metastatic castration-resistant prostate cancer (MAINSAIL): A randomised, double-blind, placebo-controlled phase 3 trial. *Lancet Oncol.* **2015**, *16*, 417–425. [CrossRef]
146. Yakes, F.M.; Chen, J.; Tan, J.; Yamaguchi, K.; Shi, Y.; Yu, P.; Qian, F.; Chu, F.; Bentzien, F.; Cancilla, B.; et al. Cabozantinib (XL184), a novel MET and VEGFR2 inhibitor, simultaneously suppresses metastasis, angiogenesis, and tumor growth. *Mol. Cancer Ther.* **2011**, *12*, 2298–2308. [CrossRef]
147. Schöffski, P.; Gordon, M.; Smith, D.C.; Kurzrock, R.; Daud, A.; Vogelzang, N.J.; Lee, Y.; Scheffold, C.; Shapiro, G.I. Phase II randomised discontinuation trial of cabozantinib in patients with advanced solid tumours. *Eur. J. Cancer* **2017**, *86*, 296–304. [CrossRef]
148. Smith, D.C.; Smith., M.R.; Sweeney, C.; Elfiky, A.A.; Logothetis, C.; Corn, P.G.; Vogelzang, N.J.; Small, E.J.; Harzstark, A.L.; Gordonet, M.S.; et al. Cabozantinib in patients with advanced prostate cancer: Results of a phase II randomized discontinuation trial. *J. Clin. Oncol.* **2013**, *31*, 412–419. [CrossRef]
149. Smith, M.; De Bono, J.; Sternberg, C.; Oudard, S.; De Giorgi, U.; Krainer, M.; Bergman, A.; Hoelzer, W.; De Wit, R.; Bögemann, M.; et al. Phase III Study of Cabozantinib in Previously Treated Metastatic Castration-Resistant Prostate Cancer: COMET-1. *J. Clin. Oncol.* **2016**, *34*, 3005–3013. [CrossRef]
150. Kluetz, P.G.; Figg, W.D.; Dahut, W.L. Angiogenesis inhibitors in the treatment of prostate cancer. *Expert Opin. Pharmacother.* **2010**, *11*, 233–247. [CrossRef]
151. Melegh, Z.; Oltean, S. Targeting Angiogenesis in Prostate Cancer. *Int. J. Mol. Sci.* **2019**, *20*, 2676. [CrossRef] [PubMed]
152. Adesunloye, B.A.; Karzai, F.H.; Dahut, W.L. Angiogenesis inhibitors in the treatment of prostate cancer. *Chem. Immunol. Allergy* **2014**, *99*, 197–215. [CrossRef] [PubMed]
153. Yu, E.M.; Jain, M.; Aragon-Ching, J.B. Angiogenesis inhibitors in prostate cancer therapy. *Discov. Med.* **2010**, *10*, 521–530. [PubMed]
154. De Bono, J.S.; Scher, H.I.; Montgomery, R.B.; Parker, C.; Miller, M.C.; Tissing, H.; Doyle, G.V.; Terstappen, L.W.; Pienta, K.J.; Raghavan, D.; et al. Circulating tumor cells predict survival benefit from treatment in metastatic castration-resistant prostate cancer. *Clin. Cancer Res.* **2008**, *14*, 6302–6309. [CrossRef] [PubMed]

155. Hlatky, L.; Hahnfeldt, P.; Folkman, J. Clinical application of antiangiogenic therapy: Microvessel density, what it does and doesn't tell us. *J. Natl. Cancer Inst.* **2002**, *94*, 883–893. [CrossRef]
156. Jain, R.K.; Schlenger, K.; Höckel, M.; Yuan, F. Quantitative angiogenesis assays: Progress and problems. *Nat. Med.* **1997**, *3*, 1203–1208. [CrossRef]
157. Jiang, J.; Chen, Y.; Zhu, Y.; Yao, X.; Qi, J. Contrast-enhanced ultrasonography for the detection and characterization of prostate cancer: Correlation with microvessel density and Gleason score. *Clin. Radiol.* **2011**, *66*, 732–737. [CrossRef]

4

Survival Outcomes of Patients with Pathologically Proven Positive Lymph Nodes at Time of Radical Cystectomy with or without Neoadjuvant Chemotherapy

Guillaume Ploussard [1,*], Benjamin Pradere [2,3], Jean-Baptiste Beauval [1], Christine Chevreau [4], Christophe Almeras [1], Etienne Suc [5], Jean-Romain Gautier [1], Anne-Pascale Laurenty [5], Mathieu Roumiguié [6], Guillaume Loison [1], Christophe Tollon [1], Loïc Mourey [4], Ambroise Salin [1], Evanguelos Xylinas [7] and Damien Pouessel [4]

1 Department of Urology, La Croix du Sud Hospital, 31130 Quint Fonsegrives, France; jbbeauval@gmail.com (J.-B.B.); c.almeras@gmail.com (C.A.); gautierjr@hotmail.fr (J.-R.G.); guillaumeloison@gmail.com (G.L.); tol@club-internet.fr (C.T.); ambroise.salin@gmail.com (A.S.)
2 Department of Urology, Bretonneau Hospital, 37000 Tours, France; benjaminpradere@gmail.com
3 Department of Urology, Comprehensive Cancer Center, Medical University of Vienna, 1090 Vienna, Austria
4 Department of Oncology, IUCT-O, 31000 Toulouse, France; chevreau.christine@iuct-oncopole.fr (C.C.); mourey.loic@iuct-oncopole.fr (L.M.); pouessel.damien@iuct-oncopole.fr (D.P.)
5 Department of Oncology, La Croix du Sud Hospital, 31130 Quint Fonsegrives, France; esucsjl@club-internet.fr (E.S.); aplaurenty@capio.fr (A.-P.L.)
6 Department of Urology, CHU-IUC, 31000 Toulouse, France; roumiguie_mathieu@yahoo.fr
7 Department of Urology, Bichat-Claude Bernard Hospital, Assistance Publique-Hopitaux de Paris, Paris University, 75018 Paris, France; evanguelosxylinas@hotmail.com
* Correspondence: g.ploussard@gmail.com

Abstract: Background: To compare overall survival (OS) outcomes in pN1-3 disease at the time of radical cystectomy (RC) for muscle invasive bladder according to the neoadjuvant chemotherapy (NAC) status. Materials and Methods: This multicenter study included 450 consecutive patients undergoing RC for muscle-invasive urothelial bladder cancer with pN1-3 pM0 disease from 2010 to 2019. NAC consisted in platinum-based chemotherapy. The primary endpoint was the comparison between NAC and non-NAC in terms of death from any cause. OS was assessed using the Kaplan–Meier method and multivariate Cox proportional hazards regression was used to estimate adjusted hazard ratios. Results: Median age was 69 years. Patients receiving NAC were younger ($p = 0.051$), and more likely had downstaging to non-muscle invasive disease (10.7% versus 4.3%, $p = 0.042$). Median OS was 26.6 months. NAC patients had poorer OS compared with those who did receive NAC (Hazard ratio (HR) 1.6; $p = 0.019$). The persistence of muscle-invasive bladder in RC specimens was also significantly associated with OS (HR 2.40). In the NAC cohort, the two factors independently correlated with OS were the number of positive lymph nodes ($p = 0.013$) and adjuvant chemotherapy (AC) (HR 0.31; $p = 0.015$). Conclusions: Persistent nodal disease in RC specimens after NAC was associated with poor prognosis and lower OS rates compared with pN1-3 disease after upfront RC. In this sub-group of NAC patients, AC was independently associated with better OS.

Keywords: bladder cancer; nodal disease; pN1; radical cystectomy; neoadjuvant; adjuvant; chemotherapy

1. Introduction

Muscle-invasive bladder cancer is a highly aggressive disease with poor oncologic outcomes in case of lymph node involvement. Neoadjuvant chemotherapy (NAC) prior to radical cystectomy

(RC) has proven to improve survival outcomes in localized muscle-invasive bladder [1–3]. Level I evidence demonstrates a survival advantage of 5% as well as complete response on both primary and nodal tumor tissues [3]. The pN0 rate after NAC in cN+ patients has been evaluated as high as 48% in a retrospective series of 304 patients [4]. However, in spite of this proven overall survival (OS) advantage, a certain proportion of patients did not respond to NAC and exhibited aggressive patterns at the time of deferred RC, including pN1-3 disease. Despite NAC, up to one-fifth of the patients harbored nodal disease involvement at the time of RC [5]. However, the differential outcomes of pN1-3 patients stratified by the use or not of NAC is not well established. Moreover, there is little evidence and no firm recommendation on how to treat patients with positive lymph nodes after RC, especially after NAC administration [6]. In that setting, the use of adjuvant chemotherapy (AC) and of platinum-based regimens could be limited by potential tumor cells resistance and cumulative toxicity. Thus, whereas the impact of NAC on survival outcomes of cN1-3 patients prior to RC has been assessed in retrospective trials, to our knowledge, no series has compared OS between NAC and non-NAC patients harboring pN1-3 disease at the time of RC, and therefore the potential benefit of AC administration in that setting [4,7]. Studies comparing oncologic outcomes of pN1-3 disease according to the NAC status are biased by the selection, in the NAC group, of patients who did not respond to chemotherapy given persistent or progressing node disease after NAC. This selection bias based on resistance to neoadjuvant therapy has to be considered but helped to understand the need for aggressive post-RC treatment or monitoring in case of NAC failure.

2. Materials and Methods

2.1. Patients

We included 450 consecutive patients that underwent radical cystectomy (RC) for muscle-invasive urothelial bladder cancer with pathologically proven nodal disease from 2010 to 2019 at two institutions. After institutional review board approval (IRB number: 00006477 2017-016; review board: CEERB Paris Nord), all patients gave their written informed consent to participate in the prospective assessment of the outcomes (personal data collection and analysis). All RC were planned for cT2-4 cM0 disease, and we only included patients with pN1-3 disease. Clinical stage showed cT3 and cT4 disease in 31% and 20% of NAC patients, and 30% and 13.8% of non-NAC patients, respectively (48.2% of missing data for that variable). Patients with distant metastases (pM1a-b) on the pre-operative computerized tomography (CT) scan were excluded from analysis. The CT scan was systematically performed at the time of diagnosis. RC was performed less than 6 weeks after the diagnosis or less than 6 weeks after the last cycle of NAC. In case of NAC, another CT scan was performed before RC to confirm the absence of progression during NAC which would contra-indicate surgery. NAC and AC consisted of platinum-based chemotherapy. All patients treated by NAC received MVAC (methotrexate-vinblastine-doxorubicine-cisplatin) or GC (gemcitabline-cisplatin) regimen. AC was defined as a chemotherapy regimen given after RC before any sign of post-surgery progression, and platinum-based chemotherapy was the regimen of choice in the absence of contra-indication. Chemotherapy regimen and number of cycles were administered at clinician discretion in accordance with institutional standards and on individual decision-making. Patients treated with adjuvant radiotherapy or a combination of radiation and chemotherapy were excluded. All pathology data, including TNM stage, tumor grade, presence of positive soft tissue margin, total number of removed lymph nodes (LN), and number of LN+ were obtained from the pathological reports. Clinicopathological characteristics, surgical and adjuvant treatments, and follow-up data were collected in medical records. The chemotherapy status (NAC, AC) was recorded.

2.2. Primary and Secondary Endpoints and Statistics

The primary endpoint was the comparison between NAC and non-NAC in terms of death from any cause. Overall survival (OS) was assessed from the date of surgery until the date of death. OS was estimated using the Kaplan–Meier method and was compared using log-rank analysis. OS rates were calculated with 95% confidence intervals. Multivariate Cox proportional hazards regression was used to estimate adjusted hazard ratios with 95% confidence interval. The limit of statistical significance was defined as $p < 0.05$. The SPSS 22.0 (IBM, Chicago, IL, USA) software was used for analysis.

3. Results

3.1. Clinical and Pathological Features of the Entire Cohort (n = 450)

Median age was 69 years with 73.1% male patients (Table 1). Downstaging to non-muscle invasive disease in RC specimens was 5.0%. Lymphovascular invasion and concomitant carcinoma in situ (CIS) were reported in 67.1% and 40.2% of cases, respectively. Soft tissue surgical margins were positive in 12.9% of the specimens. Median lymph node yield and positive lymph nodes were 16 and 2, respectively. Overall, 12.4% and 54.2% of patients received NAC +/− AC, and AC only, respectively. Among the overall cohort, 4.4% of patients received both chemo regimens. Approximately, half of patients died after a mean follow-up of 23 months. Distant systemic progression (bone and/or visceral metastases) was reported in 41.8% of patients.

Table 1. Overall cohort clinical and pathological characteristics ($n = 450$).

	***N* = 450**
Gender (*n*, %):	
Male	329 (73.1)
Female	121 (26.9)
Age (years):	
Mean	67.5
Median (range) IQR	69.0 (25–93)
Pathological stage (*n*, %):	
pT0-pTis	12 (2.6)
pT1	11 (2.4)
pT2	78 (17.3)
pT3	247 (54.9)
pT4	102 (22.7)
Presence of lymphovascular invasion (*n*, %)	302 (67.1)
Presence of concomitant CIS (*n*, %)	181 (40.2)
Presence of soft tissue surgical margins (*n*, %)	58 (12.9)
Number of lymph nodes analyzed:	
Mean	17.5
Median (range) IQR	16.0 (1–70)
Number of positive lymph nodes:	
Mean	3.9
Median (range) IQR	2.0 (1–41)
Type of chemotherapy regimen (%):	
None	170 (37.8)
Neoadjuvant without adjuvant	36 (8.0)
Neoadjuvant + adjuvant	20 (4.4)
Adjuvant only	224 (54.2)
All-cause death (%)	220 (48.9)
Follow-up (months):	
Mean	23.0
Median (range) IQR	17.3 (3–130)

IQR = interquartile range, CIS = carcinoma in situ.

3.2. Comparisons of Clinical and Pathological Features Stratified by NAC Administration

Clinical and pathological features of both cohorts were compared (Table 2). Patients receiving NAC were younger (65 versus 68 years, $p = 0.051$), and more likely had downstaging to non-muscle invasive disease (10.7% versus 4.3%, $p = 0.042$). No significant difference was seen regarding CIS, lymphovascular invasion, positive lymph nodes, and soft tissue margin. Non-NAC patients were more frequently treated by AC (56.9% versus 35.7%, $p = 0.003$) and developed fewer systemic progression (39.1% versus 60.1%, $p = 0.002$).

Table 2. Comparisons between neoadjuvant chemotherapy (NAC) and non-NAC patients.

	NAC Cohort $N = 56$	**Non-NAC Cohort** $N = 394$	***p*-Value**
Male (%) gender	46 (82.1)	283 (71.8)	0.103
Age (mean)	65.0	68.0	0.051
Pathological stage (%):			
pT0-pTis	3 (5.4)	9 (2.3)	
pT1	3 (5.4)	8 (2.0)	0.097
pT2	6 (10.7)	72 (18.3)	
pT3	29 (51.8)	218 (55.3)	
pT4	15 (26.8)	87 (22.1)	
Previous history of non-muscle-invasive bladder tumor before T2-4 diagnosis (%)	6 (10.7)	17 (4.3)	0.042
Presence of lymphovascular invasion (%)	42 (75.0)	260 (66.0)	0.179
Presence of concomitant CIS (%)	17 (30.4)	164 (41.6)	0.108
Soft tissue surgical margins (%)	7 (12.5)	51 (12.9)	0.926
Number of lymph nodes analyzed yield (mean)	17.6	17.1	0.777
Number of positive lymph nodes (mean)	3.8	4.8	0.197
Adjuvant chemotherapy administration (%)	20 (35.7)	224 (56.9)	0.003
Distant metastases (%)	34 (60.7)	154 (39.1)	0.002

NAC = neoadjuvant chemotherapy, CIS = carcinoma in situ.

3.3. Survival Analysis in the Overall Cohort

The OS curve of the overall cohort is shown in Figure 1A. Median OS was 26.6 months. The 1-, 2-, and 5-year OS rates were 75.9% (±2.1), 54.3% (±2.7), and 29.2% (±3.2) in the overall cohort.

NAC patients had poorer OS compared with those who did not receive NAC (log rank test: $p = 0.019$, Figure 1B). The 1-, 2-, and 5-year OS rates were 66.8% (±7.3), 34.6% (±8.3), and 16.3% (±7.7) in the NAC cohort, versus 76.9% (±2.2), 56.3% (±2.8), and 30.5% (±3.5) in the non-NAC cohort. Median OS in the NAC and non-NAC cohorts was 16.7 and 28.8 months, respectively.

The OS curves were then stratified according to the type of primary chemotherapy received (Figure 1C): no chemotherapy, NAC, or AC. Patients treated by AC had better OS outcomes compared with those receiving NAC or no chemotherapy (log rank test: $p < 0.001$). Median OS was 33.6 months, compared with 22.0 and 16.7 months in the no chemotherapy and NAC cohorts, respectively. Survival curves did not differ significantly between patients who did not receive any chemotherapy and NAC patients, in spite of a trend toward better outcomes during the first 18 months after RC ($p = 0.557$). Curves crossed at this time point with better long-term outcomes in patients without any neoadjuvant or adjuvant chemotherapy regimens.

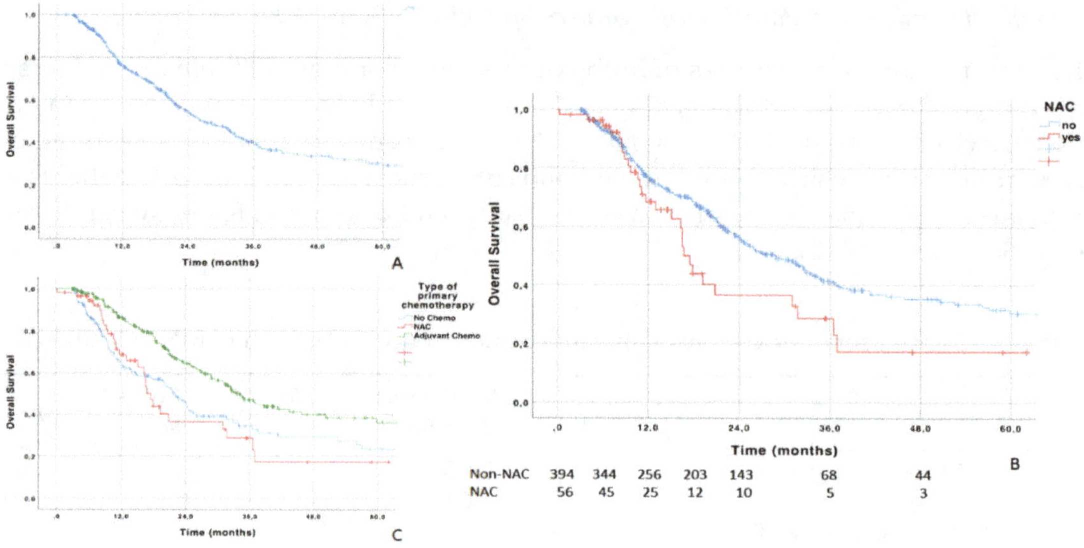

Figure 1. (**A**) Overall survival (OS) curve in the overall cohort; (**B**) OS stratified by the use of neoadjuvant chemotherapy (NAC); (**C**) OS stratified by the type of primary chemotherapy: neoadjuvant chemotherapy (NAC), adjuvant chemotherapy (AC), no chemotherapy.

3.4. Multivariable Analysis of Predictive Factors for OS in the Overall Cohort

Cox regression model confirmed that NAC was independently associated with overall mortality (Table 3). NAC patients had a 1.6-fold higher risk of death compared with non-NAC patients ($p = 0.018$; 95% confidence interval: 1.09–2.47). The persistence of muscle-invasive bladder in RC specimens was also significantly associated with OS (HR 2.40; 95% confidence interval: 1.06–5.44). This negative effect of NAC ($p = 0.072$) failed to reach significance when AC was taken into the multivariable model. AC was then positively and independently correlated with improved OS (HR 0.56; 95% confidence interval: 0.42–0.73; $p < 0.001$).

Table 3. Multivariable Cox regression analyses for predictors of overall survival (OS) in the overall cohort and in the neoadjuvant chemotherapy (NAC) cohort.

	HR	95% CI	*p*-Value
Overall cohort			
Model 1			
Gender	0.884	0.647–1.209	0.441
Age (continuous)	1.009	0.996–1.023	0.178
Muscle-invasive disease	2.404	1.062–5.442	0.035
Lymphovascular invasion	0.882	0.664–1.171	0.385
Concomitant CIS	1.088	0.830–1.427	0.540
Soft tissue surgical margin	1.338	0.910–1.965	0.138
Positive lymph nodes >3	1.283	0.959–1.717	0.093
NAC	1.638	1.089–2.465	0.018
Model 2			
NAC	1.445	0.968–2.159	0.072
Adjuvant Chemotherapy	0.557	0.426–0.728	<0.001
NAC cohort			
Muscle-invasive disease	0.296	0.060–1.470	0.137
Positive lymph nodes >3	3.281	1.287–8.365	0.013
Adjuvant chemotherapy	0.310	0.120–0.800	0.015

HR = hazard ratio; CI = confidence interval; CIS = carcinoma in situ.

3.5. *Stratified Survival Analysis in NAC Cohort*

Among NAC cohort, the administration of adjuvant chemotherapy was correlated with improved OS, without significant difference (Figure 2; $p = 0.099$). Median OS was 16.5 versus 31.7 months in patients receiving AC after NAC. The one-year OS rates were 61.9% (±9.7) versus 75.0% (±10.8) comparing patients who received AC and those who did not.

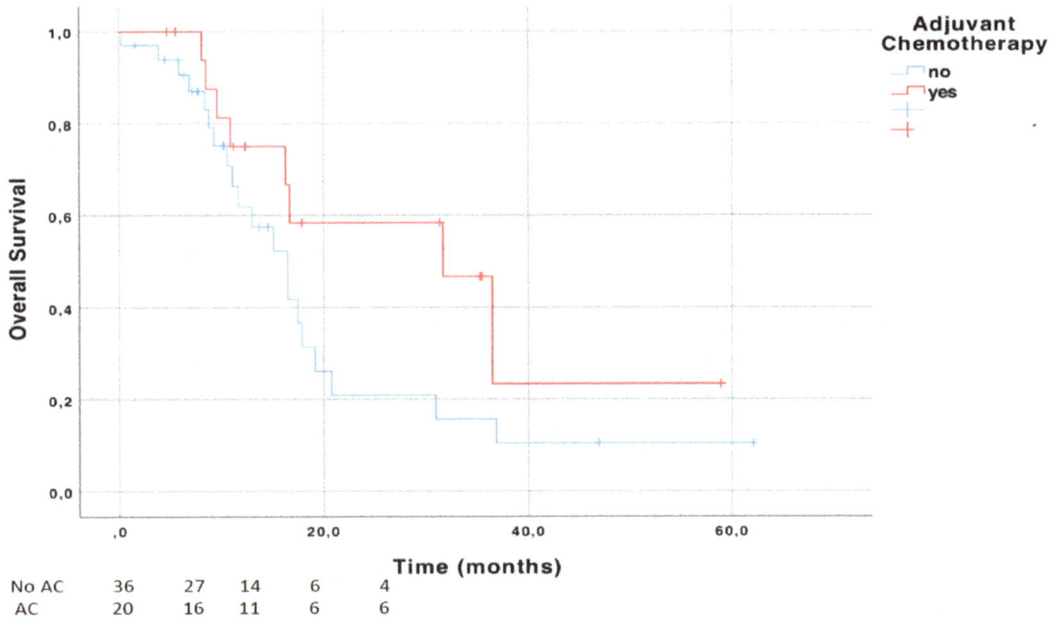

Figure 2. Survival curves for overall survival (OS) in the neoadjuvant chemotherapy (NAC) cohort stratified by the use of adjuvant chemotherapy (AC).

3.6. *Multivariable Analysis of Factors Associated with Overall Mortality in the NAC Cohort*

Cox regression analysis was performed in the subgroup of NAC patients (Table 3). Given the low number of patients ($n = 56$) and consequently the low number of events, we only included three factors which were the most correlated with overall mortality in univariable analyses. In the NAC cohort, the two factors independently correlated with overall mortality were the number of positive lymph nodes (>3 nodes; $p = 0.013$) and the administration of AC. AC was independently associated with a lower risk of overall mortality (HR 0.31; 95% confidence interval: 0.12–0.80; $p = 0.015$).

4. Discussion

NAC prior to RC has proven to improve survival outcomes in localized and locally advanced muscle-invasive bladder [1–3]. However, a non-negligible proportion of patients did not respond to NAC and exhibited aggressive patterns at the time of deferred RC including one-fifth of patients with nodal disease [5].

To date, there is little evidence on how to treat patients with positive lymph nodes after NAC and RC [6]. In a recent UK survey, 45% of oncologist responders would not give AC in patients with node disease after NAC and RC. Due to several factors, such as post-operative complications, impaired renal function, and poor performance status, the delivery of AC may be challenging even if an OS benefit is achieved [8]. Thus, the feasibility of re-challenging this group of NAC patients with AC is currently not well established, and patients are often offered salvage chemotherapy only at time of disease progression for palliation. A previous study of 37 patients with node positive disease after NAC previously suggested that patients who have persistent nodal disease have a very poor prognosis [9]. The two-year OS survival rate was 20%. The findings of this single-arm retrospective study highlighted a potential benefit from adjuvant chemotherapy. As reported in our series, there was a trend toward improved OS when AC was used.

While the rate of pT0 disease after NAC has been well assessed in the literature (approximately 30%), the complete response rate in node cannot be accurately evaluated due to the inaccuracy of preoperative evaluation. Indeed, node staging is currently performed by CT scan or pelvic magnetic resonance imaging (MRI). Both procedures are limited by poor sensitivity and specificity. In a series of clinical node-positive patients prior to NAC, Hermans et al. suggested that the rate of complete post-NAC response in pelvic lymph nodes (pN0) was 31% and 19% in cN1 and cN2-3 patients, respectively [7]. A complete response in lymph nodes has been evaluated at 48% in another retrospective study [4]. We were unable to assess this node downstaging rate given that we only included pN1-3 patients. However, even in patients having an aggressive disease with positive nodes at RC, our study suggests a positive impact of NAC on tumor tissue given that the pT0-1 rate was 10.8% in the NAC cohort, versus 4.3% only in non-NAC patients ($p = 0.042$). Unfortunately, given the limitations already evoked, the potential difference of response between primary cancer and metastatic nodal tissue cannot be relevantly evaluated.

The poorer OS achieved by NAC versus non-NAC patients with pN1-3 disease confirmed the need for adapting post-RC treatment in this high-risk sub-population. These patients will more frequently develop post-RC systemic progression (60.7% versus 39.1%) and die prematurely. Our findings suggest that the use of AC could be beneficial even after NAC. Indeed, OS was improved when AC was given, and AC was an independent protective factor in multivariable analysis, after taking into account positive lymph node burden and pT stage.

Consistently with French habits, MVAC was regarded in our experience as the first-line treatment of choice [10]. The pathological complete response rate achieved by dose dense MVAC appeared better than GC in retrospective studies [11]. Few patients received GC which could be preferred in other centers and/or countries due to a better toxicity profile. Comparable efficacy of GC has been emphasized, but in the metastatic setting [12]. Preliminary data from the VESPER trial (NCT01812369), comparing GC and MVAC as NAC, were presented recently, and the mature publication is awaited.

The role of AC after RC remains controversial. The main data come from underpowered trials due to poor recruitment, or from studies suffering from methodological issues. The advent of NAC before RC has also had a negative impact on enrollment in such trials [13]. The European Organisation for Research and Treatment of Cancer (NCT 30994) evaluated four cycles of immediate adjuvant chemotherapy versus six cycles of deferred chemotherapy at the time of relapse [14]. The benefit in OS was only seen in a small sub-group of pN0 patients ($n = 86$). Meta-analyses tend to confirm the reduction in the risk of death with AC (approximately 23%) [15,16]. Thus, although AC is no longer recommended, evidence suggests that it could be efficient, but mainly in chemotherapy-naive patients with locally advanced bladder cancer (pT3-4, pN0/pN +, pM0). Until now, no prospective trial has compared the sequence NAC versus NAC plus AC in patients with persistent locally advanced bladder cancer or lymph node involvement at the time of RC.

We did not report the detailed chemotherapy regimens in terms of number of cycles, toxicity data, palliative chemotherapy, and number of subsequent lines. The OS we showed could be impacted by all these parameters. Subsequent therapies for metastatic disease, that may have affected OS rates, were not available for all patients. Until recently, the only licensed second-line chemotherapy was vinflunine, which has demonstrated a three-month survival benefit with toxicity. However, the therapy landscape of advanced bladder cancer rapidly evolves. It is also worthy to note that this cohort was followed before the approval of immunotherapy regimens in advanced bladder cancer. The implementation of immunotherapy in the metastatic as well as in the neoadjuvant setting may modify the response to neoadjuvant treatment, as well as progression-free and overall survival [17]. In this study, we found that NAC patients treated by AC after RC achieved better OS outcomes compared with patients receiving only palliative chemotherapy. However, only one-third of NAC patients received AC due to poor performance status, post-operative complications, cumulative toxicity or various reasons.

The possibility to change AC for adjuvant immunotherapy could increase the number of NAC patients eligible for adjuvant therapy and offer life-prolonging drug options in that particular setting of pN1-3 NAC patients.

The combination of therapy could also be an interesting option in pN1-3 disease. Zaghloul et al. recently demonstrated in a phase II study that the addition of radiotherapy to AC could improve the locoregional recurrence-free survival [18]. The trend reported in terms of OS has to be confirmed in larger phase III trials. The GETUG-AFU 30 trial (NCT03333356) is ongoing to evaluate the benefit of adjuvant radiotherapy in high-risk cancers in terms of pelvic recurrence-free survival as primary endpoint, and OS as secondary endpoint.

It seemed worthy to note that we only included in this study NAC patients who did not respond to chemotherapy given persistent or progressing node disease after NAC. This sub-group selection based on first therapy resistance explained the worse prognosis of NAC patients compared with non-NAC patients who were not selected by any type of treatment resistance. This selection bias has to be considered and helps to understand the need for aggressive post-RC treatment or monitoring in case of NAC failure.

Finally, the main limitation was the difficulty to draw any firm conclusion based on a retrospective study. In addition to potential selection biases in the selection of patients for NAC, for surgery and for AC, our results could have also been limited by the relatively small sample size. Currently, it is not possible to establish with absolute certainty what is the best sequence of perioperative treatments. However, to our knowledge, this study was the first to directly compare contemporary outcomes after RC in pN1-3 patients treated or not with NAC, and it confirmed the potential of AC even in patients already treated by NAC.

5. Conclusions

Persistent nodal disease in RC specimens after NAC is associated with poor prognosis and lower OS rates compared with pN1-3 disease after upfront RC. In this sub-group of NAC patients, AC was given to one-third of NAC patients and was an independent predictive factor for better OS outcomes. Larger prospective data as well as studies assessing the impact of other adjuvant therapies such as immunotherapy or radiotherapy are awaited.

Author Contributions: Conceptualization, G.P. and M.R.; data curation, G.P., B.P., J.-B.B., A.-P.L., A.S., E.X., and D.P.; formal analysis, G.P., B.P., J.-B.B., C.C., C.A., E.S., J.-R.G., M.R., C.T., L.M., A.S., E.X., and D.P.; investigation, J.-B.B., E.S., and G.L.; methodology, B.P., J.-B.B., J.-R.G., and G.L.; supervision, C.C., A.-P.L., G.L., C.T., and L.M.; validation, C.C., C.A., E.S., J.-R.G., A.-P.L., M.R., G.L., C.T., L.M., A.S., E.X., and D.P.; visualization, C.A.; writing—original draft, G.P., B.P., E.X., and D.P.; writing—review and editing, C.C., C.A., E.S., J.-R.G., A.-P.L., M.R., C.T., L.M., and A.S. All authors have read and agreed to the published version of the manuscript.

References

1. Griffiths, G.; Hall, R.; Sylvester, R.; Raghavan, D.; Parmar, M.K.; Club Urologico Espanol de Tratamiento Oncologico Group. International phase III trial assessing neoadjuvant cisplatin, methotrexate, and vinblastine chemotherapy for muscle-invasive bladder cancer: Longterm results of the BA06 30894 trial. *J. Clin. Oncol.* **2011**, *29*, 2171. [PubMed]
2. Grossman, H.B.; Natale, R.B.; Tangen, C.M.; Speights, V.O.; Vogelzang, N.J.; Trump, D.L.; White, R.W.D.; Sarosdy, M.F.; Wood, D.P., Jr.; Raghavan, D.; et al. Neoadjuvant chemotherapy plus cystectomy compared with cystectomy alone for locally advanced bladder cancer. *N. Engl. J. Med.* **2003**, *349*, 859–866. [CrossRef] [PubMed]
3. Vale, C.L.; Advanced Bladder Cancer (ABC) Meta-analysis Collaboration. Neoadjuvant chemotherapy in invasive bladder cancer: Update of a systematic review and meta-analysis of individual patient data advanced bladder cancer (ABC) meta analysis collaboration. *Eur. Urol.* **2005**, *48*, 202–206. [CrossRef] [PubMed]

4. Zargar-Shoshtari, K.; Zargar, H.; Lotan, Y.; Shah, J.B.; van Rhijn, B.W.; Daneshmand, S.; Spiess, P.E.; Black, P.C.; Fairey, L.S.M.C.A.S.; Fairey, A.S.; et al. A Multi-Institutional Analysis of Outcomes of Patients with Clinically Node Positive Urothelial Bladder Cancer Treated with Induction Chemotherapy and Radical Cystectomy. *J. Urol.* **2016**, *195*, 53–59. [CrossRef]
5. Mertens, L.S.; Meijer, R.P.; Meinhardt, W.; Van Der Poel, H.G.; Bex, A.; Kerst, J.M.; Van Der Heijden, M.S.; Bergman, A.M.; Horenblas, S.; Van Rhijn, B.W.G. Occult lymph node metastases in patients with carcinoma invading bladder muscle: Incidence after neoadjuvant chemotherapy and cystectomy vs. after cystectomy alone. *BJU Int.* **2014**, *114*, 67–74. [CrossRef] [PubMed]
6. Tan, W.S.; Lamb, B.W.; Payne, H.; Hughes, S.; Green, J.S.; Lane, T.; Adshead, J.; Boustead, G.; Vasdev, N. Management of Node-Positive Bladder Cancer after Neoadjuvant Chemotherapy and Radical Cystectomy: A Survey of Current UK Practice. *Clin. Genitourin. Cancer* **2015**, *13*, e153–e158. [CrossRef] [PubMed]
7. Hermans, T.J.; van de Putte, E.E.F.; Horenblas, S.; Meijer, R.P.; Boormans, J.L.; Aben, K.K.H.; Van Der Heijden, M.S.; De Wit, R.; Beerepoot, L.V.; Verhoeven, R.; et al. Pathological downstaging and survival after induction chemotherapy and radical cystectomy for clinically node-positive bladder cancer-Results of a nationwide population-based study. *Eur. J. Cancer* **2016**, *69*, 1–8. [CrossRef] [PubMed]
8. Herr, H.W.; Dotan, Z.; Donat, S.M.; Bajorin, D.F. Defining optimal therapy for muscle invasive bladder cancer. *J. Urol.* **2007**, *177*, 437–443. [CrossRef] [PubMed]
9. Kassouf, W.; Agarwal, P.K.; Grossman, H.B.; Leibovici, D.; Munsell, M.F.; Siefker-Radtke, A.; Pisters, L.L.; Swanson, D.A.; Dinney, C.P.N.; Kamatbe, A.M. Outcome of patients with bladder cancer with pNþ disease after preoperative chemotherapy and radical cystectomy. *Urology* **2009**, *73*, 147–152. [CrossRef] [PubMed]
10. Zargar, H.; Shah, J.B.; van Rhijn, B.W.; Daneshmand, S.; Bivalacqua, T.J.; Spiess, P.E.; Black, P.C.; Kassouf, W.; Van De Putte, E.E.F.; Horenblas, S.; et al. Neoadjuvant Dose Dense MVAC versus Gemcitabine and Cisplatin in Patients with cT3-4aN0M0 Bladder Cancer Treated with Radical Cystectomy. *J. Urol.* **2018**, *199*, 1452–1458. [CrossRef] [PubMed]
11. Loehrer, P.J.; Einhorn, L.H.; Elson, P.J.; Crawford, E.D.; Kuebler, P.; Tannock, I.; Raghavan, D.; Stuart-Harris, R.; Sarosdy, M.F.; Lowe, B.A. A randomized comparison of cisplatin alone or in combination with methotrexate, vinblastine, and doxorubicin in patients with metastatic urothelial carcinoma: A cooperative group study. *J. Clin. Oncol.* **1992**, *10*, 1066–1073. [CrossRef] [PubMed]
12. von der Maase, H.; Hansen, S.W.; Roberts, J.T.; Dogliotti, L.; Oliver, T.; Moore, M.; Bodrogi, I.; Albers, P.; Knuth, A.; Lippert, C.; et al. Gemcitabine and cisplatin versus methotrexate, vinblastine, doxorubicin, and cisplatin in advanced or metastatic bladder cancer: Results of a large, randomized, multinational, multicenter, phase III study. *J. Clin. Oncol.* **2000**, *18*, 3068–3077. [CrossRef] [PubMed]
13. Paz-Ares, L.; Solsona, E.; Esteban, E.; Saez, A.; Gonzalez-Larriba, J.; Anton, A.; de la Rosa, F.; Guillem, V.; Bellmunt, J. On behalf of the SOGUG and GUO-AEU groups Randomized phase III trial comparing adjuvant paclitaxel/gemcitabine/cisplatin (PGC to observation in patients with resected invasive bladder cancer: Results of the SOGUG (Spanish Oncology Genito-Urinary Group) 99/01 study. *J. Clin. Oncol.* **2010**, *4518*. [CrossRef]
14. Sternberg, C.N.; Skoneczna, I.; Kerst, J.M.; Albers, P.; Fossa, S.D.; Agerbaek, M.; Dumez, H.; de Santis, M.; Théodore, C.; Leahy, M.G.; et al. Immediate versus deferred chemotherapy after radical cystectomy in patients with pT3-pT4 or N1M0 urothelial carcinoma of the bladder (EORTC 30994): An intergroup, open-label, randomised phase 3 trial. *Lancet Oncol.* **2015**, *16*, 76–86. [CrossRef]
15. Leow, J.J.; Martin-Doyle, W.; Rajagopal, P.S.; Patel, C.G.; Anderson, E.M.; Rothman, A.T.; Cote, R.J.; Urun, Y.; Chang, S.L.; Choueiri, T.K.; et al. Adjuvant chemotherapy for invasive bladder cancer: A 2013 updated systematic review and meta-analysis of randomized trials. *Eur. Urol.* **2014**, *66*, 42–54. [CrossRef] [PubMed]
16. Wosnitzer, M.S.; Hruby, G.W.; Murphy, A.M.; Barlow, L.J.; Cordon-Cardo, C.; Mansukhani, M.; Petrylak, D.P.; Benson, M.C.; McKiernan, J.M.; Cordon-Cardo, C. A comparison of the outcomes of neoadjuvant and adjuvant chemotherapy for clinical T2-T4aN0-N2M0 bladder cancer. *Cancer* **2012**, *118*, 358–364. [CrossRef] [PubMed]
17. Necchi, A.; Anichini, A.; Raggi, D.; Briganti, A.; Massa, S.; Lucianò, R.; Colecchia, M.; Giannatempo, P.; Mortarini, R.; Bianchi, M.; et al. Pembrolizumab as Neoadjuvant Therapy Before Radical Cystectomy in Patients With Muscle-Invasive Urothelial Bladder Carcinoma (PURE-01): An Open-Label, Single-Arm, Phase II Study. *J. Clin. Oncol.* **2018**, *20*, 3353–3360. [CrossRef] [PubMed]

5

CPT1A Over-Expression Increases Reactive Oxygen Species in the Mitochondria and Promotes Antioxidant Defenses in Prostate Cancer

Molishree Joshi [1], Jihye Kim [2], Angelo D'Alessandro [3,4], Emily Monk [2], Kimberley Bruce [5], Hanan Elajaili [6], Eva Nozik-Grayck [6], Andrew Goodspeed [1,4], James C. Costello [1,4] and Isabel R. Schlaepfer [2,*]

1 Department of Pharmacology, University of Colorado Anschutz Medical Campus, Aurora, CO 80045, USA; Molishree.Joshi@cuanschutz.edu (M.J.); Andrew.Goodspeed@cuanschutz.edu (A.G.); James.Costello@cuanschutz.edu (J.C.C.)
2 Division of Medical Oncology, University of Colorado Anschutz Medical Campus, Aurora, CO 80045, USA; Jihye.Kim@cuanschutz.edu (J.K.); Emily.Monk@cuanschutz.edu (E.M.)
3 Department of Biochemistry, University of Colorado Anschutz Medical Campus, Aurora, CO 80045, USA; Angelo.Dalessandro@cuanschutz.edu
4 University of Colorado Comprehensive Cancer Center, Anschutz Medical Campus, Aurora, CO 80045, USA
5 Division of Endocrinology, Metabolism and Diabetes, University of Colorado Anschutz Medical Campus, Aurora, CO 80045, USA; Kimberley.Bruce@cuanschutz.edu
6 Department of Pediatrics Critical Care, University of Colorado Anschutz Medical Campus, Aurora, CO 80045, USA; Hanan.Elajaili@cuanschutz.edu (H.E.); Eva.Nozik@cuanschutz.edu (E.N.-G.)
* Correspondence: Isabel.Schlaepfer@cuanschutz.edu

Simple Summary: Prostate cancer (PCa) is the most common cancer in men and the second highest contributor to cancer deaths. Targeting lipid catabolism enzymes in PCa may offer new avenues for therapeutic approaches. During the last decade, carnitine palmitoyl transferase I (CPT1A) has been identified as a potential therapeutic target for a growing list of cancers. In this study, we have tested the hypothesis that excess CPT1A plays a key role in supporting adaptation to stress and antioxidant defense production in PCa cells. Specifically, we have studied molecular differences between CPT1A gain and loss of function models, revealing genetic and metabolic vulnerabilities that could be targeted to avoid progression to neuroendocrine differentiation, a lethal form of the disease. Examining public datasets, we have also found that excess CPT1A expression leads to worse progression-free survival in PCa patients.

Abstract: Cancers reprogram their metabolism to adapt to environmental changes. In this study, we examined the consequences of altered expression of the mitochondrial enzyme carnitine palmitoyl transferase I (CPT1A) in prostate cancer (PCa) cell models. Using transcriptomic and metabolomic analyses, we compared LNCaP-C4-2 cell lines with depleted (knockdown (KD)) or increased (overexpression (OE)) CPT1A expression. Mitochondrial reactive oxygen species (ROS) were also measured. Transcriptomic analysis identified ER stress, serine biosynthesis and lipid catabolism as significantly upregulated pathways in the OE versus KD cells. On the other hand, androgen response was significantly downregulated in OE cells. These changes associated with increased acyl-carnitines, serine synthesis and glutathione precursors in OE cells. Unexpectedly, OE cells showed increased mitochondrial ROS but when challenged with fatty acids and no androgens, the Superoxide dismutase 2 (SOD2) enzyme increased in the OE cells, suggesting better antioxidant defenses with excess CPT1A expression. Public databases also showed decreased androgen response correlation with increased serine-related metabolism in advanced PCa. Lastly, worse progression free survival was observed with increased lipid catabolism and decreased androgen response. Excess CPT1A is associated with a ROS-mediated stress phenotype that can support PCa disease progression. This study provides a rationale for targeting lipid catabolic pathways for therapy in hormonal cancers.

Keywords: CPT1A; prostate cancer; fatty acids; serine; androgen response; ROS; oxidative stress

1. Introduction

Prostate cancer (PCa) is the most common cancer in men and the second highest contributor to cancer deaths [1]. Although initially highly effective as a treatment for metastatic PCa, androgen deprivation therapy is characterized by a predictable emergence of resistance, a disease state termed castration-resistant prostate cancer (CRPC) [2]. An important feature of CRPC is the reactivation of androgen receptor (AR) signaling, an event reflected by progressive rises in serum prostate-specific antigen (PSA), a gene product regulated by the androgen receptor (AR) [3]. Substantial evidence has documented that the majority of AR-regulated genes (androgen-response hallmark genes) are re-expressed in most CRPCs, and several mechanisms capable of maintaining AR activity have been established [4,5]. Alternatively, disease progression can arise in the absence of a functional AR as an extremely aggressive and metastatic variant called small cell or neuroendocrine PCa [6,7]. Although genetic alterations are known to promote this aggressive state of the disease [8], we currently lack mechanistic insight as to which metabolic pathways play important roles in PCa plasticity, resistance and progression to lethal disease.

Mitochondrial fatty acid β-oxidation is the major pathway for the catabolism of fatty acids, and it plays an essential role in maintaining whole body energy homeostasis. The transfer of fatty acids into the mitochondria for oxidation happens in an organized, controlled way. The enzyme carnitine palmitoyl transferase I (CPT1A) resides in the outer mitochondrial membrane and catalyzes the reversible transfer of acyl groups between coenzyme A (CoA) and L-carnitine, converting acyl-CoA esters into acyl-carnitine esters. These acyl-carnitines can then enter the matrix where β-oxidation takes place [9]. The activity of CPT1A produces a greater number of acetyl groups, which can be used for energy, de novo lipid synthesis and acetylation reactions, including histone acetylation in the nucleus [10].

Support for a strong association between specific dietary lipids and PCa is still unclear. For example, a recent paper showed that a high fat diet promotes metastatic prostate cancer [11]. Although this is a great step forward in understanding the clinical role of dietary lipids promoting metastatic PCa, it does not address how tumor cells use the lipids to their benefit. Particularly, it is not clear how CPT1A activity could promote a metabolic environment conducive to cell transformation, cancer progression and drug resistance [12].

Targeting lipid catabolism enzymes in PCa may offer new avenues for therapeutic approaches [13]. During the last decade, CPT1A has been identified as a potential therapeutic target for a growing list of cancers [14]. In these cancers, CPT1A expression is increased, and/or its inhibition has been reported to have antitumor effects. Our group has shown that fatty acid oxidation is an important pathway in cancer metabolism in PCa cells when using the CPT1 inhibitor etomoxir [15–17]. The blockade of CPT1A with etomoxir produced unresolved endoplasmic reticulum (ER) stress leading to cell apoptosis and decreased tumor growth in vivo. Indeed, lipid oxidation in the mitochondria of aggressive cancer cells can provide adaptation to stress by promoting the generation of antioxidant molecules, like Nicotinamide adenine dinucleotide phosphate (NADPH) [18].

Loss of balance between the antioxidant defense and oxidant production in the cells, which commonly occurs as a secondary feature in many diseases, is loosely termed "oxidative stress". This balance is important because the intracellular redox environment must be more reducing than oxidizing to maintain optimal cell function. Oxidative stress and ER stress are linked to multiple pathologies, including metabolic, neurodegenerative, immune, and neoplastic diseases. Studies on these two cellular stresses have not only contributed to our understanding of disease, but also opened new avenues to next-generation therapies for these illnesses [19,20]. Their exact role in supporting cancer survival and drug resistance remains unknown.

Since oxidative stress is usually coupled with ER stress [21], the unfolded protein response (UPR) has evolved to handle both proteins folding defects and oxidative challenge. In fact, excess nutrients are proposed to induce ER stress and oxidative stress in pancreatic beta-cells, including glucotoxicity and lipotoxicity. For example, chronic excess glucose induces the pro-apoptotic UPR and oxidative stress in beta-cells cells in vitro and in mice models [22]. In addition, free fatty acids, such as palmitate, induce ER stress and oxidative stress and cause apoptosis in β cells [23]. Cancer cells, especially hormone-dependent cancers, like PCa, exploit these stress responses to deal with the oncogenic and metabolic reprograming, making them more adaptable to affront the insults from drug cancer therapies. Indeed, conditional knockout of the ER chaperone GRP78 (HSPA5) in the prostate of mice with PTEN inactivation suppressed prostate cancer growth [24]. The role of CPT1A in supporting adaptive ER stress responses and redox regulation has not been studied.

In this study, we have tested the hypothesis that excess CPT1A plays a key role in supporting adaptation to stress and antioxidant defense production in CRPC cells. We have used the LNCap-C4-2 model as it represents advanced CRPC that can grow in androgen depleted conditions and form metastasis [25]. We have also explored publicly available clinical databases to support our findings. Specifically, we have studied molecular differences between CPT1A gain and loss of function C4-2 models, revealing metabolic vulnerabilities that could be targeted to avoid progression to neuroendocrine differentiation.

2. Results

2.1. *Cells with Overexpression of CPT1A Show a Lipid Catabolic Phenotype and Increased Growth When Supplemented with Fatty Acids*

CPT1A fuels lipid beta-oxidation in PCa cells by producing acyl-carnitines in the mitochondria [9]. To characterize the biochemical changes in the newly described knockdown (KD) and overexpression (OE) C4-2 models [10], we used lipid-based assays and metabolomics. Figure 1A shows that CPT1A is significantly increased in the OE cells and this is associated with a significant increase in intracellular lipase activity, a step which liberates fatty acids from triglyceride stores which can then be used for beta oxidation [26] (Figure 1B). Metabolomic analysis of the OE versus KD C4-2 cells showed significant increases in most of the acyl-carnitine identified, from the short and medium-chain (Figure 1C) to the long-chain species (Figure 1D). Furthermore, the KD cells (blue bars) showed decreased production of the abundant long-chain C16:0 (palmitic) and C18:1 (Oleic) species as expected from the decreased activity of CPT1A in these cells. The use of the CPT1 inhibitor etomoxir, also resulted in decreased production of acyl carnitines in C4-2 parental cells treated with the inhibitor for 48 h (Figure 1E). We next studied the effects of fatty acid availability on the colony growth of OE and KD cells (Figure 1F–I). Fatty acids were conjugated to bovine serum albumin (BSA) and growth was normalized to BSA-only treatment for each cell line. Dodecanoate (C12) treatment showed increased growth in OE compared to empty virus (EV) control cells (Figure 1G), and this effect was not observed in the KD cells (Figure 1F). Similar results were obtained with C16:0 supplementation, where OE cells increased in growth (Figure 1I) but not in KD cells (Figure 1H). The addition of other medium- and long-chain fatty acids also produced significant increases in growth in OE cells compared to controls (Figure S1), except for C18:1, which promoted growth in both KD and EV cells. These results may reflect the lipid droplet-inducing effects of oleic acid supplementation in cancer cells, promoting growth and survival [27,28].

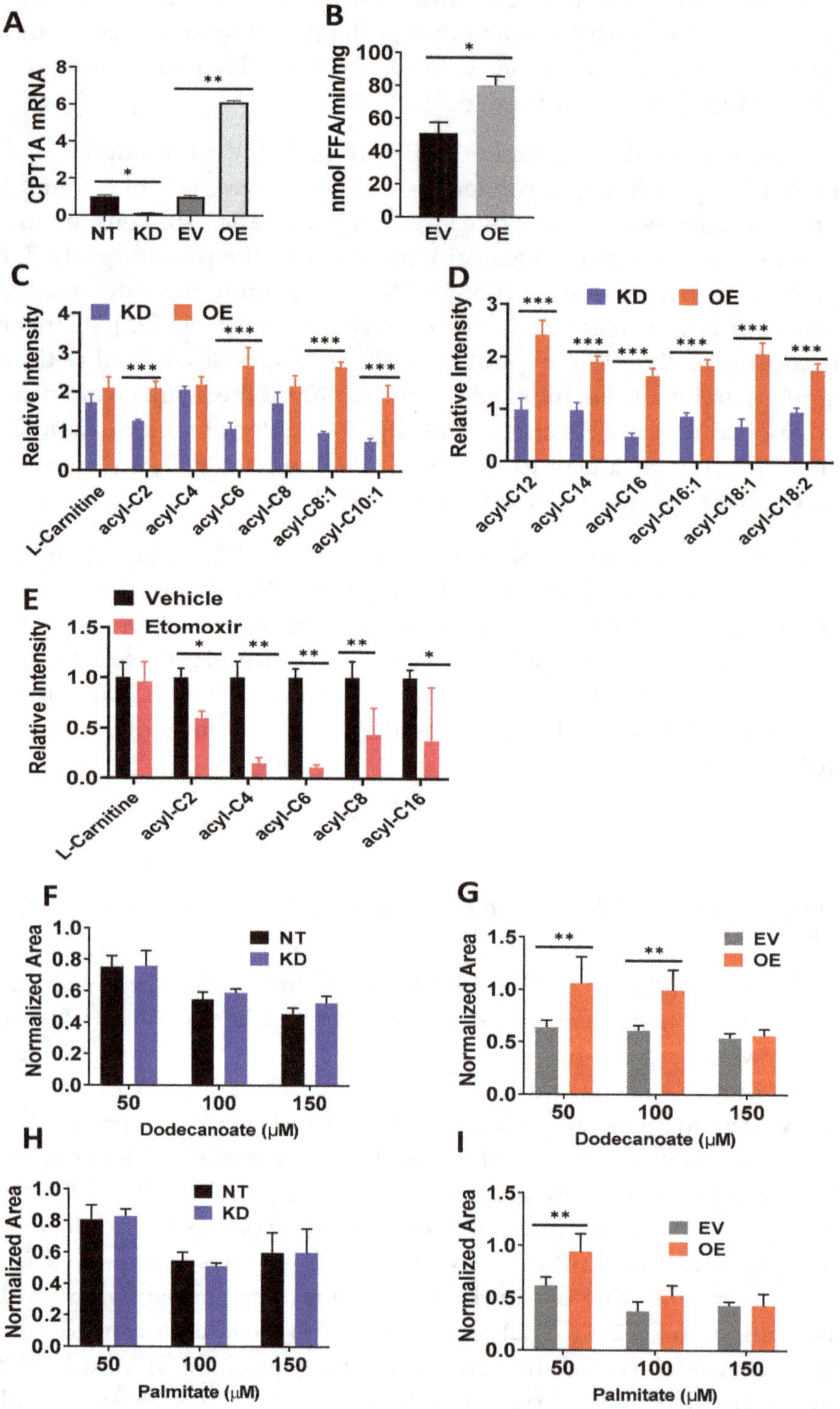

Figure 1. Cells with overexpression of carnitine palmitoyl transferase I (CPT1A) show a lipid catabolic phenotype and increased growth when supplemented with fatty acids. (**A**) mRNA expression of C4-2 cells with decreased (knockdown (KD)) and overexpression (OE) of CPT1A cells and their respective controls (non-targeting (NT) and empty virus (EV)). (**B**) Intracellular triglyceride lipase assay in OE cells. (**C**,**D**) Short and medium (**C**) and long chain (**D**) acyl carnitine content in OE (red) versus KD (blue), normalized to their own controls. (**E**) Acyl carnitine changes in C4-2 parental cells treated with etomoxir (100 μM) for 48 h. (**F**,**G**) Colony growth after treatment with C12:0 fatty acid conjugated to BSA for 14 days and normalized to BSA-only treatment. (**H**,**I**) Colony growth after treatment with C16:0 fatty acid conjugated to BSA for 14 days and normalized to BSA-only treatment. * $p < 0.05$, ** $p < 0.01$, *** $p < 0.001$.

2.2. RNAseq Analysis of CPT1A OE Cells Shows Increased ER Stress Response, Serine Metabolism and Less AR Signaling

To identify the molecular signatures associated with CPT1A expression, we performed RNAseq in the C4-2 KD and OE cells. Figure 2 and Table S1 show the results of our analysis comparing the OE cells to the KD cells. Briefly, we normalized each cell line to its respective control (Figure 2A), and then we used limma to compare the gene expression differences between OE and KD [29]. Overall, we found 1157 genes upregulated and 1385 genes downregulated when comparing the OE cells to the KD cells. Genes were filtered by an adjusted p-value of 0.0001. Using gene set enrichment analysis (GSEA), we found that ER stress and UPR response were some of the most significant pathways increased in the OE cells, pointing to possible lipid-mediated oxidative stress (Figure 2B). Cell division, mitosis and E2F targets pathways were significantly decreased in OE cells, which is in agreement with their decreased growth rate compared to their control line [10]. The androgen response hallmark gene set was significantly decreased in the OE cells and it reflects less dependency of OE cells on AR signaling, which is something we have observed and reported previously [10]. As expected from our metabolic observations, the lipid catabolic process pathway, including the CPT1A gene, was significantly increased in OE cells compared to KD cells. Figure 2C shows a heatmap of genes from the leading-edge analysis in Figure 2B associated with lipid catabolism, response to cellular stress and androgen response pathways. Enrichment plots for these pathways are shown in Figure S2. Examination of the significant genes in these pathways (Figure 2D–F), showed opposite directions of change between OE and KD cells. For most of the genes, the KD cells showed decreases in gene expression when compared to OE cells.

2.3. Excess CPT1A Is Associated with Serine and Glycine Metabolism and Glutathione Homeostasis Metabolites

To understand the type of stress imposed in the CPT1A OE cells, we performed global, non-targeted metabolomics in the four cells lines: non-targeting (NT), KD, EV, and OE cells. In parallel to the RNAseq analysis, we focused on the metabolic pathway differences between OE and KD cells after controlling for their respective control lines (EV and NT respectively). Analysis of the top 25 significant pathways revealed that lipid metabolism, glycine and serine metabolism, and glutathione homeostasis were the most significantly changed pathways (Figure 3A and Figure S3). Glycolysis was also significantly different across groups, with the OE cells showing less glycolysis compared to KD cells (Figure S3).

Considering the RNAseq data, we next analyzed the metabolites corresponding to the serine/glycine metabolism. The serine, glycine and one carbon metabolism pathway are a metabolic network upregulated in tumors and of high clinical relevance [30,31]. Except glucose, individual metabolites of the serine/glycine pathway were not changed significantly in OE versus KD (Figure 3B). However, the OE cells showed more intracellular glucose being shunted towards de novo serine biosynthesis compared to control EV cells (Figure S3A). In fact, less glucose seemed to be used for glycolysis in the OE cells. These results correlated with significantly increased expression of key serine/glycine pathway genes: D-3-phosphoglycerate dehydrogenase (PHGDH), phosphohydroxythreonine aminotransferase (PSAT1), and Serine hydroxymethyltransferase (SHMT2) (Figures 2E and 3B). SHMT2 is a mitochondrial enzyme that converts serine (3 carbons) into glycine (2 carbons), transferring one carbon to tetrahydrofolate (mitochondrial folate cycle). The increased dimethylglycine and cystathionine levels in OE cells compared to KD cells supports a higher folate cycle activity in these cells (Figure 3B,C).

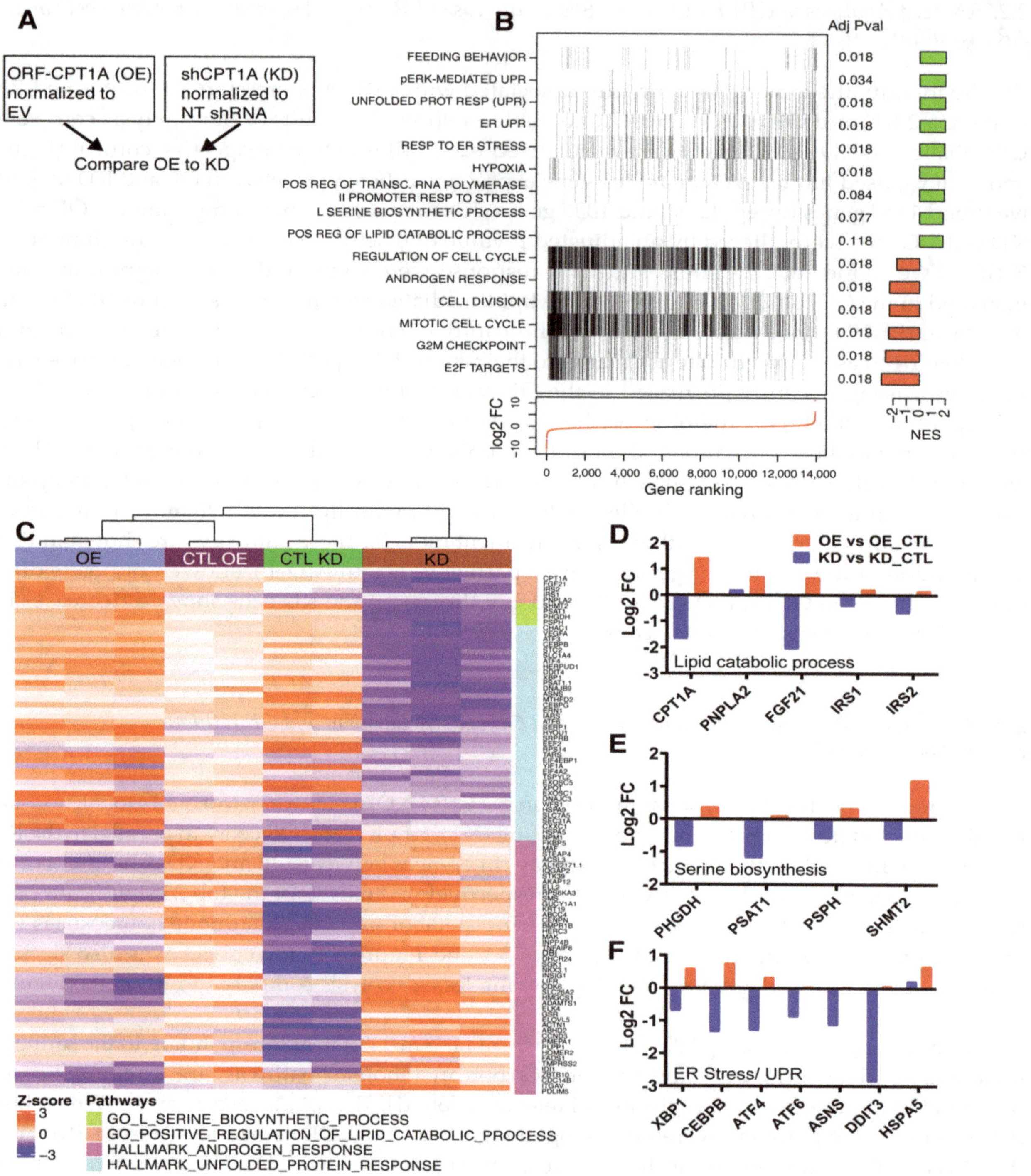

Figure 2. RNAseq analysis of CPT1A OE cells shows increased endoplasmic reticulum (ER) stress response, serine metabolism, and less androgen receptor (AR) signaling. (**A**) Schematic of the RNAseq analysis paradigm with the CPT1A-KD and OE cells. (**B**) Gene set enrichment analysis was performed on the fold change of the comparison. Normalized Enrichment Scores (NES) and False discovery rate (FDR) adjusted *p*-values are shown for select pathways, as well as the rank of those genes in fold change ranking, are plotted. (**C**) Heatmap of the leading-edge genes for select pathways. (**D**–**F**) Gene expression graphs of significant genes associated with lipid catabolism (**D**), serine biosynthesis (**E**) and ER stress (**F**) in OE versus KD comparison after adjustment to their respective control cell lines. Adj p value < 0.001.

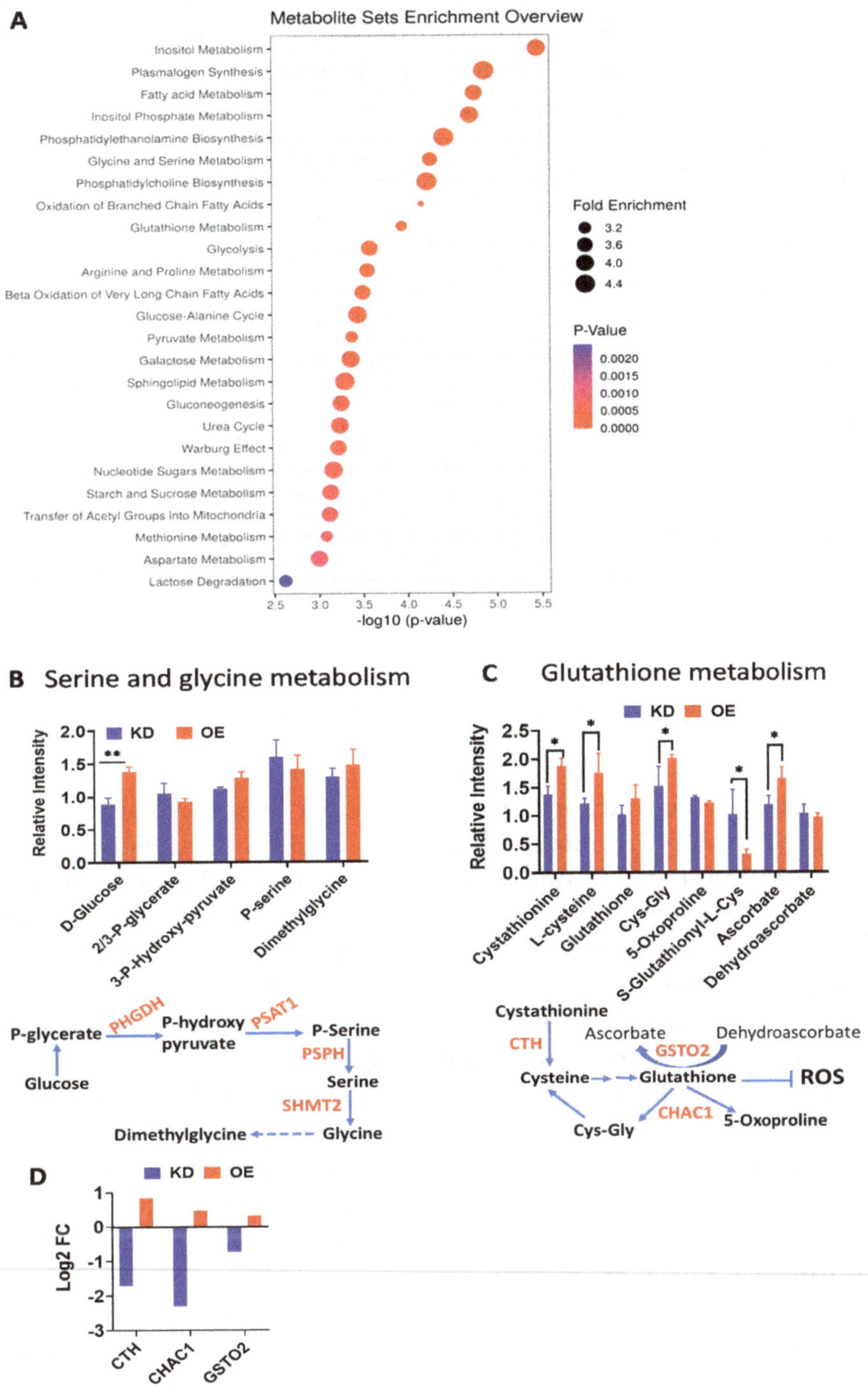

Figure 3. Excess CPT1A is associated with serine and glycine metabolism pathway and glutathione homeostasis metabolites. (**A**) Metabolite set enrichment analysis of OE metabolites versus KD cell metabolites after normalization to their own controls. The p-value is defined by the color scale, and the enrichment by the size of the circle. (**B**) Relative abundance of metabolites associated with the serine and glycine biosynthesis via the SHMT2 gene in the mitochondria. A scheme of the pathway is shown under the graphs, highlighting the sequence of events from glucose to synthesis of serine, glycine and the one carbon metabolism compound dimethylglycine. The genes significantly altered in OE cells from the RNAseq analysis involved in the pathway are shown in red. (**C**) Relative abundance of metabolites associated glutathione (GSH) homeostasis. The S-glutathionyl-L-Cys metabolite is associated with ineffective handling of oxidative stress. A scheme to the pathway is shown below. * $p < 0.05$, ** $p < 0.01$. (**D**) Gene expression analysis of OE versus KD cells for CTH ($p = 6.29 \times 10^{-13}$), CHAC1 ($p = 3.6 \times 10^{-12}$) and GSTO2 ($p = 0.003$) genes (adj p-value).

Metabolites involved in Glutathione (GSH) homeostasis were also significantly changed in the OE cells compared to the KD cells (Figure 3C), suggesting better antioxidant defense. Particularly, cystathionine and cysteine were significantly increased in OE versus KD cells, and between OE cells and controls, suggesting increased cysteine synthesis and availability to generate glutathione. These increases are associated with increased expression of CTH, a cystathionine gamma lyase that breaks down cystathionine to generate cysteine [32], Figure 3D. Unexpectedly, we also observed increased generation of two breakdown products of glutathione via the ChaC Glutathione Specific Gamma-Glutamylcyclotransferase 1 (CHAC1) enzyme. These enzymes are gamma-glutamyl cyclotransferases, which are induced by ER stress and have specific activity towards glutathione [33]. CHAC1 has been shown to break glutathione into 5-oxoproline and cysteinyl-glycine (Cys-Gly), promoting the depletion of glutathione and stress-induced apoptosis in cysteine deprived cancer cells [34]. However, we did not observe a depletion of glutathione in OE cells with higher CHAC1 expression (Figure 3C), suggesting that metabolite recycling mechanisms or compensatory increased production of glutathione may exist in OE cells [35]. Another indication that OE may have more antioxidant defense than KD cells comes from the increased ratio of ascorbate to dehydroascorbate, which is likely maintained by the dehydroascorbate activity of Glutathione S-Transferase Omega 2 (GSTO2) [36], which is significantly upregulated in the OE cells and can recycle the glutathione to a reduced state, Figure 3C,D.

2.4. *Mitochondrial Reactive Oxygen Species (ROS) Are Increased in CPT1A-OE Cells*

Since GSH homeostasis was significantly changed in OE cells, we reasoned that mitochondrial ROS production could be altered in response to increased CPT1A expression. Thus, we next studied the amount of ROS produced in the mitochondria of the cell models. Figure 4A shows the stacked traces of the Electron Paramagnetic Resonance (EPR) assay, highlighting the increased amplitude of the signal in the OE cells compared to all the other samples. Quantification of the signals is shown in Figure 4B, with the OE cells having a 4-fold increase in mitochondrial ROS production compared to KD cells. Examination of the RNAseq data indicated that SOD2, the mitochondrial superoxide dismutase, was significantly decreased in OE cells compared to KD cells (1.4-fold less $p < 0.0007$, Figure 4C). The cytosolic counterpart SOD1 was not significantly changed between OE and KD cells, while the extracellular SOD3 mRNA was significantly increased in the KD compared to the OE cells ($p = 0.01$). Thus, less SOD2 expression in the OE cells likely accounted for the increase in mitochondrial ROS in these cells. Since the OE cells did not show signs of apoptosis induced by excess ROS we next challenged the cells with long chain lipids (oleic and palmitate mixture at 25 μM each) in the presence or absence of androgens, using regular fetal bovine serum (FBS) or charcoal stripped serum (CSS) devoid of steroid hormones. This fatty acid mixture was used because it represents the most common fatty acids circulating in blood and they are substrates for CPT1A activity (Figure 1D). Figure 4D,E and Figure S4, show that SOD2 did not change in response to the lipid stimulation (Figure 4D), but it decreased in the KD cells compared to the OE cells with androgen withdraw conditions (Figure 4E). Thus, in the presence of lipids and androgen deprivation conditions, CPT1A OE cells are likely to cope with the excess mitochondrial ROS from fat oxidation (Figure 4F).

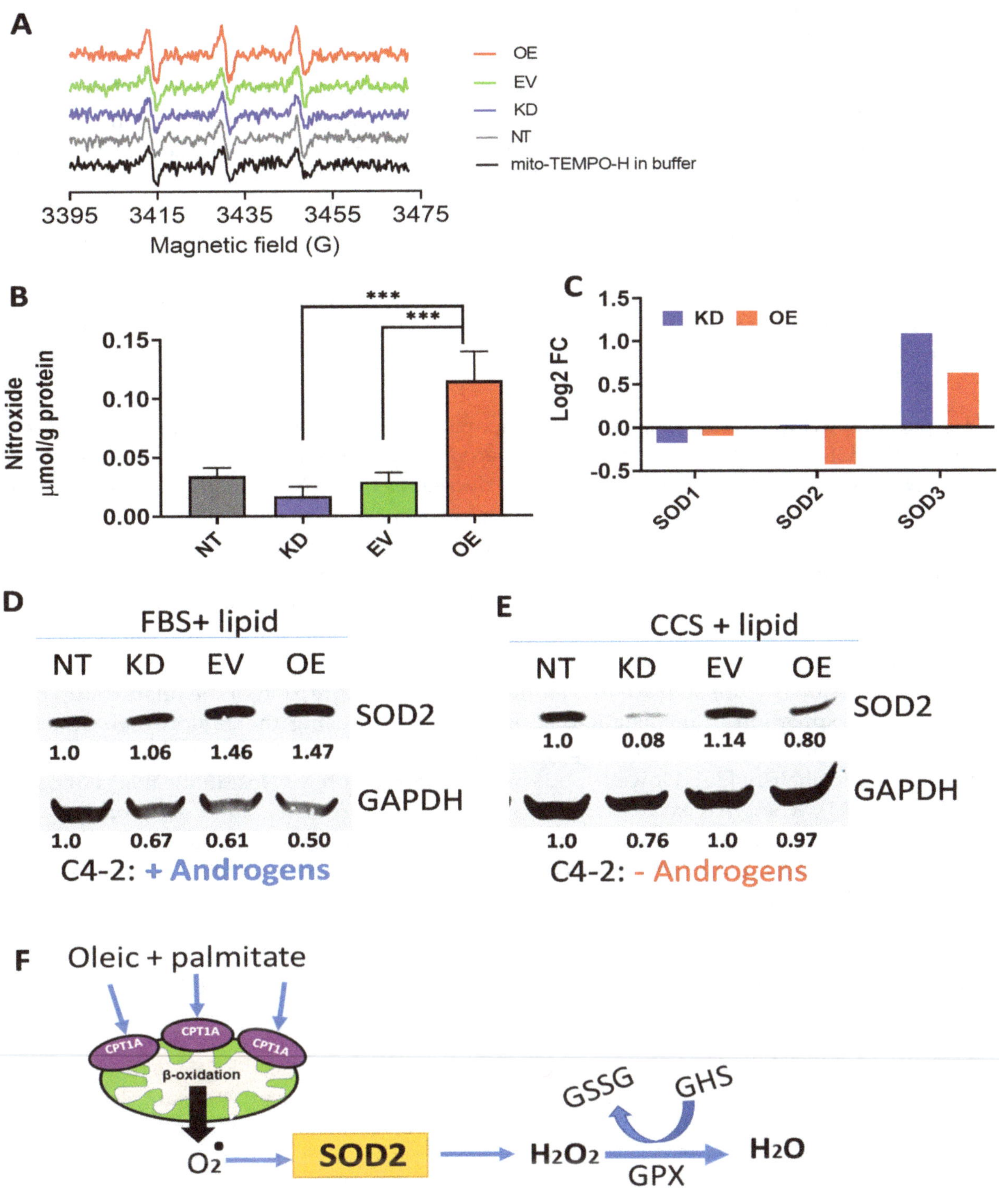

Figure 4. Mitochondrial reactive oxygen species (ROS) are increased in CPT1A-OE cells. (**A**) Electron paramagnetic resonance spectroscopy (EPR) traces of the four cell lines tested, including the mitochondrial probe by itself. Amplitude and linewidth provide information of the amount of ROS. The concentration was acquired by Spin Fit followed by SpinCount module (Bruker). (**B**) Quantification of the EPR traces normalized to protein content. *** $p < 0.001$. (**C**) Gene expression analysis of OE versus KD cells for SOD1 ns), SOD2 ($p = 6.9 \times 10^{-4}$), and SOD3 ($p = 0.015$). Only SOD2 is a mitochondrial enzyme. (**D**,**E**) Western blots of SOD2 expression after incubation with fatty acids (Oleic and palmitate mixture; 25 μM each) in FBS (**D**) or charcoal stripped serum (CSS) (**E**) for 48 h. (**F**) Schematic of the role of SOD2 in metabolizing superoxide and the role of glutathione in eliminating H_2O_2. GPX = Glutathione peroxide. GSSG = oxidized glutathione.

2.5. Lipid and Serine Metabolism Genes Are Associated with Less Androgen Signaling and a More Neuroendocrine Phenotype

Gene set enrichment analysis of our RNAseq showed decreased expression of androgen response genes CPT1A OE cells (Figure 5A). Since decreased AR signaling is associated with changes to a neuroendoendocrine phenotype [7], we next looked for markers of neuronal-like differentiation and identified Enolase 2 (ENO2), Synaptophysin (SYP), Neural Cell Adhesion Molecule 2 (NCAM2), and Neurexophilin 4 (NXPH4) genes significantly upregulated in OE versus KD cells. The ENO2 and SYP genes are markers associated with neuroendocrine PCa (NEPC). To investigate the possibility that CPT1A overexpression (OE) is associated with more aggressive disease, we searched previous transcriptome analysis in the public databases. Particularly, we searched for studies that compared adenocarcinoma with aggressive disease like small cell NEPC and focused on serine and one carbon metabolism, CPT1A and AR expression in clinical data.

Using the dataset from GSE32967 [37], we compared gene expression between small cell carcinoma (a subset of NEPC) and adenocarcinoma patient derived PCa xenografts. GSE Analysis showed that the androgen response hallmark was significantly decreased in the NEPC samples, while significant increases were observed in the serine metabolism and one carbon (tetrahydrofolate) metabolism pathways (Figure 5C). Several of serine and tetrahydrofolate leading-edge genes increased in our RNAseq analysis were also increased in the GSE32967 dataset (Figure 5D). Addition of CPT1A and AR gene expression to the heatmap showed that one NEPC sample had low AR as expected, but modest increased CPT1A associated with increased SHMT2, MTHFD2 and PSPH expression. Conversely, one sample with adenocarcinoma features showed less CPT1A associated with less SHMT2, MTHFD2, and PSAT1 expression (Figure 5D). We further investigated the direction of the relationship between CPT1A and AR expression in metastatic disease (Figure S5), using the Taylor et al. dataset [38]. A positive correlation was observed in the primary tumors, as expected from the role of androgens in regulating lipid metabolism [39]. However, this positive correlation was lost in the metastatic samples ($R = -0.28$, $p = 0.25$), where AR expression was significantly increased compared to primary tumors (Wilcoxon $p = 1.1 \times 10^{-7}$). The possibility that a strong anti-androgen blockade in these metastatic samples could reverse the correlation to less AR and more CPT1A expression, as it happens in NEPC, warrants further investigation.

2.6. Increased Lipid Catabolism and Decreased Androgen Response Is Associated with Poorer Progression-Free Survival

To further validate the role of CPT1A and lipid catabolism in advanced PCa, we turned to publicly accessible TCGA (The Cancer Genome Atlas) Firehose Legacy dataset (492 samples). Pathways were scored in each patient using GSEA and grouped according by median split of each pathway. Examination of the same GSEA pathways identified in our RNAseq data (Figure 2C) showed that the lipid catabolic process (Figure 6A), and the androgen response hallmark (Figure 6B), were significantly associated with progression free survival (PFS) but in opposite directions. The increase in lipid catabolism genes and the decrease in androgen response genes shortened the PFS. We did not observe significant PFS changes with the GO serine metabolism and the unfolded protein response hallmark pathways (Figure S6).

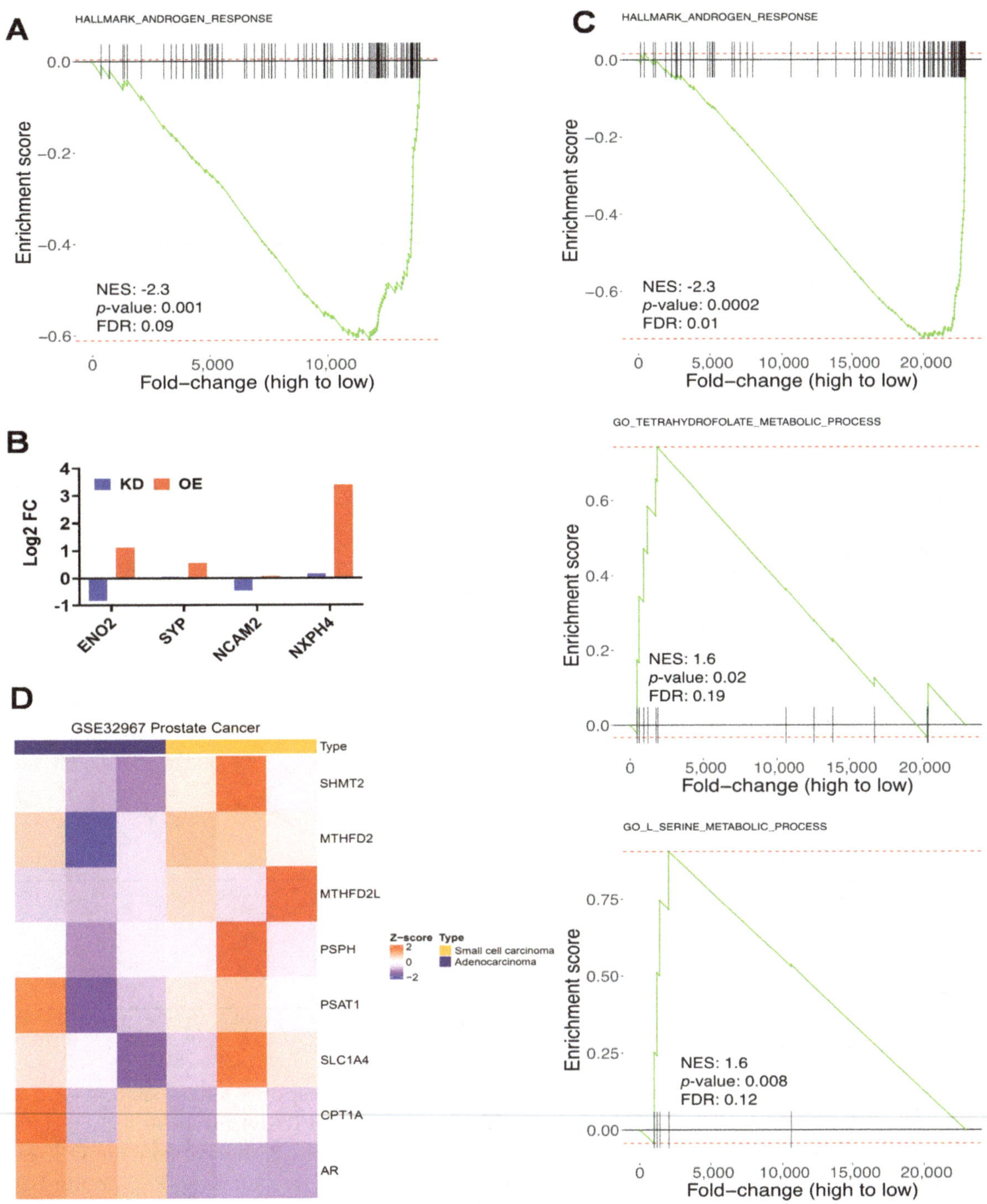

Figure 5. Lipid and serine metabolism genes are associated with less androgen signaling and a neuroendocrine phenotype. (**A**) Gene set enrichment analysis (GSEA) plot of the OE versus KD analysis showing the decrease in the androgen response hallmark in OE cells. (**B**) Gene expression analysis of OE versus KD cells for neuronal-like markers like ENO2 ($p = 6.1 \times 10^{-10}$), SYP (p = ns), NCAM2 ($p = 4.14 \times 10^{-5}$), NXPH4 ($p = 1.6 \times 10^{-17}$). (**C**) GSEA plots of the public GSE32967 dataset showing the comparison between small cell carcinoma ($n = 3$) versus adenocarcinoma ($n = 3$) patient xenografts for the Hallmark Androgen Response; GO_Serine and GO_Tetrahydrofolate pathways. Normalized enrichment scores (NES) and statistical significance are indicated in the plots. (**D**) Heatmap of the leading-edge genes from the serine and tetrahydrofolate functional GSEA plots shown in panel C, which are also genes increased in the OE cells compared to KD cells. CPT1A and AR are also included and show an inverse correlation in one of the samples of each subtype of PCa studied.

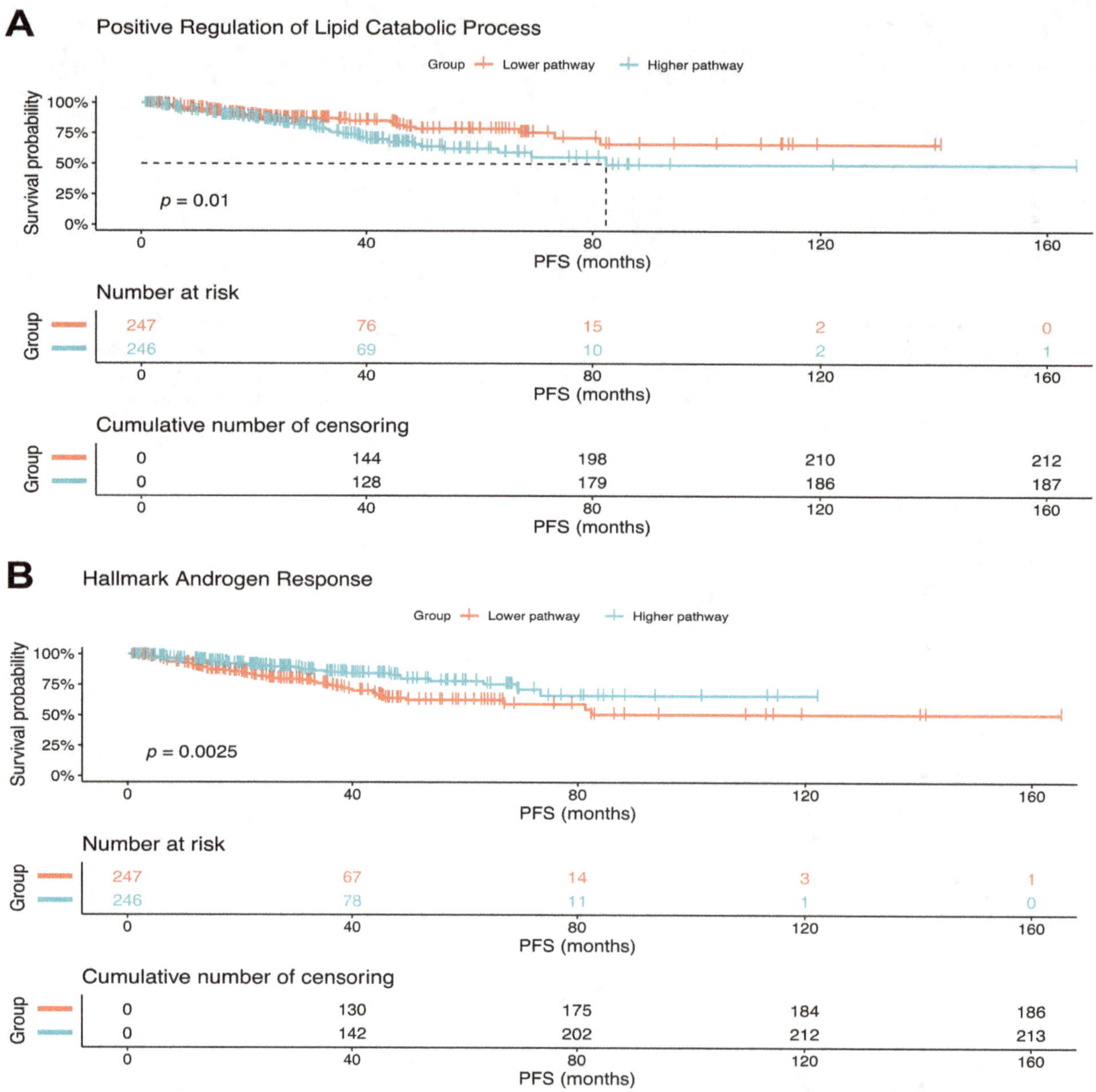

Figure 6. Increased lipid catabolism and decreased androgen response is associated with less progression-free survival. The TCGA prostate adenocarcinoma (PRAD) Firehose legacy dataset ($n = 492$) was divided by median split into high and low pathway scores. Pathways from our OE versus KD RNAseq analyses (Figure 2C) were then studied for progression free survival (PFS) in the TCGA PRAD dataset. Kaplan–Meier (KM) plots for Lipid Catabolism Process (**A**) and Androgen Response Hallmark (**B**), with the number at risk and p-value (logrank test) are shown.

3. Discussion

This study reports on the connection between CPT1A overexpression (OE) and the metabolic and genetic consequences of its increased activity. Particularly, we found that CPT1A OE cells produced a significant number of acyl-carnitines that promote growth and resistance to stress insults, like excess lipids and androgen withdrawal. These later conditions are characteristic of advanced PCa, where androgen deprivation and excess circulating lipids frequently exists [40].

At the molecular level, this work provides insights into the metabolic changes precipitated by the excess use of lipid oxidation in the mitochondria, particularly the upregulation of the overall lipid catabolic process. As expected, not only CPT1A was increased, but also the ability to hydrolyze lipid stores via PNPLA2 (triglyceride lipase or ATGL) to increase the supply of fatty acids for the mitochondria (Figures 1B and 2D). It is possible that new inhibitors for ATGL could be of therapeutic value for cancers with increased CPT1A activity [41]. Another molecular aspect of the increased CPT1A activity was the re-wiring of metabolism towards the serine biosynthesis pathway, which has been recently shown to be important in supporting mitochondrial function [30], and a driver in NEPC [42]. These unexpected amino acid metabolism changes are likely promoted by the strong activation of the adaptive ER Stress response, as indicated by the transcriptional upregulation of genes linked to the ER stress response, Figure 2. In fact, ATF4 is a key transcription factor translationally induced upon activation of the unfolded protein response or UPR [43]. This induction triggers an anti-stress response that promotes adaptation, or in the case of a chronic unresolved stress, it can promote cell death. Increased ATF4 regulates serine and glycine metabolism genes to drive de novo serine and glycine production, which can be used for antioxidant defense and glutathione production [44]. In the CPT1A-OE cells, the mitochondrial SHMT2 gene was significantly increased in OE versus KD cells, suggesting a strong induction of serine/glycine synthesis in the mitochondria. This is likely to provide antioxidant defense via the mitochondrial folate cycle that can generate NADPH [45], and carbon units to produce cystathionine, an intermediate in the synthesis of cysteine and ultimately glutathione (Figure 3).

The ER stress observed in the OE cells compared to the KD cells is likely a response to the high ROS production in the mitochondria and low SOD2 expression. This is a known mechanism to promote cancer growth [46]. This was an unexpected result considering the OE cells did not show signs of distressed or fragmented mitochondria. A possible explanation is the upregulation of the glutathione homeostasis pathway. We found that the glutathione-degrading and ER response gene CHAC1 (cation transport regulator homolog1) was increased in OE cells. This gene was discovered in a co-regulated group of genes enriched for components of the ATF4 pathway, including CCAAT/enhancer-binding protein beta (CEBPB), which also binds to the CHAC1 promoter [47,48]. All this evidence would suggest that increased expression of a glutathione-degrading enzyme and activation of the ER stress pathway will lead to cancer cell death. However, we did not observe such changes in the OE cells as the levels of glutathione did not change and cells were able to grow in the presence of exogenously added lipids (Figures 1 and 4). Other studies in breast and ovarian cancer have shown that CHAC1 expression correlates with tumor differentiation and survival [49], suggesting that the observed ER stress in our models is likely stress-resolving and can promote disease progression. In fact, when we challenged the cells with commonly circulating fatty acids in the absence of androgens (a stressful environment), more SOD2 expression was observed in the OE cells and less on the KD cells. This underscores the increased antioxidant response capabilities of the OE cells and potential for survival and growth. This environment may promote adaptation of the OE cells to androgen deprivation, supporting progression to lethal disease. Recent studies have also shown that increased SOD2 activity can protect prostate cells when exposed to radiation [50].

How oxidative changes in the mitochondria connect with ER stress remains unknown. ER and oxidative stress have overlapping and intertwined functions in cancer [21]. Both promote epithelial mesenchymal transition, a key step of metastasis and tissue invasion of many tumor cells. In addition, detachment from the extracellular matrix activates the ATF4-HSPA5 branch of the UPR, which protects from anoikis by stimulating both autophagy and antioxidative stress responses [51]. As the CPT1A-OE cells prefer to grow in suspension [10], they might be using the ER stress response and the mitochondrial oxidative environment to transform to more aggressive tumors [52].

This study and the public databases provide evidence that lipid catabolism driven by CPT1A is associated with more aggressive disease. CPT1A-OE cells showed more SYP and ENO2 neuroendocrine marker expression compared to the KD cells. This suggests that in CRPC tumors, CPT1A activity can rewire metabolism to promote growth and transformation via activation of serine biosynthesis, folate cycle, and glutathione homeostasis, all geared to maintain an adequate redox balance in the cancer cells. The role of mitochondrial ROS in activating these pro-tumor antioxidant pathways warrants further investigation.

4. Materials and Methods

4.1. Cell Lines Fatty Acids and Drugs

LNCaP-C4-2 cells were purchased from the University of Texas MD Anderson Cancer Center (Houston, TX, USA). Cells were used at low passage number and grown in RPMI containing 10% FBS supplemented with amino acids and Insulin (Gibco, ThermoFisher, Walthman, MA, USA). Charcoal stripped serum (CSS) was used for androgen-deprived conditions. Lentiviral particles for shRNA and complete cDNA specific to CPT1A were prepared at the Functional Genomics facility at the University of Colorado. For transfection, the following shRNAs from the Sigma (St. Louis, MO, USA) library were used: For knockdown (KD), TRCN0000036279 (CPT1A-sh1, [17]) and control shRNA (NTshRNA) SHC202 were used. This specific shRNA has been used by us successfully in several models of cancer [10,15–17,52,53]. For CPT1A overexpression (OE), we used the ccsbBroad304-00359 clone from the CCSB-Broad lentiviral library as described [10]. Lentiviral transduction and selection were performed according to Sigma's MISSION protocol. Puromycin (1 μg/mL) and blasticidin (5 μg/mL) from Sigma were used for KD and OE cell line drug selection, respectively. Fatty acids were purchased from Sigma, resuspended in ethanol for a stock solution of 10 mM and stored at −80 °C. Fatty acids were conjugated to albumin, (A7030, Sigma), before use at a 2 mM: 5% (Fatty acid:BSA) ratio in RPMI media. Etomoxir-HCL (CPT1 inhibitor) was purchased from Sigma and resuspended in PBS to 33.4 mM and stored at −20 °C.

4.2. Reverse-Transcriptase-PCR

For RT-PCR analysis, cDNA was synthesized (Applied Biosystems, Foster City, CA, USA) and quantified by real-time PCR using SYBR green (BioRad, Hercules, CA, USA) detection. Results were normalized to the housekeeping gene RPL13A mRNA and expressed as arbitrary units of $2^{-\Delta\Delta CT}$ relative to the control group. Primer sequences:

RPL13A-F: 5-CCTGGAGGAGAAGAGGAAAGAGA.
RPL13A-R 5-TTGAGGACCTCTGTGTATTTGTCAA.
CPT1A-F: 5-TGGATCTGCTGTATATCCTTC.
CPT1A-R: 5-AATTGGTTTGATTTCCTCCC.

4.3. Western Blot Analysis

Protein extracts of 20 μg were separated on a 4–20% SDS-PAGE gel and transferred to nitrocellulose membranes as described [10]. Band signals were obtained and visualized with the LI-COR Biosciences system (Lincoln, NE, USA). Antibodies: CPT1A: 15184-1-AP, (Proteintech, Rosemont, IL, USA); GAPDH: CST 5174, (Cell Signaling Technology, Beverly, MA, USA); SOD2: CST 13141, Cell Signaling Technology.

4.4. Metabolomics and Acyl Carnitine Analysis

Cells were grown to 80% confluency before trypsinization and collection in 2×10^6 aliquots. Samples were processed at Biological Mass Spectrometry Facility at the University of Colorado AMC (Aurora, CO, USA) using standard protocols. For the measurement of acyl-carnitines, samples were extracted in a solution of methanol, acetonitrile, and water (5:3:2) at a concentration of 1 million cells/mL in presence of acyl-carnitines, deuterated standards (NSK-B, Cambridge Isotope Laboratories, Tewksbury, MA, USA). Samples were analyzed via UHPLC-MS (Vanquish-Q Exactive, ThermoFisher, Walthman, MA, USA) as previously described [54]. Analysis of the most significant pathways was performed with the MetaboAnalyst web-based analytical program [55].

4.5. Intracellular Lipase Analysis

The enzymatic activity of intracellular lipase was measured using a substrate containing 3H Triolein (Perkin Elmer, Waltham, MA, USA) and human serum as a source of ApoC2 as described previously [56]. In brief, LNCaP-C4-2 cells overexpressing CPT1A (OE) and controls (EV) were grown to 80% confluence. Intracellular lipase was made accessible by lysing the cells in heparin containing M-PER cell lysis buffer (Pierce, Rockford, IL, USA). Intracellular lipase activity was determined by incubation with 3H Triolein substrate for 45 min at 37 °C. The protein concentration of the lysate was determined to calculate the Lipase-dependent hydrolysis (FFA release) of 3H Triolein per mg, per min.

4.6. Electron Paramagnetic Resonance Spectroscopy

Mitochondrial ROS production was measured by EPR using the mitochondrial-targeted spin probe 1-hydroxy-4-[2-triphenylphosphonio)-acetamido]-2,2,6,6-tetramethyl-piperidine,1-hydroxy-2,2,6,6-tetramethyl-4-[2-(triphenylphosphonio)acetamido] piperidinium dichloride (mito-TEMPO-H) as previously reported [57]. Cells were grown to 80% confluency prior to the EPR measurements. The mito-TEMPO-H probe was prepared in deoxygenated 50 mM phosphate buffer. Cells were washed and treated with mito-TEMPO-H 0.25 mM in Krebs-HEPES buffer (KHB) containing 100 μM of a metal chelator DTPA to avoid direct oxidation with metal ion or hydroxyl radical generation by Fenton reaction. Cells were incubated for 50 min at 37 °C, placed on ice, then gently scraped. 50 μL of cell suspension was loaded in an EPR capillary tube and EPR measurements were performed at room temperature using Bruker EMXnano X-band spectrometer [57]. EPR acquisition parameters were: microwave frequency = 9.6 GHz; center field = 3432 G; modulation amplitude = 2.0 G; sweep width = 80 G; microwave power = 19.9 mW; total number of scans = 10; sweep time = 12.11 s; and time constant = 20.48 ms. mito-TEMPO. Nitroxide radicals concentration was obtained by simulating the spectra using the SpinFit module incorporated in the Xenon software of the bench-top EMXnano EPR spectrometer followed by the SpinCount module (Bruker, Billerica, MA, USA).Total protein was extracted from analyzed samples and quantified with a Bio-Rad DC protein assay kit (Bio-Rad, Hercules, CA, USA), and nitroxide concentrations were normalized to total protein.

4.7. Statistics

Student *t*-tests or ANOVA tests were used to compare between groups, followed by post hoc tests when appropriate, alpha = 0.05. Analysis was carried out with GraphPad Prism software v8 (GraphPad Software, San Diego, CA, USA). All data represent mean ± SD, unless otherwise indicated.

4.8. RNAseq and Pathway Analysis

All cells (KD, OE, and their respective controls) were grown to 80% confluency before RNA isolation. RNA was extracted using a RNeasy Plus Mini Kit (Qiagen, Valencia, CA, USA). RNA quality was verified using a High Sensitivity ScreenTape Assay on the Tape Station 4200 (Agilent Technologies, Santa Clara, CA, USA) and measured with a Tecan Plate Reader (Thermo Fisher Scientific, Waltham, MA, USA). Library construction was performed using the Universal Plus mRNA Library Kit (NuGen Technologies, Redwood City, CA, USA), and sequencing was performed on the NovaSeq 6000 instrument (Illumina, San Diego, CA, USA) using paired-end sequencing (150 bp) by the University of Colorado Cancer Center Genomics and Microarray Core. Illumina adapters were removed using BBDuk (sourceforge.net/projects/bbmap) and reads <50 bp after trimming were discarded. Reads were aligned and quantified using STAR (2.6.0a) [58]) to the Ensembl human transcriptome (hg38.p12, release 96). Normalization and differential expression were calculated using the limma R package [29]. An interaction model within limma used to directly compare the OE and the KD. Gene set enrichment analysis was performed using the fGSEA R package (v1.10.0) with 10,000 permutations and the Hallmarks and GO Biological Processes gene set collections from the Molecular Signatures Database [59]. Heatmaps were generated with the ComplexHeatmap R package [60] following *z*-score transformation. RNA-sequencing data have been deposited into the NCBI Gene Expression Omnibus database (accession number GSE161243).

4.9. Public Database Analysis

RMA normalized prostate cancer microarray data was downloaded from GEO (GSE32967, [37]). Only the first replicate for each sample was used for the analysis to deal with uneven sample replicates. The most variable probe was selected to represent each gene. The limma R package was used to compare small cell carcinoma ($n = 4$) to adenocarcinoma ($n = 3$) prostate cancer. TPM normalized gene expression and clinical data from The Cancer Genome Atlas PRAD dataset (Firehose Legacy) [61], was downloaded from cBioPortal [62]. Gene Set Variation Analysis (GSVA) was performed using the GSVA R package [63], to score several gene sets with a Poison distribution. Patients were classified into high and low pathway groups by median score splitting. The survival (https://cran.r-project.org/web/packages/survival/citation.html) and survminer R packages (https://rpkgs.datanovia.com/survminer/index.html) were used to generate Kaplan-Meier curves and perform log rank tests. For the CPT1A and AR gene expression correlations, Log2 normalized whole transcript mRNA expression values from Taylor et al. [38] prostate cancer samples were downloaded from cBioPortal [62]. Expression of AR and CPT1A between primary and metastatic samples were compared using a Wilcoxon rank sum test. Pearson correlation was calculated for the correlation between AR and CPT1A expression in either primary or metastatic tumors.

5. Conclusions

The overall goal of this study is to understand the lipid metabolic underpinnings of advanced prostate cancer so that metabolic therapies can be designed effectively. Overall, we provide evidence that CPT1A activity may have a relevant role in advanced PCa, including transformation to NEPC. Etomoxir is a potent inhibitor of CPT1 that has been used in clinical trials in Europe [64], but it is not currently being used in the USA. Considering all the toxic chemotherapeutic agents used in cancer treatments, the potential for drugs like etomoxir to impact cancer growth and drug response warrants investigation.

Author Contributions: Conceptualization, I.R.S.; Formal analysis, J.K., K.B., E.N.-G., A.G., J.C.C. and I.R.S.; Funding acquisition, I.R.S. and J.C.C.; Investigation, H.E. and A.G.; Methodology, A.D., E.M., K.B., and H.E.; Software, A.G. and J.C.C.; Supervision, I.R.S.; Writing–original draft, I.R.S.; Writing–review & editing, M.J., A.D., A.G., E.N.-G., J.C.C., and I.R.S. All authors have read and agreed to the published version of the manuscript.

Acknowledgments: We are grateful from the technical support from Maren Salzmann-Sullivan, Gergana Stoykova, and Juliana Oviedo. We are also thankful to Kristofer Fritz for the advice on SOD2 antibodies.

References

1. Auchus, R.J.; Sharifi, N. Sex hormones and prostate cancer. *Annu. Rev. Med.* **2020**, *71*, 33–45. [CrossRef] [PubMed]
2. Sharp, A.; Coleman, I.; Yuan, W.; Sprenger, C.; Dolling, D.; Rodrigues, D.N.; Russo, J.W.; Figueiredo, I.; Bertan, C.; Seed, G.; et al. Androgen receptor splice variant-7 expression emerges with castration resistance in prostate cancer. *J. Clin. Investig.* **2019**, *129*, 192–208. [CrossRef] [PubMed]
3. Nevedomskaya, E.; Baumgart, S.J.; Haendler, B. Recent advances in prostate cancer treatment and drug discovery. *Int. J. Mol. Sci.* **2018**, *19*, 1359. [CrossRef] [PubMed]
4. Carver, B.S.; Chapinski, C.; Wongvipat, J.; Hieronymus, H.; Chen, Y.; Chandarlapaty, S.; Arora, V.K.; Le, C.; Koutcher, J.; Scher, H.; et al. Reciprocal feedback regulation of PI3K and androgen receptor signaling in PTEN-deficient prostate cancer. *Cancer Cell* **2011**, *19*, 575–586. [CrossRef]
5. Dehm, S.M.; Tindall, D.J. Alternatively spliced androgen receptor variants. *Endocr. Relat. Cancer* **2011**, *18*, R183–R196. [CrossRef]
6. Beltran, H.; Prandi, D.; Mosquera, J.M.; Benelli, M.; Puca, L.; Cyrta, J.; Marotz, C.; Giannopoulou, E.; Chakravarthi, B.V.; Varambally, S.; et al. Divergent clonal evolution of castration-resistant neuroendocrine prostate cancer. *Nat. Med.* **2016**, *22*, 298–305. [CrossRef]

7. Conteduca, V.; Oromendia, C.; Eng, K.W.; Bareja, R.; Sigouros, M.; Molina, A.; Faltas, B.M.; Sboner, A.; Mosquera, J.M.; Elemento, O.; et al. Clinical features of neuroendocrine prostate cancer. *Eur. J. Cancer* **2019**, *121*, 7–18. [CrossRef]
8. Ku, S.Y.; Rosario, S.; Wang, Y.; Mu, P.; Seshadri, M.; Goodrich, Z.W.; Goodrich, M.M.; Labbé, D.P.; Gomez, E.C.; Wang, J.; et al. Rb1 and Trp53 cooperate to suppress prostate cancer lineage plasticity, metastasis, and antiandrogen resistance. *Science* **2017**, *355*, 78–83. [CrossRef]
9. Schlaepfer, I.R.; Joshi, M. CPT1A-mediated fat oxidation, mechanisms, and therapeutic potential. *Endocrinology* **2020**, *161*, 161. [CrossRef]
10. Joshi, M.; Stoykova, G.E.; Salzmann-Sullivan, M.; Dzieciatkowska, M.; Liebman, L.N.; Deep, G.; Schlaepfer, I.R. CPT1A supports castration-resistant prostate cancer in androgen-deprived conditions. *Cells* **2019**, *8*, 1115. [CrossRef]
11. Chen, M.; Zhang, J.; Sampieri, K.; Clohessy, J.G.; Mendez, L.; Gonzalez-Billalabeitia, E.; Liu, X.S.; Lee, Y.R.; Fung, J.; Katon, J.M.; et al. An aberrant SREBP-dependent lipogenic program promotes metastatic prostate cancer. *Nat. Genet.* **2018**, *50*, 206–218. [CrossRef]
12. Yao, C.H.; Liu, G.Y.; Wang, R.; Moon, S.H.; Gross, R.W.; Patti, G.J. Identifying off-target effects of etomoxir reveals that carnitine palmitoyltransferase I is essential for cancer cell proliferation independent of beta-oxidation. *PLoS Biol.* **2018**, *16*, e2003782. [CrossRef] [PubMed]
13. Carracedo, A.; Cantley, L.C.; Pandolfi, P.P. Cancer metabolism: Fatty acid oxidation in the limelight. *Nat. Rev. Cancer* **2013**, *13*, 227–232. [CrossRef] [PubMed]
14. Qu, Q.; Zeng, F.; Liu, X.; Wang, Q.J.; Deng, F. Fatty acid oxidation and carnitine palmitoyltransferase I: Emerging therapeutic targets in cancer. *Cell Death Dis.* **2016**, *7*, e2226. [CrossRef] [PubMed]
15. Schlaepfer, I.R.; Glode, L.M.; Hitz, C.A.; Pac, C.T.; Boyle, K.E.; Maroni, P.; Deep, G.; Agarwal, R.; Lucia, S.M.; Cramer, S.D.; et al. Inhibition of lipid oxidation increases glucose metabolism and enhances 2-deoxy-2-[f]fluoro-d-glucose uptake in prostate cancer mouse xenografts. *Mol. Imaging Biol.* **2015**, *17*, 529–538. [CrossRef]
16. Schlaepfer, I.R.; Nambiar, D.K.; Ramteke, A.; Kumar, R.; Dhar, D.; Agarwal, C.; Bergman, B.; Graner, M.; Maroni, P.; Singh, R.P.; et al. Hypoxia induces triglycerides accumulation in prostate cancer cells and extracellular vesicles supporting growth and invasiveness following reoxygenation. *Oncotarget* **2015**, *6*, 22836–22856. [CrossRef] [PubMed]
17. Schlaepfer, I.R.; Rider, L.; Rodrigues, L.U.; Gijon, M.A.; Pac, C.T.; Romero, L.; Cimic, A.; Sirintrapun, S.J.; Glode, L.M.; Eckel, R.H.; et al. Lipid catabolism via CPT1 as a therapeutic target for prostate cancer. *Mol. Cancer Ther.* **2014**, *13*, 2361–2371. [CrossRef]
18. Pike, L.S.; Smift, A.L.; Croteau, N.J.; Ferrick, D.A.; Wu, M. Inhibition of fatty acid oxidation by etomoxir impairs NADPH production and increases reactive oxygen species resulting in ATP depletion and cell death in human glioblastoma cells. *Biochim. Biophys. Acta* **2011**, *1807*, 726–734. [CrossRef]
19. Yun, J.; Mullarky, E.; Lu, C.; Bosch, K.N.; Kavalier, A.; Rivera, K.; Roper, J.; Chio, I.I.C.; Giannopoulou, E.G.; Rago, C.; et al. Vitamin C selectively kills KRAS and BRAF mutant colorectal cancer cells by targeting GAPDH. *Science* **2015**, *350*, 1391–1396. [CrossRef]
20. Schafer, Z.T.; Grassian, A.R.; Song, L.; Jiang, Z.; Gerhart-Hines, Z.; Irie, H.Y.; Gao, S.; Puigserver, P.; Brugge, J.S. Antioxidant and oncogene rescue of metabolic defects caused by loss of matrix attachment. *Nature* **2009**, *461*, 109–113. [CrossRef]
21. Cao, S.S.; Kaufman, R.J. Endoplasmic reticulum stress and oxidative stress in cell fate decision and human disease. *Antioxid. Redox Signal.* **2014**, *21*, 396–413. [CrossRef] [PubMed]
22. Scheuner, D.; Vander Mierde, D.; Song, B.; Flamez, D.; Creemers, J.W.; Tsukamoto, K.; Ribick, M.; Schuit, F.C.; Kaufman, R.J. Control of mRNA translation preserves endoplasmic reticulum function in beta cells and maintains glucose homeostasis. *Nat. Med.* **2005**, *11*, 757–764. [CrossRef] [PubMed]
23. Lin, N.; Chen, H.; Zhang, H.; Wan, X.; Su, Q. Mitochondrial reactive oxygen species (ROS) inhibition ameliorates palmitate-induced INS-1 beta cell death. *Endocrine* **2012**, *42*, 107–117. [CrossRef] [PubMed]
24. Fu, Y.; Wey, S.; Wang, M.; Ye, R.; Liao, C.P.; Roy-Burman, P.; Lee, A.S. Pten null prostate tumorigenesis and AKT activation are blocked by targeted knockout of ER chaperone GRP78/BiP in prostate epithelium. *Proc. Natl. Acad. Sci. USA* **2008**, *105*, 19444–19449. [CrossRef] [PubMed]

25. Thalmann, G.N.; Anezinis, P.E.; Chang, S.M.; Zhau, H.E.; Kim, E.E.; Hopwood, V.L.; Pathak, S.; von Eschenbach, A.C.; Chung, L.W. Androgen-independent cancer progression and bone metastasis in the LNCaP model of human prostate cancer. *Cancer Res.* **1994**, *54*, 2577–2581.
26. Das, S.K.; Eder, S.; Schauer, S.; Diwoky, C.; Temmel, H.; Guertl, B.; Gorkiewicz, G.; Tamilarasan, K.P.; Kumari, P.; Trauner, M.; et al. Adipose triglyceride lipase contributes to cancer-associated cachexia. *Science* **2011**, *333*, 233–238. [CrossRef]
27. Englinger, B.; Laemmerer, A.; Moser, P.; Kallus, S.; Röhrl, C.; Pirker, C.; Baier, D.; Mohr, T.; Niederstaetter, L.; Meier-Menches, S.M.; et al. Lipid droplet-mediated scavenging as novel intrinsic and adaptive resistance factor against the multikinase inhibitor ponatinib. *Int. J. Cancer* **2020**, *147*, 1680–1693. [CrossRef]
28. Schlaepfer, I.R.; Hitz, C.A.; Gijon, M.A.; Bergman, B.C.; Eckel, R.H.; Jacobsen, B.M. Progestin modulates the lipid profile and sensitivity of breast cancer cells to docetaxel. *Mol. Cell. Endocrinol.* **2012**, *363*, 111–121. [CrossRef]
29. Ritchie, M.E.; Phipson, B.; Wu, D.; Hu, Y.; Law, C.W.; Shi, W.; Smyth, G.K. Limma powers differential expression analyses for RNA-sequencing and microarray studies. *Nucleic Acids Res.* **2015**, *43*, e47. [CrossRef]
30. Gao, X.; Lee, K.; Reid, M.A.; Sanderson, S.M.; Qiu, C.; Li, S.; Liu, J.; Locasale, J.W. Serine availability influences mitochondrial dynamics and function through lipid metabolism. *Cell Rep.* **2018**, *22*, 3507–3520. [CrossRef]
31. Gao, X.; Locasale, J.W.; Reid, M.A. Serine and methionine metabolism: Vulnerabilities in lethal prostate cancer. *Cancer Cell* **2019**, *35*, 339–341. [CrossRef] [PubMed]
32. Wang, Y.H.; Huang, J.T.; Chen, W.L.; Wang, R.H.; Kao, M.C.; Pan, Y.R.; Chan, S.H.; Tsai, K.W.; Kung, H.J.; Lin, K.T.; et al. Dysregulation of cystathionine γ-lyase promotes prostate cancer progression and metastasis. *EMBO Rep.* **2019**, *20*, e45986. [CrossRef] [PubMed]
33. Kumar, A.; Tikoo, S.; Maity, S.; Sengupta, S.; Sengupta, S.; Kaur, A.; Bachhawat, A.K. Mammalian proapoptotic factor $ChaC_1$ and its homologues function as γ-glutamyl cyclotransferases acting specifically on glutathione. *EMBO Rep.* **2012**, *13*, 1095–1101. [CrossRef] [PubMed]
34. Chen, M.S.; Wang, S.F.; Hsu, C.Y.; Yin, P.H.; Yeh, T.S.; Lee, H.C.; Tseng, L.M. CHAC1 degradation of glutathione enhances cystine-starvation-induced necroptosis and ferroptosis in human triple negative breast cancer cells via the GCN2-eIF2α-ATF4 pathway. *Oncotarget* **2017**, *8*, 114588–114602. [CrossRef] [PubMed]
35. Bachhawat, A.K.; Yadav, S. The glutathione cycle: Glutathione metabolism beyond the γ-glutamyl cycle. *IUBMB Life* **2018**, *70*, 585–592. [CrossRef]
36. Schmuck, E.M.; Board, P.G.; Whitbread, A.K.; Tetlow, N.; Cavanaugh, J.A.; Blackburn, A.C.; Masoumi, A. Characterization of the monomethylarsonate reductase and dehydroascorbate reductase activities of Omega class glutathione transferase variants: Implications for arsenic metabolism and the age-at-onset of Alzheimer's and Parkinson's diseases. *Pharm. Genom.* **2005**, *15*, 493–501. [CrossRef]
37. Tzelepi, V.; Zhang, J.; Lu, J.F.; Kleb, B.; Wu, G.; Wan, X.; Hoang, A.; Efstathiou, E.; Sircar, K.; Navone, N.M.; et al. Modeling a lethal prostate cancer variant with small-cell carcinoma features. *Clin. Cancer Res.* **2012**, *18*, 666–677. [CrossRef]
38. Taylor, B.S.; Schultz, N.; Hieronymus, H.; Gopalan, A.; Xiao, Y.; Carver, B.S.; Arora, V.K.; Kaushik, P.; Cerami, E.; Reva, B.; et al. Integrative genomic profiling of human prostate cancer. *Cancer Cell* **2010**, *18*, 11–22. [CrossRef]
39. Mah, C.Y.; Nassar, Z.D.; Swinnen, J.V.; Butler, L.M. Lipogenic effects of androgen signaling in normal and malignant prostate. *Asian J. Urol.* **2020**, *7*, 258–270. [CrossRef]
40. Collier, A.; Ghosh, S.; McGlynn, B.; Hollins, G. Prostate cancer, androgen deprivation therapy, obesity, the metabolic syndrome, type 2 diabetes, and cardiovascular disease: A review. *Am. J. Clin. Oncol.* **2012**, *35*, 504–509. [CrossRef]
41. Schweiger, M.; Romauch, M.; Schreiber, R.; Grabner, G.F.; Hütter, S.; Kotzbeck, P.; Benedikt, P.; Eichmann, T.O.; Yamada, S.; Knittelfelder, O.; et al. Pharmacological inhibition of adipose triglyceride lipase corrects high-fat diet-induced insulin resistance and hepatosteatosis in mice. *Nat. Commun.* **2017**, *8*, 14859. [CrossRef] [PubMed]
42. Reina-Campos, M.; Linares, J.F.; Duran, A.; Cordes, T.; L'Hermitte, A.; Badur, M.G.; Bhangoo, M.S.; Thorson, P.K.; Richards, A.; Rooslid, T.; et al. Increased serine and one-carbon pathway metabolism by PKCλ/ι deficiency promotes neuroendocrine prostate cancer. *Cancer Cell* **2019**, *35*, 385–400. [CrossRef] [PubMed]

43. Balsa, E.; Soustek, M.S.; Thomas, A.; Cogliati, S.; García-Poyatos, C.; Martín-García, E.; Jedrychowski, M.; Gygi, S.P.; Enriquez, J.A.; Puigserver, P. ER and nutrient stress promote assembly of respiratory chain supercomplexes through the PERK-eIF2α axis. *Mol. Cell* **2019**, *74*, 877–890. [CrossRef] [PubMed]
44. DeNicola, G.M.; Chen, P.H.; Mullarky, E.; Sudderth, J.A.; Hu, Z.; Wu, D.; Tang, H.; Xie, Y.; Asara, J.M.; Huffman, K.E.; et al. NRF2 regulates serine biosynthesis in non-small cell lung cancer. *Nat. Genet.* **2015**, *47*, 1475–1481. [CrossRef]
45. Fan, J.; Ye, J.; Kamphorst, J.J.; Shlomi, T.; Thompson, C.B.; Rabinowitz, J.D. Quantitative flux analysis reveals folate-dependent NADPH production. *Nature* **2014**, *510*, 298–302. [CrossRef]
46. Zhu, C.H.; Huang, Y.; Oberley, L.W.; Domann, F.E. A family of AP-2 proteins down-regulate manganese superoxide dismutase expression. *J. Biol. Chem.* **2001**, *276*, 14407–14413. [CrossRef]
47. Crawford, R.R.; Prescott, E.T.; Sylvester, C.F.; Higdon, A.N.; Shan, J.; Kilberg, M.S.; Mungrue, I.N. Human $CHAC_1$ protein degrades glutathione, and mRNA induction is regulated by the transcription factors ATF_4 and ATF_3 and a bipartite ATF/CRE regulatory element. *J. Biol. Chem.* **2015**, *290*, 15878–15891. [CrossRef]
48. Gargalovic, P.S.; Imura, M.; Zhang, B.; Gharavi, N.M.; Clark, M.J.; Pagnon, J.; Yang, W.P.; He, A.; Truong, A.; Patel, S.; et al. Identification of inflammatory gene modules based on variations of human endothelial cell responses to oxidized lipids. *Proc. Natl. Acad. Sci. USA* **2006**, *103*, 12741–12746. [CrossRef]
49. Goebel, G.; Berger, R.; Strasak, A.M.; Egle, D.; Müller-Holzner, E.; Schmidt, S.; Rainer, J.; Presul, E.; Parson, W.; Lang, S.; et al. Elevated mRNA expression of $CHAC_1$ splicing variants is associated with poor outcome for breast and ovarian cancer patients. *Br. J. Cancer* **2012**, *106*, 189–198. [CrossRef]
50. Shrishrimal, S.; Chatterjee, A.; Kosmacek, E.A.; Davis, P.J.; McDonald, J.T.; Oberley-Deegan, R.E. Manganese porphyrin, MnTE-2-PyP, treatment protects the prostate from radiation-induced fibrosis (RIF) by activating the NRF2 signaling pathway and enhancing SOD2 and sirtuin activity. *Free Radic. Biol. Med.* **2020**, *152*, 255–270. [CrossRef]
51. Avivar-Valderas, A.; Salas, E.; Bobrovnikova-Marjon, E.; Diehl, J.A.; Nagi, C.; Debnath, J.; Aguirre-Ghiso, J.A. PERK integrates autophagy and oxidative stress responses to promote survival during extracellular matrix detachment. *Mol. Cell. Biol.* **2011**, *31*, 3616–3629. [CrossRef] [PubMed]
52. Sawyer, B.T.; Qamar, L.; Yamamoto, T.M.; McMellen, A.; Watson, Z.L.; Richer, J.K.; Behbakht, K.; Schlaepfer, I.R.; Bitler, B.G. Targeting fatty acid oxidation to promote anoikis and inhibit ovarian cancer progression. *Mol. Cancer Res.* **2020**, *18*, 1088–1098. [CrossRef] [PubMed]
53. Flaig, T.W.; Salzmann-Sullivan, M.; Su, L.J.; Zhang, Z.; Joshi, M.; Gijon, M.A.; Kim, J.; Arcaroli, J.J.; Van Bokhoven, A.; Lucia, M.S.; et al. Lipid catabolism inhibition sensitizes prostate cancer cells to antiandrogen blockade. *Oncotarget* **2017**, *8*, 56051–56065. [CrossRef] [PubMed]
54. Reisz, J.A.; Zheng, C.; D'Alessandro, A.; Nemkov, T. Untargeted and semi-targeted lipid analysis of biological samples using mass spectrometry-based metabolomics. In *Methods in Molecular Biology*; Humana Press: Totowa, NJ, USA, 2019; Volume 1978, pp. 121–135. [CrossRef]
55. Xia, J.; Wishart, D.S. Web-based inference of biological patterns, functions and pathways from metabolomic data using MetaboAnalyst. *Nat. Protoc.* **2011**, *6*, 743–760. [CrossRef]
56. Bruce, K.D.; Gorkhali, S.; Given, K.; Coates, A.M.; Boyle, K.E.; Macklin, W.B.; Eckel, R.H. Lipoprotein lipase is a feature of alternatively-activated microglia and may facilitate lipid uptake in the CNS during demyelination. *Front. Mol. Neurosci.* **2018**, *11*, 57. [CrossRef]
57. Elajaili, H.B.; Hernandez-Lagunas, L.; Ranguelova, K.; Dikalov, S.; Nozik-Grayck, E. Use of electron paramagnetic resonance in biological samples at ambient temperature and 77 K. *J. Vis. Exp. JoVE* **2019**, e58461. [CrossRef]
58. Dobin, A.; Davis, C.A.; Schlesinger, F.; Drenkow, J.; Zaleski, C.; Jha, S.; Batut, P.; Chaisson, M.; Gingeras, T.R. STAR: Ultrafast universal RNA-seq aligner. *Bioinformatics* **2013**, *29*, 15–21. [CrossRef]
59. Liberzon, A.; Subramanian, A.; Pinchback, R.; Thorvaldsdóttir, H.; Tamayo, P.; Mesirov, J.P. Molecular signatures database (MSigDB) 3.0. *Bioinformatics* **2011**, *27*, 1739–1740. [CrossRef]
60. Gu, Z.; Eils, R.; Schlesner, M. Complex heatmaps reveal patterns and correlations in multidimensional genomic data. *Bioinformatics* **2016**, *32*, 2847–2849. [CrossRef]
61. The Cancer Genome Atlas Research Network. The molecular taxonomy of primary prostate cancer. *Cell* **2015**, *163*, 1011–1025. [CrossRef]

62. Cerami, E.; Gao, J.; Dogrusoz, U.; Gross, B.E.; Sumer, S.O.; Aksoy, B.A.; Jacobsen, A.; Byrne, C.J.; Heuer, M.L.; Larsson, E.; et al. The cBio cancer genomics portal: An open platform for exploring multidimensional cancer genomics data. *Cancer Discov.* **2012**, *2*, 401–404. [CrossRef] [PubMed]
63. Hänzelmann, S.; Castelo, R.; Guinney, J. GSVA: Gene set variation analysis for microarray and RNA-Seq data. *BMC Bioinform.* **2013**, *14*, 7. [CrossRef] [PubMed]
64. Holubarsch, C.J.; Rohrbach, M.; Karrasch, M.; Boehm, E.; Polonski, L.; Ponikowski, P.; Rhein, S. A double-blind randomized multicentre clinical trial to evaluate the efficacy and safety of two doses of etomoxir in comparison with placebo in patients with moderate congestive heart failure: The ERGO (etomoxir for the recovery of glucose oxidation) study. *Clin. Sci.* **2007**, *113*, 205–212. [CrossRef] [PubMed]

6

A Multiplex Test Assessing *MiR663a*$_{me}$ and *VIM*$_{me}$ in Urine Accurately Discriminates Bladder Cancer from Inflammatory Conditions

Sara Monteiro-Reis [1], Ana Blanca [2], Joana Tedim-Moreira [1], Isa Carneiro [1,3], Diana Montezuma [1,3], Paula Monteiro [1,3], Jorge Oliveira [4], Luís Antunes [5], Rui Henrique [1,2,6], António Lopez-Beltran [7,8] and Carmen Jerónimo [1,6,*]

1 Cancer Biology and Epigenetics Group—Research Center (CI-IPOP), Portuguese Oncology Institute of Porto (IPO Porto), and Porto Comprehensive Cancer Center (P.CCC), Maimonides Biomedical Research Institute of Cordoba, 14004 Cordoba, Spain; sara.raquel.reis@ipoporto.min-saude.pt (S.M.-R.); joana.matos@ua.pt (J.T.-M.); isa.carneiro@ipoporto.min-saude.pt (I.C.); dianafelizardo@gmail.com (D.M.); paula.monteiro@ipoporto.min-saude.pt (P.M.); henrique@ipoporto.min-saude.pt (R.H.)

2 Department of Urology, University Hospital of Reina Sofia, Maimonides Biomedical Research Institute of Cordoba, 14004 Cordoba, Spain; anblape78@hotmail.com

3 Department of Pathology, Portuguese Oncology Institute of Porto (IPO Porto), 4200-072 Porto, Portugal

4 Department of Urology, Portuguese Oncology Institute of Porto (IPO-Porto), 4200-072 Porto, Portugal; jorge.oliveira@ipoporto.min-saude.pt

5 Department of Epidemiology, Portuguese Oncology Institute of Porto (IPO Porto) & Cancer Epidemiology Group—Research Center (CI-IPOP), 4200-072 Porto, Portugal; luis.antunes@ipoporto.min-saude.pt

6 Department of Pathology and Molecular Immunology, Institute of Biomedical Sciences Abel Salazar (ICBAS)—University of Porto, 4050-313 Porto, Portugal

7 Department of Surgery and Pathology, Faculty of Medicine, University of Cordoba, 14071 Cordoba, Spain; em1lobea@uco.es

8 Champalimaud Clinical Center, 1400-038 Lisbon, Portugal

* Correspondence: carmenjeronimo@ipoporto.min-saude.pt

Abstract: Bladder cancer (BlCa) is a common malignancy with significant morbidity and mortality. Current diagnostic methods are invasive and costly, showing the need for newer biomarkers. Although several epigenetic-based biomarkers have been proposed, their ability to discriminate BlCa from common benign conditions of the urinary tract, especially inflammatory diseases, has not been adequately explored. Herein, we sought to determine whether VIM$_{me}$ and miR663a$_{me}$ might accurately discriminate those two conditions, using a multiplex test. Performance of VIM$_{me}$ and miR663a$_{me}$ in tissue samples and urines in testing set confirmed previous results (96.3% sensitivity, 88.2% specificity, area under de curve (AUC) 0.98 and 92.6% sensitivity, 75% specificity, AUC 0.83, respectively). In the validation sets, VIM$_{me}$-miR663a$_{me}$ multiplex test in urine discriminated BlCa patients from healthy donors or patients with inflammatory conditions, with 87% sensitivity, 86% specificity and 80% sensitivity, 75% specificity, respectively. Furthermore, positive likelihood ratio (LR) of 2.41 and negative LR of 0.21 were also disclosed. Compared to urinary cytology, VIM$_{me}$-miR663a$_{me}$ multiplex panel correctly detected 87% of the analysed cases, whereas cytology only forecasted 41%. Furthermore, high miR663a$_{me}$ independently predicted worse clinical outcome, especially in patients with invasive BlCa. We concluded that the implementation of this panel might better stratify patients for confirmatory, invasive examinations, ultimately improving the cost-effectiveness of BlCa diagnosis and management. Moreover, miR663a$_{me}$ analysis might provide relevant information for patient monitoring, identifying patients at higher risk for cancer progression.

Keywords: bladder cancer; methylation; biomarkers

1. Introduction

Bladder cancer (BlCa) is one of the most incident cancers, ranking ninth in prevalence worldwide [1,2]. In men, which are more prone to develop BlCa, it represents the second most frequent urological malignancy after prostate cancer [1,2]. Moreover, it is expected that, by 2040, the number of estimated new cases and cancer-related deaths will almost double the 549,393 newly diagnosed cases and 199,922 deaths recorded in 2018 [1,2]. Most BlCa cases correspond to urothelial carcinoma, generally presenting as non-muscle invasive BlCa (NMIBC), accounting for 75–80% of all new cases, characterised by frequent recurrences and eventual progression to more aggressive, deeply invasive and metastatic disease, or muscle-invasive BlCa (MIBC), an aggressive, locally invading carcinoma, corresponding to 20–25% of all cases, with propensity for metastisation [3,4]. Haematuria is the most common clinical sign of BlCa, although it also occurs in several common benign disease such as urinary tract infections and non-infectious inflammatory conditions. Presently, BlCa diagnosis generally involves cytoscopic examination, an expensive and invasive procedure, complemented by urine cytology [5–7]. However, the latter has limited accuracy, particularly for identification of low-grade papillary tumours, and the invasive nature of cystoscopic examination entails patient discomfort and, in some cases, infection [5]. Moreover, because of the high incidence, recurrence and progression rate, active long follow-up is required, making BlCa the costliest malignancy [8]. Thus, early, accurate and non-invasive BlCa detection is the determinant to improve both patients and healthcare financial management.

Epigenetic changes, including DNA methylation, have been largely investigated for cancer detection [9]. Owing to chemical and biological stability, DNA methylation-based biomarkers have potential clinical applications in early cancer detection, diagnosis, follow-up and targeted therapies [10]. Previously, two independent DNA methylation-based biomarker panels have been reported as promising tests for accurate early detection of BlCa [11,12]. In 2010, a three-gene panel comprised *GDF15, TMEFF2* and *VIM* methylation identified BlCa with 94% sensitivity and 100% specificity in urine samples from 51 BlCa patients [11]. More recently, a panel testing the promoter methylation of two microRNAs—*miR129-2* and *miR663a*—identified urothelial carcinoma (from upper and lower urinary tracts) with a sensitivity of 87.8% and specificity of 82.7% in 49 urine samples from patients with urothelial carcinoma [12]. Furthermore, the same panels could discriminate BlCa from other common genitourinary cancers (i.e., from kidney and prostate). Nonetheless, both studies used a singleplex approach, and the ability of these tests to discriminate BlCa from common benign conditions of the urinary tract with overlapping manifestations, especially inflammatory diseases, has not been adequately explored, thus far. Indeed, inflammatory conditions of the urinary tract may negatively impact the specificity of urinary-based biomarkers for BlCa detection, increasing false positive results and entailing unnecessary complementary invasive tests [6,13,14].

Thus, we sought to assess whether the most promising markers in each published panel—*miR-663a* ($miR663a_{me}$) and *Vimentin* (VIM_{me})—might accurately discriminate BlCa from inflammatory conditions in voided urine, allowing for the development of a multiplex test that could be used for early detection in clinical practice.

2. Experimental Section

2.1. Patients and Tumour Sample Collection

Ninety-four primary BlCa tissue samples were obtained from a consecutive series of patients diagnosed, treated with transurethral resection (TUR) or radical cystectomy, between 1994 and 2011, and followed at Portuguese Oncology Institute of Porto (IPO Porto), Portugal (Table 1). Briefly, tumour samples were obtained during surgery and immediately snap-frozen, stored at −80 °C and subsequently macrodissected for tumours' cells enrichment and cut in cryostat for DNA extraction. Routine collection and processing of tissue samples allowed for pathological examination, classification, grading and staging [15]. For control purposes, an independent set of 19 normal bladder mucosae

(NB) samples were also collected from BlCa-free individuals (prostate cancer patients submitted to radical prostatectomy) (Table 1).

Table 1. Clinical and histopathological characteristics of patients with bladder carcinoma (BlCa), normal bladder mucosae (NB), healthy donors (HD) and inflammatory controls (IC).

	Tissues		Urines				
			Testing Set		Validation Sets		
Clinicopaphological Features	Bladder UC	Normal Bladder Mucosae	Bladder UC	Healthy Donors	Bladder UC	Healthy Donors (#1)	Inflammatory Controls (#2)
Patients, n	94	19	27	24	100	57	174
Gender, n							
Males	78	19	20	13	79	16	132
Females	16	0	7	12	21	41	42
Median age, yrs	69	63	69	45	68	49	64
(range)	(45–91)	(48–75)	(47–88)	(39–61)	(38–91)	(41–64)	(18–92)
Grade, n							
Papillary, low-grade	34	n.a.	13	n.a.	51	n.a.	n.a.
Papillary, high-grade	33	n.a.	8	n.a.	26	n.a.	n.a.
Invasive, high-grade	27	n.a.	6	n.a.	23	n.a.	n.a.
Invasion of Muscular Layer, n							
NMIBC	67	n.a.	19	n.a.	77	n.a.	n.a.
MIBC	27	n.a.	8	n.a.	23	n.a.	n.a.

#1—Validation Set #1; #2—Validation Set #2; yrs—years; n.a.—non applicable; NMIBC—Non-Muscle Invasive Bladder Cancer; MIBC—Muscle Invasive Bladder Cancer, UC—Urothelial Carcinoma.

2.2. *Urine Sample Collection and Processing*

For the "Testing sets", 27 voided urine samples (one per patient) were collected from BlCa patients, diagnosed and treated between 2006 and 2016 at IPO Porto, as well as a set of 24 voided urine samples from healthy donors (HD), also from IPO Porto, with no personal or familial history of cancer, used as controls (Table 1). The "Validation sets" comprised: (1) 100 urine samples from BlCa patients, diagnosed and treated between 2002 and 2016 at IPO Porto, and 57 urine samples from HD collected at IPO Porto, and (2) an independent set of control urine sediments (n = 174) from patients diagnosed with urinary tract inflammatory conditions (IC), diagnosed between 2008 and 2014 at the University Hospital of Cordoba (UHC). All BlCa patients' urines were obtained before treatment. Moreover, all sets of samples were collected from different cohorts of patients. Informed consent was obtained from patients and controls after approval from the ethics committees of IPO Porto and UHC (CES-IPO 019/08, approval date: 16th January 2008). All urine samples were processed by immediate centrifugation at 4000 rpm for 10 min; the respective pellet was washed twice with phosphate-buffered saline (PBS) and stored at −80 °C.

2.3. *Nucleic Acids Isolation, Bisulfite Modification and Multiplex qMSP Analysis*

DNA was extracted from frozen BlCa and NB tissues, and all urine sample sets, using a standard phenol-chloroform protocol [16], and its concentration determined using a Qubit 3 Fluorometer (Thermo Fisher Scientific, Waltham, MA, USA). Bisulfite modification was performed through sodium bisulfite, using the EZ DNA Methylation-Gold™ Kit (Zymo Research, Irvine, CA, USA), according to manufacturer's protocol. For this, 1000 ng and 50 ng of DNA were converted for tissues and urine sediments, respectively. Quantitative methylation levels were performed using Xpert Fast Probe Master Mix (GRiSP, Porto, Portugal), and multiplex reactions were run in triplicates in 96-well plates using an Applied Biosystems 7500 Sequence Detector (Perkin Elmer, Waltham, CA, USA), with Beta-Actin (ACTB) as internal reference gene for normalization. Primer and probe sequences were designed using Methyl Primer Express 1.0 and purchased from Sigma-Aldrich (St. Louis, MO, USA) (Supplementary Table S1). Additionally, six serial dilutions (dilution factor of 5×) of a fully methylated bisulphite modified universal DNA control were included in each plate to generate a standard curve. In each sample and for each gene, the relative DNA methylation levels were determined using the following formula: ((target gene/ACTB) ×1000). A run was considered valid when previously reported criteria were met [11].

2.4. Statistical Analysis

Differences in quantitative methylation values were assessed with the non-parametric Mann-Whitney *U* (MW) and Kruskal-Wallis (KW) tests. Associations between age, gender, grade, invasion of muscular layer and methylation levels were carried out using Spearman's correlation, MW or KW tests, as appropriate. For multiple comparisons, Bonferroni's correction was applied in pairwise comparisons.

Biomarker performance parameters, including sensitivity, specificity, positive predictive value (PPV), negative predictive value (NPV), accuracy and positive and negative likelihood ratios (LR), were estimated [17]. Receiver operator characteristics (ROC) curves were constructed by plotting the true positive (sensitivity) against false positive (1-specificity) rate, and the area under the curve (AUC) was calculated. The higher value obtained from the sum of sensitivity and 1-specificity in each ROC-curve was used as cut-off to categorise samples as methylated or non-methylated. ROC curves were constructed using logistic regression model for DNA methylation panel. Disease-specific and disease-free survival curves (Kaplan-Meier with log rank test) were computed for standard variables and for categorised genes' promoter methylation status. A Cox-regression model comprising all significant variables (univariable and multivariable model) was computed to assess the relative contribution of each variable to the follow-up status. All two-tailed p values were derived from statistical tests, using a computer-assisted program (SPSS Version 26.0, IBM, Armonk, NY, EUA) and the results were considered statistically significant at $p < 0.05$. Bonferroni's correction for multiple comparisons was used when applicable.

3. Results

3.1. Methylation Analysis and Performance of the Multiplex Panel in BlCa Tissue Series

To confirm the previously published performance of *miR663a* and *VIM* promoter methylation as BlCa biomarkers, tissue samples were tested. As expected, both *miR663a* and *VIM* were found hypermethylated (76.6% and 94.4%, respectively) in most BlCa tissue samples, and methylation levels were significantly higher compared to NB ($p < 0.0001$ and $p < 0.0001$, respectively) (Figure 1A). The two genes independently performed well as BlCa detection biomarkers in tissues, with an AUC of 0.979 for VIM_{me} (95% confidence interval (CI): 0.956–1.002, $p < 0.0001$), and of 0.897 for $miR663a_{me}$ (95% CI: 0.836–0.959, $p < 0.0001$). Moreover, in combination as multiplex panel, it accurately discriminated BlCa from NB with 96.3% sensitivity and 88.2% specificity, corresponding to an AUC of 0.982 (Figure 1B; Supplementary Table S2).

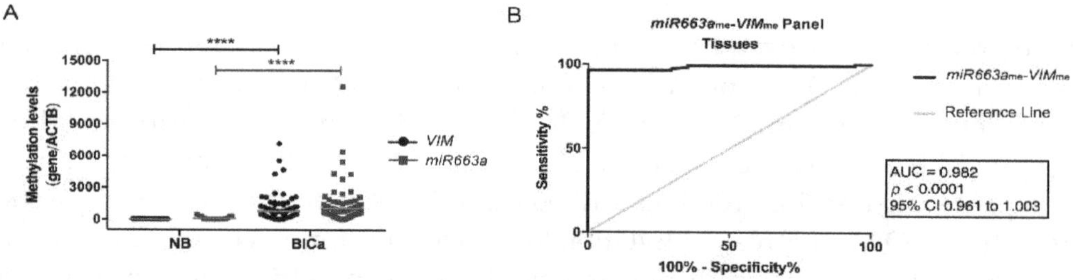

Figure 1. (**A**) Distribution of VIM_{me} and $miR663a_{me}$ levels in normal bladder mucosae (NB; $n = 19$) and bladder carcinoma (BlCa; $n = 94$) tissue samples. Mann-Whitney U test, **** $p < 0.0001$. Median is represented by the red line. (**B**) Receiver operator characteristic (ROC) curve evaluating the performance of the VIM_{me}-$miR663a_{me}$ panel for the identification of BlCa in tissue samples. (AUC—Area under the curve; CI—Confidence interval; ACTB—Beta-Actin; VIM—Vimentin).

3.2. Methylation Analysis and Performance of Multiplex Panel in BlCa Testing Set

Paralleling the previous observations in tissues, *miR663a*$_{me}$ and *VIM*$_{me}$ levels were significantly higher in BlCa urine samples than in those of controls ($p < 0.0001$ and $p < 0.0001$, Figure 2A), and the multiplex panel discriminated BlCa from HD with 92.6% sensitivity and 90% NPV (Supplementary Table S2), corresponding to an AUC of 0.83 (Figure 2B).

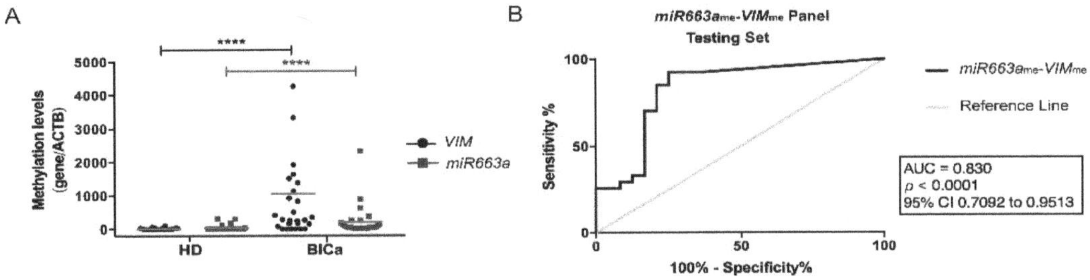

Figure 2. (**A**) Distribution of *VIM*$_{me}$ and *miR663a*$_{me}$ levels in the Testing Cohort, composed by healthy donors (HD; $n = 24$) and bladder carcinoma (BlCa; $n = 27$) urine samples. Mann-Whitney U test, **** $p < 0.0001$. Median is represented by the red line. (**B**) Receiver operator characteristic (ROC) curve evaluating the performance of the *VIM*$_{me}$-*miR663a*$_{me}$ panel for the identification of BlCa in urine samples of the Testing Cohort. (AUC—Area under the curve; CI—Confidence interval; ACTB—Beta-Actin; VIM—Vimentin).

3.3. Methylation Analysis and Performance of VIM$_{me}$ and miR663$_{me}$ Multiplex Panel for BlCa vs. HD

In line with the testing set results, a higher number of malignant samples disclosed significantly higher *VIM*$_{me}$ and *miR663*$_{me}$ levels than HDs ($p < 0.0001$ and $p < 0.0001$, respectively) in the validation sets (Figure 3A). ROC curve analysis confirmed a high discriminative ability of *VIM*$_{me}$-miR663$_{me}$ panel, with an AUC of 0.91 (Figure 3B). Indeed, the multiplex panel discriminated BlCa from HD subjects with 87% sensitivity and 86% specificity (Table 2).

Table 2. Performance of *VIM*$_{me}$-*miR663a*$_{me}$ panel for the detection of bladder cancer in Validation Cohorts #1 and #2. (PPV—positive predictive value; NPV—negative predictive value).

Samples	Biomarker Performance	*miR663a*$_{me}$-*VIM*$_{me}$ (%)
Validation #1	Sensitivity	87.0
	Specificity	86.0
	PPV	91.6
	NPV	79.0
	Accuracy	86.6
Validation #2	Sensitivity	80.0
	Specificity	75.3
	PPV	65.0
	NPV	86.8
	Accuracy	77.0

PPV—Positive Predictive Value; NPV—Negative Predictive Value.

Remarkably, the proportion of true positive cases detected by the *VIM*$_{me}$-miR663$_{me}$ multiplex panel was significantly higher than that of urine cytology ($p < 0.001$). Indeed, of 46 BlCa cases with valid urine cytology results, only 19 were classified as positive, 17 as negative and 10 as "inconclusive/suspicious", corresponding to 41% sensitivity (Figure 4). Contrarily, the *VIM*$_{me}$-miR663$_{me}$ multiplex panel correctly identified 40/46 cases as BlCa, corresponding to an overall sensitivity of 87% (Figure 4). Importantly, 12 of 14 low-grade papillary carcinomas were accurately identified by *VIM*$_{me}$-*miR663*$_{me}$ multiplex panel, whereas cytology merely identified four cases.

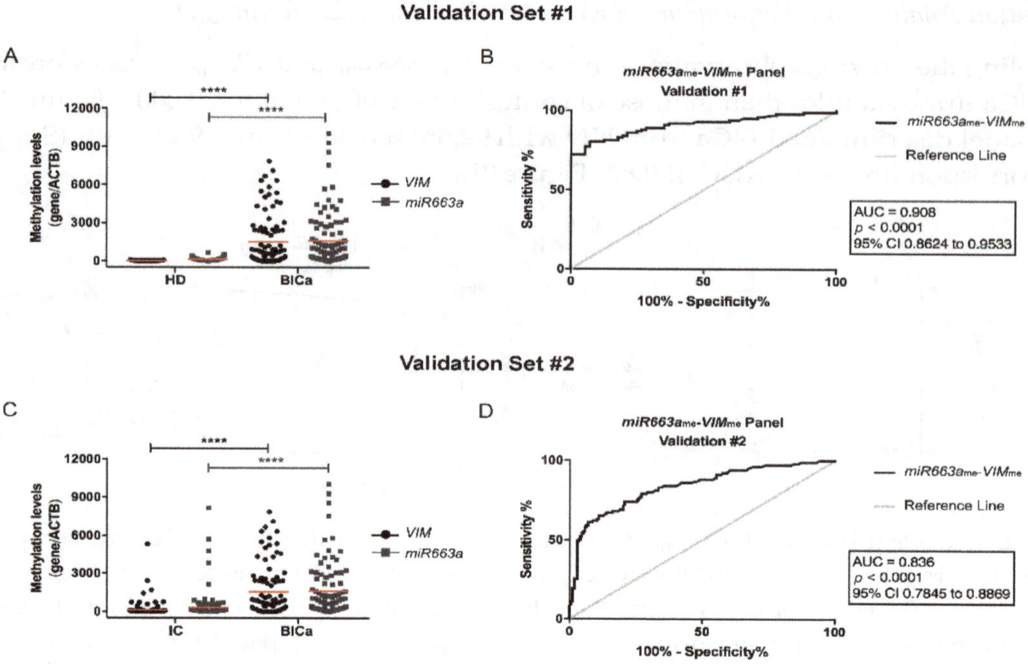

Figure 3. (**A**) Distribution of VIM_{me} and $miR663a_{me}$ levels in the Validation Cohort #1, composed by healthy donors (HD; $n = 57$) and bladder carcinoma (BlCa; $n = 100$) urine samples. Mann-Whitney U (MW) test, **** $p < 0.0001$. Median is represented by the red line. (**B**) Receiver operator characteristic (ROC) curve evaluating the performance of the VIM_{me}-$miR663a_{me}$ panel for the identification of BlCa in urine samples of the Validation Cohort #1. (**C**) Distribution of VIM_{me} and $miR663a_{me}$ levels in the Validation Cohort #2, composed by inflammatory controls (IC; $n = 174$) and bladder carcinoma (BlCa; $n = 100$) urine samples. MW test, **** $p < 0.0001$. (**D**) ROC curve evaluating the performance of the VIM_{me}-$miR663a_{me}$ panel for the identification of BlCa in urine samples of the Validation Cohort #2. (AUC—Area under the curve; CI—Confidence interval; ACTB—Beta-Actin; VIM—Vimentin).

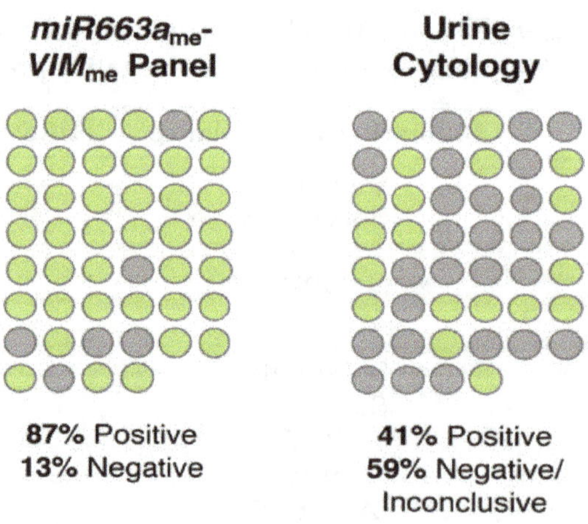

Figure 4. Representation of the percentage of bladder cancer (BlCa) cases correctly identified with the VIM_{me}-$miR663a_{me}$ panel and a standard urine cytology analysis. Green circles represent positive cases, grey circles represent negative/inconclusive cases.

3.4. Methylation Analysis and Performance of VIM_{me} and $miR663_{me}$ Multiplex Panel for BlCa vs. IC

In urine samples, VIM_{me}-$miR663_{me}$ levels discriminated BlCa from IC patients (Figure 3C), with 80% sensitivity, 75.3% specificity and, importantly, 86.8% NPV (Table 2), corresponding to an AUC of 0.836 (Figure 3D). Remarkably, a 2.86 Positive LR and a Negative LR of 0.21 were also disclosed by VIM_{me}-$miR663_{me}$ multiplex panel in this setting.

3.5. Clinicopathologic Correlations and Survival Analyses

High-grade papillary BlCa showed significantly higher $miR663a_{me}$ levels than low-grade papillary BlCa ($p = 0.007$), in tissue samples. The same was observed in urine samples from the validation set ($p = 0.0072$), a result which was extensive to VIM_{me} ($p = 0.0052$) (Supplementary Figure S1). No additional associations were disclosed between VIM_{me} and $miR663a_{me}$ levels and other standard clinical variables, including patients' age and gender.

Follow-up data was available for 91 (out of 94) IPO Porto's BlCa patients that provided tissue samples. The median follow-up time was 66 months (range: 1–203 months). At the last follow-up timepoint, 30 patients were alive with no evidence of cancer, 12 patients were alive with disease, 29 had deceased due to BlCa and 23 died from other causes. Univariable and multivariable Cox regression analysis were performed, including the variables grade, invasion of muscular layer, gender and age. As expected, a poor outcome was depicted for patients with higher grade and muscle invasive BlCa ($p = 0.001$ and $p < 0.0001$, respectively) (Table 3). In the multivariate model for disease-specific survival, $miR663a_{me}$ levels, higher grade and muscle invasion were independent predictors of outcome ($p = 0.04$, $p = 0.035$ and $p = 0.031$, respectively; Table 3). Moreover, after categorization into NMIBC *vs.* MIBC, tumours with higher $miR663a_{me}$ levels implied a 3.7-fold increased risk of cancer-related death among patients with MIBC (95% CI: 1.32–10.25, $p = 0.013$; Supplementary Figure S2). Contrarily, no associations were found for $miR663a_{me}$ or VIM_{me} levels concerning disease-free survival.

Table 3. Cox regression models assessing the potential of clinical and VIMme and miR663ame levels in the prediction of disease-specific survival for bladder carcinoma (BlCa) patients.

Disease-specific Survival	Variables	Hazard Ratio (HR)	95% CI for OR	*p*
Univariate	Invasion of muscular layer	6.15	2.76–13.72	0.0001
	Grade			
	PLG vs. PHG	15.59	2.03–119.94	0.008
	PLG vs. IHG	32.83	4.31–250.06	0.001
	Age	2.34	0.98–5.59	0.060
	Gender	1.02	0.39–2.70	0.970
	miR663a methylation ≤ median	1.61	0.75–3.48	0.225
	VIM methylation ≤ median	1.07	0.50–2.28	0.861
Multivariate	Invasion of muscular layer	3.54	1.12–11.19	0.031
	Grade			
	PLG vs. PHG	8.03	0.97–66.32	0.053
	PLG vs. IHG	11.89	1.18–119.37	0.035
	miR663a methylation ≤ median	2.67	1.05–6.81	0.040
	VIM methylation ≤ median	1.12	0.51–2.42	0.783

CI—confidence interval; OR—odds ratio; PLG—papillary low-grade; PHG—papillary high-grade; IHG—invasive high-grade.

4. Discussion

Bladder cancer is a major health concern worldwide, with an expected significant increase in incidence and mortality within the next two decades [1,2]. Early detection is critical for adequate management, aiming to reduce disease-specific mortality, as well as the economic burden imposed by BlCa treatment and follow-up. Because currently available diagnostic tools require invasive examination [13,14], development of non-invasive and less costly tests for early detection and monitoring are likely to have a significant impact in clinical practice. Although several molecular biomarkers, including epigenetic-based, have been developed for that end, discrimination of BlCa from other urinary tract malignancies and, more importantly, from benign conditions causing haematuria, including inflammatory diseases, remains a challenge. Indeed, most control samples used in biomarker discovery studies, including our own, mostly comprise normal/healthy donors, disregarding the fact that a biomarker-based test would be offered to an "at-risk" population, including patients experiencing suspicious symptoms. Therefore, based on two previously published studies by our research team [11,12], we tested whether a $miR663a_{me}$ and VIM_{me} multiplex panel could accurately discriminate BlCa from normal individuals and those afflicted with inflammatory conditions of the genitourinary tract.

Because both *miR663a*$_{me}$ and *VIM*$_{me}$ were previously assessed using two different "simplex" multi-gene biomarker panels, we firstly tested *miR663a*$_{me}$ and *VIM*$_{me}$ in multiplex in a consecutive series of primary BlCa tissue samples and normal urothelial mucosae to confirm those previous results. Indeed, employing a multiplex reaction allows for downscaling the initial tissue/body fluid sample requirements, but also the quantity of DNA required for each test [18]. Remarkably, as expected, the *miR663a*$_{me}$-*VIM*$_{me}$ multiplex panel discriminated BlCa from NB tissues with high sensitivity and specificity (96.3% and 88.2%, respectively), confirming the previous observations for the two markers separately [11,12]. In urine samples from the testing set, although the performance of the multiplex panel was slightly inferior to that of tissues, 92.6% sensitivity and 90% NPV was reached. Indeed, it should be recalled that a relatively small number of cancer cells are exfoliated into urine, which are subsequently "diluted" among a larger population of normal-looking urothelial cells. Thus, the tumour DNA content in urine is actually minute [19] and sensitivity over 90% should be regarded as a very encouraging result. Furthermore, in the validation set, comprising a larger independent cohort, specificity of the *miR663a*$_{me}$-*VIM*$_{me}$ multiplex panel increased to 86%, further increasing the potential usefulness of the test.

It should be emphasised, however, that the foremost aim of this study was to assess the multiplex panel ability to discriminate BlCa from IC, since this panel is envisaged to be tested in an "at-risk" population, including individuals complaining of haematuria, many of which will be found to harbour urinary tract inflammatory conditions. Although, in this setting, sensitivity and specificity were slightly reduced, NPV increased (86.8%), which is an important finding [20]. Indeed, it is expected that among tested individuals, most will not have a neoplastic condition and, thus, the higher the NPV, the larger the proportion of those subjects that will not be submitted to confirmatory, invasive, procedures, supporting the good performance of the test in discriminating patients negative for malignant condition. Importantly, an LR (+) of 2.86 and an LR (−) of 0.21 values were observed, indicating that a negative result decreases by 30% the probability of misdiagnosis [17].

Despite the fact that several studies suggest various genomic mutations and/or proteins' expression deregulation as biomarkers for BlCa detection and prognostication [21], the search for novel epigenetic biomarkers, mostly DNA methylation-based, for BlCa detection has been attempted by several research teams, probably due to the stability of the markers and the possibility of high-throughput tests. Although some of those previous studies report an apparently superior performance to the panel reported herein, it should be recalled that in most cases the patients' series were smaller, only healthy donors were included as controls or these were comprised of a mixed group of healthy donors and patients with diverse urological diseases, and/or did not use a multiplex approach, which might impact in sample availability, testing time length and cost [22–28]. Roperch et al. proposed a three gene multiplex methylation panel (*HS3ST2*, *SEPTIN9* and *SLIT2*) combined with *FGFR3* mutations assessment, age and smoking-status at time of diagnosis in a multivariate model, for diagnosis of NMIBC in urine samples, disclosing 97.6% sensitivity and 84.8% specificity, in a smaller control cohort [29]. Nonetheless, this strategy might be more difficult to implement in clinical practice, since it requires both mutation and methylation analyses, in which the multiplex is performed in two distinct gene duplex reactions. Similarly, Dahmcke et al. proposed a six gene methylation panel (*SALL3*, *ONECUT2*, *CCNA1*, *BCL2*, *EOMES* and *VIM*) combined with the mutational analysis of *TERT* and *FGFR3*, for early detection of BlCa, in urine samples, comparing BlCa patients and patients with gross haematuria [30]. Although this panel disclosed higher sensitivity (97%), specificity was similar (76.9%) [30], and, once again, our test uses a single technique in a single reaction, requiring less amount of sample, enabling shorter response time, reduced technical skills and lower cost.

Although urine cytology and UroVysion™ fluorescence in situ hybridization (FISH) assay are the two most commonly used urine-based tests in daily practice, they present important limitations. On one hand, UroVysion™ presents a not-negligible rate of false positive results; on the other hand, urine cytology has limited accuracy, especially in low grade tumours detection [6,31,32]. Although no direct comparison can be done with UroVysion™, the 91.6% PPV obtained for the multiplex panel clearly demonstrates higher accuracy in identifying true positive BlCa cases. In the present study, urine cytology reached 41% sensitivity, which was easily surpassed by the 86% displayed by $miR663a_{me}$-VIM_{me} multiplex panel. Notwithstanding, urine cytology remains an easy-to-perform and informative test, as it allows pathologists to have the first look at exfoliated neoplastic cells in urine. Having that in mind, we propose an algorithm where a urine cytology and the $miR663a_{me}$-VIM_{me} multiplex panel could be combined as first-line diagnostic tests in patients with common urinary complaints, with the ultimate goal of reducing the number of unnecessary cystoscopies, which are invasive, uncomfortable and costly procedures (Figure 5).

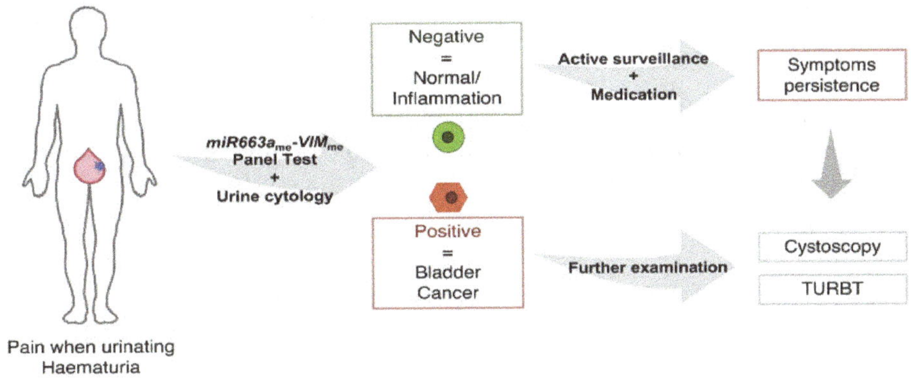

Figure 5. Proposed algorithm for the combination of urine cytology and VIM_{me}-$miR663a_{me}$ panel as a first-line diagnostic tests in patients with common urinary complaints. (TURBT—Transurethral Resection of Bladder Tumour).

In this work, we further explored the prognostic ability of the gene methylation markers, aiming to strengthen its clinical potential. Interestingly, survival analysis revealed that high $miR663a_{me}$ levels independently predicted poor disease-specific survival in BlCa patients, especially those with MIBC. Thus, the $miR663a_{me}$-VIM_{me} multiplex panel not only conveys diagnostic, but also prognostic information.

Taking into account the promising results obtained, unveiling the putative biological relevance of *miR663a* and *VIM* promoter methylation in bladder carcinogenesis may provide new important insights. VIM encodes for vimentin, an intermediate filament characteristic of cells with mesenchymal phenotype, not expressed in most normal epithelia (including urothelium), nor in most carcinomas [33]. *VIM* de-novo expression or overexpression has been reported in various epithelial cancers, including those of prostate [34], breast [35] and lung [36], associating with increased tumour growth and invasion. In these instances, vimentin expression has been associated with epithelial to mesenchymal transition (EMT), a biological process associated with tumour invasiveness [33]. Although *VIM* promoter methylation has been proposed as a detection and/or prognostic marker for other malignancies, biological functions are yet to be truly explored. Moreover, microRNAs have been extensively implicated in urological malignancies [37]. Interestingly, a dual role has already been described for miR663a, having a tumour suppressive activity in thyroid carcinoma [38] and glioblastoma [39], whereas an oncogenic function was reported in prostate cancer [40] and osteosarcoma [41]. Additionally, miR663a's downregulation fostered cell proliferation by JunD overexpression in small-cell lung carcinoma [42], and HMGA2 in hepatocellular carcinoma [43], while Transforming Growth Factor-1 (TGF-β1) [44] overexpression was linked with invasion in the tumour type. Nevertheless, it should be recalled that not all biomarkers require to have a relevant biological role in tumorigenesis.

Importantly, to assure accuracy and validity of the proposed methylation multiplex test, additional validation by others, with larger sets of samples from prospectively collected data (from both BlCa and inflammatory conditions) is warrant.

5. Conclusions

In summary, we demonstrated that a $miR663a_{me}$-VIM_{me} multiplex panel accurately identifies BlCa, allowing for precise identification of this common neoplasm in urine samples. Importantly, it also discriminates BlCa patients from those with urinary tract inflammatory conditions, although with inferior performance comparatively to healthy subjects. Thus, the implementation of this panel might assist clinicians in better stratifying patients for confirmatory, invasive examinations, ultimately improving the cost-effectiveness of BlCa diagnosis and management. Moreover, in the same analysis, $miR663a_{me}$ analysis would identify patients at higher risk for cancer progression, further highlighting the promise of this panel for patient monitoring.

Author Contributions: Conceptualization, S.M.-R., R.H. and C.J.; methodology, S.M.-R., A.B., J.T.-M., I.C., D.M., P.M. and J.O.; formal analysis, S.M.-R. and L.A.; writing—original draft preparation, S.M.-R.; review and editing, R.H., C.J. and A.L.-B.; supervision, R.H. and C.J. All authors have read and agreed to the published version of the manuscript.

Acknowledgments: The authors are grateful to the patients that volunteered to provide samples and to all the personnel of the Departments of Pathology (section of Cytopathology) and of Urology of Portuguese Oncology Institute of Porto that kindly collaborated in this study.

References

1. Ferlay, J.; Ervik, M.; Lam, F.; Colombet, M.; Mery, L.; Piñeros, M.; Znaor, A.; Soerjomataram, I.; Bray, F. Global Cancer Observatory: Cancer Tomorrow. Available online: https://gco.iarc.fr/tomorrow/home (accessed on 26 October 2019).
2. Antoni, S.; Ferlay, J.; Soerjomataram, I.; Znaor, A.; Jemal, A.; Bray, F. Bladder Cancer Incidence and Mortality: A Global Overview and Recent Trends. *Eur. Urol.* **2017**, *71*, 96–108. [CrossRef]
3. Sanli, O.; Dobruch, J.; Knowles, M.A.; Burger, M.; Alemozaffar, M.; Nielsen, M.E.; Lotan, Y. Bladder cancer. *Nat. Rev. Dis. Primers* **2017**, *3*, 17022. [CrossRef]
4. International Agency for Cancer Research. *WHO Classification of Tumours of the Urinary System and Male Genital Organs*, 4th ed.; Moch, H., Ulbright, T., Humphrey, P., Reuter, V., Eds.; IARC: Lyon, France, 2016.
5. Kaufman, D.S.; Shipley, W.U.; Feldman, A.S. Bladder cancer. *Lancet (London, England)* **2009**, *374*, 239–249. [CrossRef]
6. Babjuk, M.; Burger, M.; Comperat, E.M.; Gontero, P.; Mostafid, A.H.; Palou, J.; van Rhijn, B.W.G.; Roupret, M.; Shariat, S.F.; Sylvester, R.; et al. European Association of Urology Guidelines on Non-muscle-invasive Bladder Cancer (TaT1 and Carcinoma In Situ)—2019 Update. *Eur. Urol.* **2019**, *76*, 639–657. [CrossRef]
7. Alfred Witjes, J.; Lebret, T.; Comperat, E.M.; Cowan, N.C.; De Santis, M.; Bruins, H.M.; Hernandez, V.; Espinos, E.L.; Dunn, J.; Rouanne, M.; et al. Updated 2016 EAU Guidelines on Muscle-invasive and Metastatic Bladder Cancer. *Eur. Urol.* **2017**, *71*, 462–475. [CrossRef]
8. Leal, J.; Luengo-Fernandez, R.; Sullivan, R.; Witjes, J.A. Economic Burden of Bladder Cancer Across the European Union. *Eur. Urol.* **2016**, *69*, 438–447. [CrossRef]
9. Esteller, M. Epigenetics in cancer. *N. Engl. J. Med.* **2008**, *358*, 1148–1159. [CrossRef] [PubMed]
10. Costa-Pinheiro, P.; Montezuma, D.; Henrique, R.; Jeronimo, C. Diagnostic and prognostic epigenetic biomarkers in cancer. *Epigenomics* **2015**, *7*, 1003–1015. [CrossRef] [PubMed]
11. Costa, V.L.; Henrique, R.; Danielsen, S.A.; Duarte-Pereira, S.; Eknaes, M.; Skotheim, R.I.; Rodrigues, A.; Magalhaes, J.S.; Oliveira, J.; Lothe, R.A.; et al. Three epigenetic biomarkers, GDF15, TMEFF2, and VIM, accurately predict bladder cancer from DNA-based analyses of urine samples. *Clin. Cancer Res.* **2010**, *16*, 5842–5851. [CrossRef] [PubMed]
12. Padrao, N.A.; Monteiro-Reis, S.; Torres-Ferreira, J.; Antunes, L.; Leca, L.; Montezuma, D.; Ramalho-Carvalho, J.; Dias, P.C.; Monteiro, P.; Oliveira, J.; et al. MicroRNA promoter methylation: A new tool for accurate detection of urothelial carcinoma. *Br. J. Cancer* **2017**, *116*, 634–639. [CrossRef]
13. Heller, M.T.; Tublin, M.E. In search of a consensus: Evaluation of the patient with hematuria in an era of cost containment. *Am. J. Roentgenol.* **2014**, *202*, 1179–1186. [CrossRef] [PubMed]
14. Grover, S.; Srivastava, A.; Lee, R.; Tewari, A.K.; Te, A.E. Role of inflammation in bladder function and interstitial cystitis. *Ther. Adv. Urol.* **2011**, *3*, 19–33. [CrossRef] [PubMed]

15. Humphrey, P.A.; Moch, H.; Cubilla, A.L.; Ulbright, T.M.; Reuter, V.E. The 2016 WHO Classification of Tumours of the Urinary System and Male Genital Organs-Part B: Prostate and Bladder Tumours. *Eur. Urol.* **2016**, *70*, 106–119. [CrossRef] [PubMed]
16. Pearson, H.; Stirling, D. DNA extraction from tissue. In *PCR Protocols*, 2nd ed.; Bartlett, J.M.S., Stirling, D., Eds.; Humana Press: Totowa, NJ, USA, 2003.
17. McGee, S. Simplifying likelihood ratios. *J. Gen. Intern. Med.* **2002**, *17*, 646–649. [CrossRef]
18. Guest, P.C. Multiplex Biomarker Approaches to Enable Point-of-Care Testing and Personalized Medicine. *Methods Mol. Biol.* **2017**, *1546*, 311–315. [CrossRef]
19. Larsen, L.K.; Lind, G.E.; Guldberg, P.; Dahl, C. DNA-Methylation-Based Detection of Urological Cancer in Urine: Overview of Biomarkers and Considerations on Biomarker Design, Source of DNA, and Detection Technologies. *Int. J. Mol. Sci.* **2019**, *20*, 2657. [CrossRef]
20. Anna K Füzéry, D.W.C. Cancer Biomarker Assays: Performance Standards. In *Biomarkers in Cancer Screening and Early Detection*, 1st ed.; Srivastava, S., Ed.; John Wiley & Sons: Hoboken, NJ, USA, 2017; pp. 267–276.
21. Tan, W.S.; Tan, W.P.; Tan, M.Y.; Khetrapal, P.; Dong, L.; de Winter, P.; Feber, A.; Kelly, J.D. Novel urinary biomarkers for the detection of bladder cancer: A systematic review. *Cancer Treat. Rev.* **2018**, *69*, 39–52. [CrossRef]
22. Chihara, Y.; Kanai, Y.; Fujimoto, H.; Sugano, K.; Kawashima, K.; Liang, G.; Jones, P.A.; Fujimoto, K.; Kuniyasu, H.; Hirao, Y. Diagnostic markers of urothelial cancer based on DNA methylation analysis. *BMC Cancer* **2013**, *13*, 275. [CrossRef]
23. Wang, Y.; Yu, Y.; Ye, R.; Zhang, D.; Li, Q.; An, D.; Fang, L.; Lin, Y.; Hou, Y.; Xu, A.; et al. An epigenetic biomarker combination of PCDH17 and POU4F2 detects bladder cancer accurately by methylation analyses of urine sediment DNA in Han Chinese. *Oncotarget* **2016**, *7*, 2754–2764. [CrossRef]
24. Yegin, Z.; Gunes, S.; Buyukalpelli, R. Hypermethylation of TWIST1 and NID2 in tumor tissues and voided urine in urinary bladder cancer patients. *DNA Cell Biol.* **2013**, *32*, 386–392. [CrossRef]
25. Renard, I.; Joniau, S.; van Cleynenbreugel, B.; Collette, C.; Naome, C.; Vlassenbroeck, I.; Nicolas, H.; de Leval, J.; Straub, J.; Van Criekinge, W.; et al. Identification and validation of the methylated TWIST1 and NID2 genes through real-time methylation-specific polymerase chain reaction assays for the noninvasive detection of primary bladder cancer in urine samples. *Eur. Urol.* **2010**, *58*, 96–104. [CrossRef] [PubMed]
26. Yu, J.; Zhu, T.; Wang, Z.; Zhang, H.; Qian, Z.; Xu, H.; Gao, B.; Wang, W.; Gu, L.; Meng, J.; et al. A novel set of DNA methylation markers in urine sediments for sensitive/specific detection of bladder cancer. *Clin. Cancer Res.* **2007**, *13*, 7296–7304. [CrossRef] [PubMed]
27. Sun, J.; Chen, Z.; Zhu, T.; Yu, J.; Ma, K.; Zhang, H.; He, Y.; Luo, X.; Zhu, J. Hypermethylated SFRP1, but none of other nine genes "informative" for western countries, is valuable for bladder cancer detection in Mainland China. *J. Cancer Res. Clin. Oncol.* **2009**, *135*, 1717–1727. [CrossRef]
28. Chan, M.W.; Chan, L.W.; Tang, N.L.; Tong, J.H.; Lo, K.W.; Lee, T.L.; Cheung, H.Y.; Wong, W.S.; Chan, P.S.; Lai, F.M.; et al. Hypermethylation of multiple genes in tumor tissues and voided urine in urinary bladder cancer patients. *Clin. Cancer Res.* **2002**, *8*, 464–470. [PubMed]
29. Roperch, J.P.; Grandchamp, B.; Desgrandchamps, F.; Mongiat-Artus, P.; Ravery, V.; Ouzaid, I.; Roupret, M.; Phe, V.; Ciofu, C.; Tubach, F.; et al. Promoter hypermethylation of HS3ST2, SEPTIN9 and SLIT2 combined with FGFR3 mutations as a sensitive/specific urinary assay for diagnosis and surveillance in patients with low or high-risk non-muscle-invasive bladder cancer. *BMC Cancer* **2016**, *16*, 704. [CrossRef]
30. Dahmcke, C.M.; Steven, K.E.; Larsen, L.K.; Poulsen, A.L.; Abdul-Al, A.; Dahl, C.; Guldberg, P. A Prospective Blinded Evaluation of Urine-DNA Testing for Detection of Urothelial Bladder Carcinoma in Patients with Gross Hematuria. *Eur. Urol.* **2016**, *70*, 916–919. [CrossRef]
31. Brimo, F.; Vollmer, R.T.; Case, B.; Aprikian, A.; Kassouf, W.; Auger, M. Accuracy of urine cytology and the significance of an atypical category. *Am. J. Clin. Pathol.* **2009**, *132*, 785–793. [CrossRef]
32. Lavery, H.J.; Zaharieva, B.; McFaddin, A.; Heerema, N.; Pohar, K.S. A prospective comparison of UroVysion FISH and urine cytology in bladder cancer detection. *BMC Cancer* **2017**, *17*, 247. [CrossRef]
33. Satelli, A.; Li, S. Vimentin in cancer and its potential as a molecular target for cancer therapy. *Cell Mol. Life Sci.* **2011**, *68*, 3033. [CrossRef]
34. Singh, S.; Sadacharan, S.; Su, S.; Belldegrun, A.; Persad, S.; Singh, G. Overexpression of vimentin: Role in the invasive phenotype in an androgen-independent model of prostate cancer. *Cancer Res.* **2003**, *63*, 2306–2311.

35. Kokkinos, M.I.; Wafai, R.; Wong, M.K.; Newgreen, D.F.; Thompson, E.W.; Waltham, M. Vimentin and Epithelial-Mesenchymal Transition in Human Breast Cancer—Observations in vitro and in vivo. *Cells Tissues Organs* **2007**, *185*, 191–203. [CrossRef] [PubMed]
36. Al-Saad, S.; Al-Shibli, K.; Donnem, T.; Persson, M.; Bremnes, R.M.; Busund, L.T. The prognostic impact of NF-kappaB p105, vimentin, E-cadherin and Par6 expression in epithelial and stromal compartment in non-small-cell lung cancer. *Br. J. Cancer* **2008**, *99*, 1476–1483. [CrossRef] [PubMed]
37. Jerónimo, C.; Henrique, R. Epigenetic biomarkers in urological tumors: A systematic review. *Cancer Lett.* **2014**, *342*, 264–274. [CrossRef] [PubMed]
38. Wang, Z.; Zhang, H.; Zhang, P.; Dong, W.; He, L. MicroRNA-663 suppresses cell invasion and migration by targeting transforming growth factor beta 1 in papillary thyroid carcinoma. *Tumour Biol.* **2015**, *37*, 7633–7644. [CrossRef]
39. Shi, Y.; Chen, C.; Yu, S.; Liu, Q.; Rao, J.; Zhang, H.R.; Xiao, H.L.; Fu, T.W.; Long, H.; He, Z.; et al. MiR-663 suppresses oncogenic function of CXCR4 in glioblastoma. *Clin. Cancer Res.* **2015**, *21*, 4004–4013. [CrossRef]
40. Jiao, L.; Deng, Z.; Xu, C.; Yu, Y.; Li, Y.; Yang, C.; Chen, J.; Liu, Z.; Huang, G.; Li, L.C.; et al. MiR-663 induces castration-resistant prostate cancer transformation and predicts clinical recurrence. *J. Cell Physiol.* **2014**, *229*, 834–844. [CrossRef]
41. Huang, C.; Sun, Y.; Ma, S.; Vadamootoo, A.S.; Wang, L.; Jin, C. Identification of circulating miR-663a as a potential biomarker for diagnosing osteosarcoma. *Pathol. Res. Pract.* **2019**, *215*, 152411. [CrossRef]
42. Zhang, Y.; Xu, X.; Zhang, M.; Wang, X.; Bai, X.; Li, H.; Kan, L.; Zhou, Y.; Niu, H.; He, P. MicroRNA-663a is downregulated in non-small cell lung cancer and inhibits proliferation and invasion by targeting JunD. *BMC Cancer* **2016**, *16*, 315. [CrossRef]
43. Huang, W.; Li, J.; Guo, X.; Zhao, Y.; Yuan, X. MiR-663a inhibits hepatocellular carcinoma cell proliferation and invasion by targeting HMGA2. *Biomed. Pharmacother.* **2016**, *81*, 431–438. [CrossRef]
44. Zhang, C.; Chen, B.; Jiao, A.; Li, F.; Sun, N.; Zhang, G.; Zhang, J. MiR-663a inhibits tumor growth and invasion by regulating TGF-β1 in hepatocellular carcinoma. *BMC Cancer* **2018**, *18*, 1179. [CrossRef]

7

Role of Microtubule-Associated Protein 1b in Urothelial Carcinoma: Overexpression Predicts Poor Prognosis

Tsu-Ming Chien [1,2,3], Ti-Chun Chan [4,5], Steven Kuan-Hua Huang [6], Bi-Wen Yeh [3,5], Wei-Ming Li [1,2,3,7], Chun-Nung Huang [2,3], Ching-Chia Li [1,2,3,8], Wen-Jeng Wu [1,2,3,8,9,10] and Chien-Feng Li [4,5,11,12,13,*]

1 Graduate Institute of Clinical Medicine, College of Medicine, Kaohsiung Medical University, Kaohsiung 807, Taiwan; u108801005@kmu.edu.tw (T.-M.C.); u8401067@yahoo.com.tw (W.-M.L.); ccli1010@hotmail.com (C.-C.L.); wejewu@kmu.edu.tw (W.-J.W.)
2 Department of Urology, Kaohsiung Medical University Hospital, Kaohsiung 807, Taiwan; cnhuang.uro@gmail.com
3 Department of Urology, School of Medicine, College of Medicine, Kaohsiung Medical University, Kaohsiung 807, Taiwan; bewen90@yahoo.com.tw
4 Institute of Biomedical Science, National Sun Yat-sen University, Kaohsiung 80424, Taiwan; ibosaa@mail.nsysu.edu.tw
5 Department of Pathology, Chi Mei Medical Center, Tainan 710, Taiwan
6 Department of Urology, Chi Mei Medical Center, Tainan 710, Taiwan; skhsteven@gmail.com
7 Department of Urology, Ministry of Health and Welfare Pingtung Hospital, Pingtung 900, Taiwan
8 Department of Urology, Kaohsiung Municipal Ta-Tung Hospital, Kaohsiung 801, Taiwan
9 Center for Infectious Disease and Cancer Research, Kaohsiung Medical University, Kaohsiung 807, Taiwan
10 Center for Stem Cell Research, Kaohsiung Medical University, Kaohsiung 807, Taiwan
11 Institute of Medical Science and Technology, National Sun Yat-sen University, Kaohsiung 80424, Taiwan
12 Department of Biotechnology, Southern Taiwan University of Science and Technology, Tainan 71005, Taiwan
13 National Cancer Research Institute, National Health Research Institutes, Tainan 70456, Taiwan
* Correspondence: angelo.p@yahoo.com.tw

Abstract: We sought to examine the relationship between microtubule-associated proteins (MAPs) and the prognosis of urothelial carcinoma by assessing the microtubule bundle formation genes using a reappraisal transcriptome dataset of urothelial carcinoma (GSE31684). The result revealed that microtubule-associated protein 1b (*MAP1B*) is the most significant upregulated gene related to cancer progression. Real-time reverse-transcription polymerase chain reaction was used to measure *MAP1B* transcription levels in urothelial carcinoma of the upper tract (UTUC) and the bladder (UBUC). Immunohistochemistry was conducted to detect *MAP1B* protein expression in 340 UTUC and 295 UBUC cases. Correlations of *MAP1B* expression with clinicopathological status, disease-specific survival, and metastasis-free survival were completed. To assess the oncogenic functions of *MAP1B*, the RTCC1 and J82 cell lines were stably silenced against their endogenous *MAP1B* expression. Study findings indicated that *MAP1B* overexpression was associated with adverse clinical features and could independently predict unfavorable prognostic effects, indicating its theranostic value in urothelial carcinoma.

Keywords: urothelial carcinoma; transcriptome; microtubule; MAP1B; prognosis

---

1. Introduction

Urothelial carcinoma (UC) is the most common malignancy of the urinary tract and includes UC of the urinary bladder (UBUC) and upper urinary tract (UTUC). UBUC is a major UC, with an estimated

429,800 new cases and 165,100 deaths annually worldwide [1]. When first diagnosed, UBUC presents in most patients as a non–muscle-involved invasive disease with an estimated five-year survival rate of 88%, but this rate dramatically decreases to 15% in patients with tumor metastasis [2]. The prevalence of UTUC accounts for approximately 5% to 10% of all UC cases [3]; however, in Taiwan, the rate of UTUC is as high as 30% of affected cases. Furthermore, there is a slight predominance toward females, and ureteral tumors are attributed to greater than half of all cases of UTUC [4,5].

Transurethral resection of the bladder and radical nephroureterectomy with bladder cuff excision remain the gold-standard treatments in UBUC and UTUC for adequate local tumor control and improved long-term survival. However, despite proper surgical treatment, the mortality rate remains high [2,6,7]. Clinical prognostic factors, such as pathological tumor stage and grade, have diverse impacts in patients with identical findings; therefore, they are insufficient means for detailed risk stratification and are difficult to define before treatment [5].

UBUC staging starts from papillary (Ta) and superficial (T1) stages and extends to muscle-invasive advanced stages (T2–T4). Although the recurrence rate of superficial tumors following surgical resection of the bladder is high, it is associated with a markedly better prognosis than that of muscle-invasive tumors [8]. There is a growing pool of evidence to suggest a pathophysiological distinction exists between superficial and muscle-invasive cases of UBUC [9]. It is also important to distinguish a particular variant that may be associated with the administration of a therapy distinctive from that used in conventional invasive UC [10]. A previous study demonstrated that the gene expression profiles of UC from renal pelvis, ureter and bladder were highly similar, indicating that a common functional molecular pathway likely underlies the carcinogenesis [11]. A larger, follow-up study to elucidate better genomics-based predictors for UC is warranted, the results of which could lead to improvements in neoadjuvant/adjuvant therapy and provide suitable follow-up strategies.

Microtubules are a critical component of the cytoskeleton and are important and indispensable in several cellular processes. They are located throughout the cytoplasm and are dynamically unstable (i.e., coexisting in a state of assembly and disassembly). Microtubule-associated proteins (MAPs) are a large family of proteins involved in microtubule assembly, which is an essential step in stabilizing microtubules. MAPs are divided into two classical families: type I, which includes the MAP1 (MAP1A, MAP1B, and MAP1S) proteins [12] and type II, which includes MAP2, MAP4, and MAPT/TAU proteins [13]. Disrupting microtubule dynamics is one of the most successful and widely considered targets of cancer chemotherapy agents [14,15]. Microtubule agents target the aberrant expression of MAPs in a variety of malignancies, and their resistant phenotypes have been documented. Herein, we aimed to examine the relationship between MAPs and the prognosis of urothelial carcinoma by assessing the microtubule bundle formation genes using a reappraisal transcriptome dataset of urothelial carcinoma (GSE31684). Moreover, to our knowledge, this study is the first to examine *MAP1B* expression and the prognosis and intrinsic biologic aggressiveness of UC.

2. Results

2.1. MAP1B Is the Most Significantly Upregulated Gene Associated with Microtubule Bundle Formation in UBUC Transcriptomes

The UBUC transcriptome dataset includes 93 tissue samples, with 78 categorized as deeply invasive tissues (pT2–pT4) and 15 categorized as noninvasive or superficial (pTa and pT1) tissues. Metastasis was detected in 28 patients and absent in 49 patients. Through transcriptome profiling, we identified 11 probes spanning six transcripts associated with microtubule bundle formation (GO:0001578). Among these expressed genes, we found that tumors with increased *MAP1B* expression and decreased *MARK4* had a more advanced pT status and a higher incidence of metastatic events (Figure 1A). Our main goal was to find the most significant upregulated genes associated with advanced disease. Therefore, we choose *MAP1B* for further validation. Table 1 shows the *MAP1B* gene (Probe: 226084_at, 214577_at) upregulation with up to 1.2832-, 0.3773- and 0.9436-, 0.3943- fold log ratios in advanced and metastatic UC, respectively. Furthermore, we found through survival analysis that increased *MAP1B* expression was significantly related to poor prognosis in patients with UBUC (Figure 1B). As shown in Figure 1c,d, the *MAP1B* transcripts level was significantly higher among tumors with high pT status (pT2–pT4) than in noninvasive tumors (pTa–pT1) in both the UTUC and UBUC groups (both $p < 0.01$). Our findings indicate that *MAP1B* is associated with tumor aggressiveness.

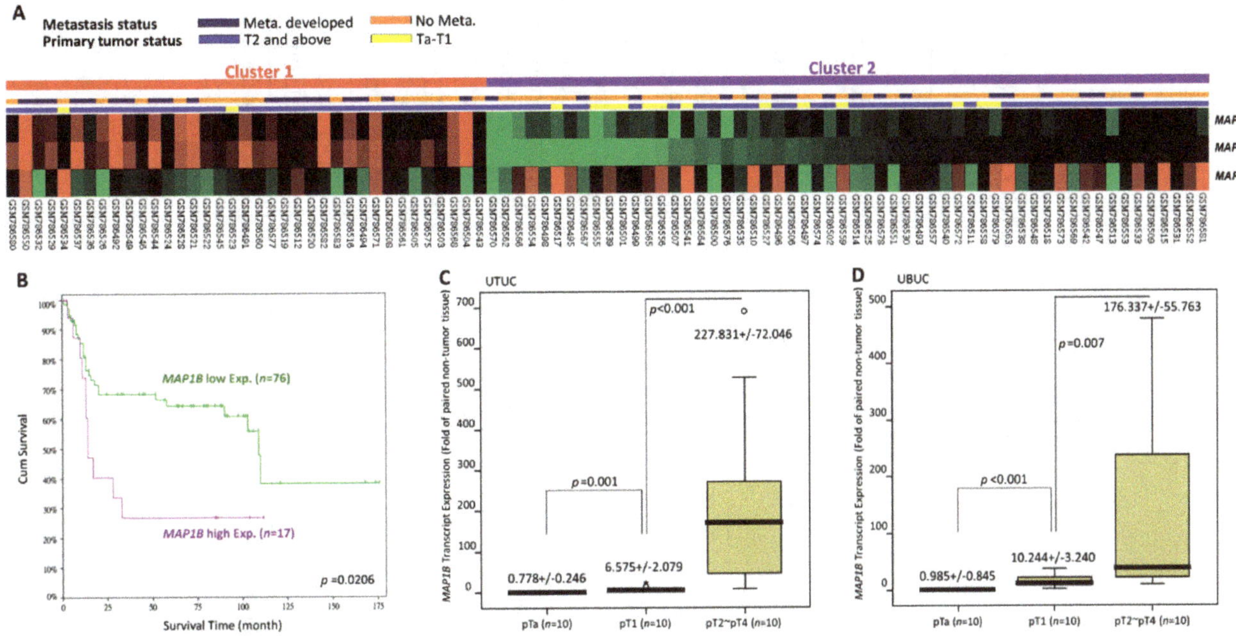

Figure 1. Analysis of gene expression in urinary bladder urothelial carcinoma (UBUC) using a published transcriptome dataset (GSE31684). (**A**) Cluster analysis of genes focusing on the GO microtubule bundle formation class (GO:0001578) revealed that *MAP1B* was one of the most significantly upregulated genes associated with more advanced pT status and metastatic disease. Tissue specimens from cancers with a distinct pT status are illustrated at the top of the heat map, and the expression levels of upregulated and downregulated genes are represented as a continuum of brightness of red or green, respectively. Specimens with no change in messenger RNA (mRNA) expression are shown in black. (**B**) Kaplan–Meier plots showing the prognostic significance of *MAP1B* expression for the survival of UBUC. Using a QuantiGene assay, *MAP1B* mRNA expression was significantly increased in both (**C**) upper tract urothelial carcinoma (UTUC) and (**D**) UBUC at advanced primary pT stages.

Table 1. Summary of differentially expressed genes associated with microtubule bundle formation (GO: 0001578) and showing positive associations to cancer invasiveness and metastasis in the transcriptome of UBUC (GSE31684).

Probe Title 1	Comparing T2-4 to Ta-T1		Comparing Meta. to Non-Meta. #		Gene Symbol	Gene Title	Biological Process	Molecular Function
	Log ratio	*p*-Value	Log ratio	*p*-Value				
214577_at	0.3773	0.0029	0.3943	< 0.0001	*MAP1B*	Microtubule-associated protein 1B	Dendrite development, microtubule bundle formation	Protein binding, structural molecule activity
221560_at	−0.3436	0.0058	−0.0115	0.9048	*MARK4*	MAP/microtubule affinity-regulating kinase 4	G1/S transition of mitotic cell cycle, G2/M transition of mitotic cell cycle, Wnt receptor signaling pathway, microtubule bundle formation, microtubule cytoskeleton organization and biogenesis, nervous system development, positive regulation of cell proliferation, positive regulation of programmed cell death, protein amino acid phosphorylation	ATP binding, gamma-tubulin binding, kinase activity, microtubule-binding, nucleotide-binding, protein-binding, protein kinase activity, protein serine/threonine kinase activity, protein-tyrosine kinase activity, tau-protein kinase activity, transferase activity, ubiquitin-binding
226084_at	1.2832	< 0.0001	0.9436	< 0.0001	*MAP1B*	Microtubule-associated protein 1B	Dendrite development, microtubule bundle formation	Protein-binding, structural molecule activity

#, Meta., distal metastasis developed during follow-up; Non-Meta.: no metastatic event developed.

2.2. MAP1B Immunoexpression and Clinicopathological and Genomic Correlations in UTUC and UBUC

The association of clinicopathological characteristics with *MAP1B* immunoreactivity is shown in Table 2. We found, in UTUC cases, that high *MAP1B* expression was markedly associated with synchronous multiple tumors ($p = 0.024$), advanced pT status ($p = 0.005$) (Figure 2A–C), positive lymph node metastasis ($p = 0.002$), the presence of vascular invasion ($p < 0.001$), and an increased mitotic rate ($p < 0.001$) (Table 2 and Figure 2D). Similarly, in cases with UBUC, we found evidence of associations between increased *MAP1B* expression and advanced pathological tumor stage ($p < 0.001$), positive lymph node metastasis ($p = 0.012$), a high histological tumor grade ($p = 0.016$), the presence of vascular invasion ($p = 0.045$), and an increased mitotic rate ($p = 0.006$) (Table 2 and Figure 2E). Of note, none of the 30 cases displaying high *MAP1B* expression enrolled for mutational analysis were positive for *MAP1B* mutation, suggesting a mutation-independent expression of *MAP1B*.

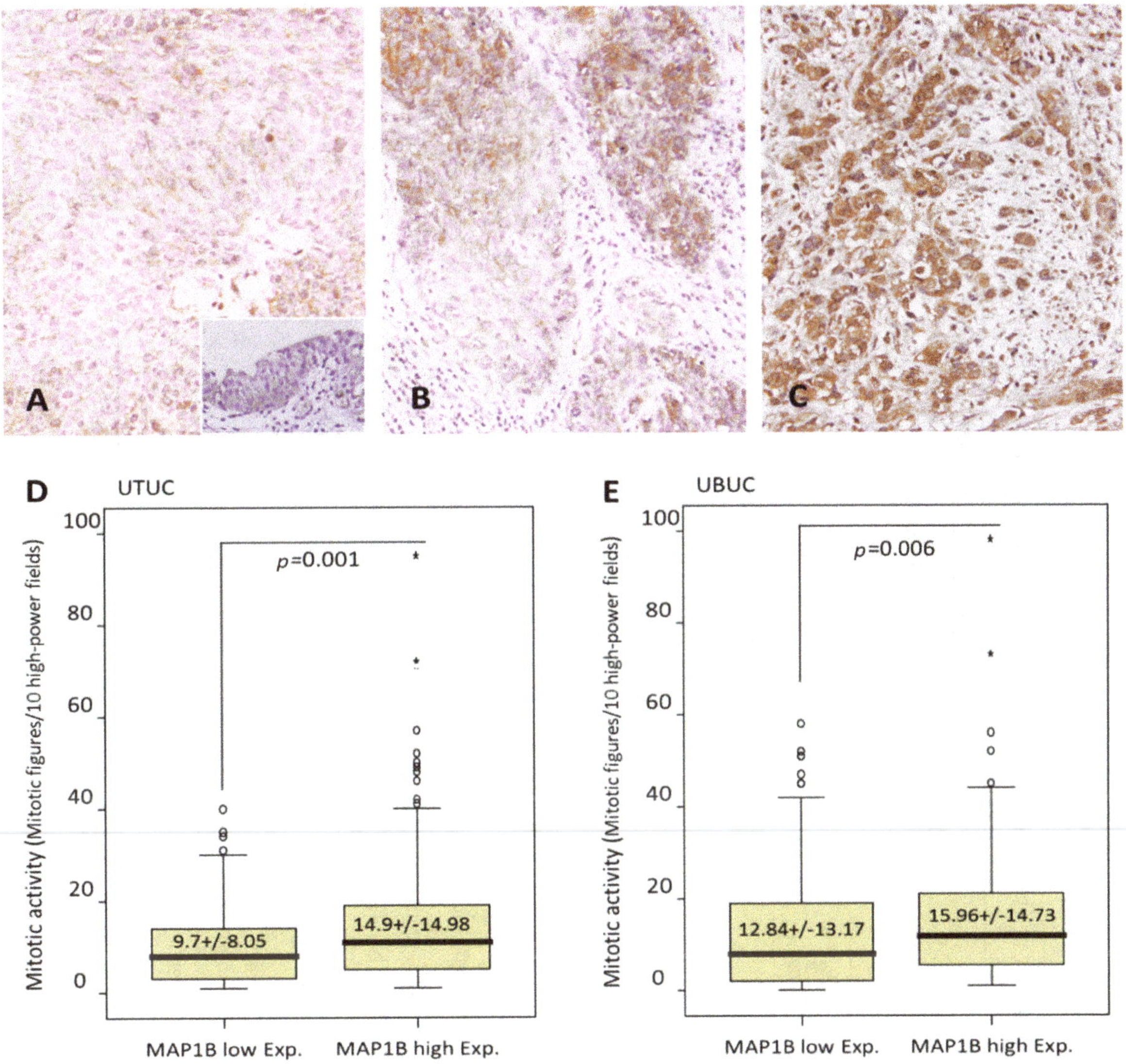

Figure 2. Representative sections of *MAP1B* immunostaining. Note the stepwise increments in *MAP1B* immunoreactivity from the nontumoral urothelial epithelium (inlet) and (**A**) noninvasive papillary UCs to (**B**) non–muscle-invasive (pT1), and (**C**) muscle-invasive (pT2–pT4) UCs. A comparison of mitotic activity showed significantly higher mitotic rates in (**D**) UTUC and (**E**) UBUC cells with increased *MAP1B* expression than in cells with low expression.

Table 2. Correlations between *MAP1B* expression and other important clinicopathological parameters in UCs.

Parameter	Category	Upper Urinary Tract Urothelial Carcinoma				Urinary Bladder Urothelial Carcinoma			
		Case no.	*MAP1B* Expression		*p*-value	Case no.	*MAP1B* Expression		*p*-value
			Low	High			Low	High	
Gender &	Male	158	79	79	1.000	216	103	113	0.223
	Female	182	91	91		79	44	35	
Age (years) #		340	65.2+/−9.87	65.9+/−9.92	0.409	295	65.76+/−12.02	66.33+/−12.44	0.759
Tumor location	Renal pelvis	141	64	77	0.023 *	-	-	-	-
	Ureter	150	87	63		-	-	-	-
	Renal pelvis & ureter	49	19	30		-	-	-	-
Multifocality&	Single	278	144	134	0.160	-	-	-	-
	Multifocal	62	26	36		-	-	-	-
Primary tumor (T) &	Ta	89	54	35	0.005 *	84	56	28	<0.001 *
	T1	92	5′	41		88	45	43	
	T2	159	65	94		123	46	77	
Nodal metastasis &	Negative (N0)	312	164	148	0.002 *	266	139	127	0.012 *
	Positive (N1–N2)	28	6	22		29	8	21	
Histological grade &	Low grade	56	34	22	0.079	56	36	20	0.016 *
	High grade	284	136	148		239	111	128	
Vascular invasion &	Absent	234	132	102	< 0.001 *	246	129	117	0.045 *
	Present	106	38	68		49	18	31	
Perineural invasion &	Absent	321	162	159	0.479	275	140	135	0.169
	Present	19	8	11		20	7	13	

&, Chi-squared test; #, Mann–Whitney U test; * Statistically significant.

2.3. *Survival Analysis in UTUC and UBUC*

During follow-up, we found in our UTUC cohort that 61 (17.9%) patients died because of their cancer and 70 (20.6%) patients experienced disease progression. During univariate analysis, we observed that multifocal tumors, advanced pathological tumor stage, positive lymph node metastasis, high histological tumor grade, the presence of vascular invasion, perineural invasion, and high MAP1B expression (Figure 3A,B) were associated with worse disease-specific survival (DSS) and metastasis-free survival (MFS) (all $p < 0.05$). In multivariate analysis, multifocal tumors, advanced pathological tumor stage, positive lymph node metastasis, high histological tumor grade, perineural invasion, and MAP1B expression were independently predictive for both DSS and MFS (all $p < 0.05$) (Table 3).

In our follow-up of UBUC patients, we found that 52 (17.6%) patients died due to the cancer and 76 (25.8%) patients experienced disease progression. During univariate analysis, we determined that advanced pT status, positive lymph node metastasis, high histological tumor grade, the presence of vascular invasion, perineural invasion, an increased mitotic rate, and increment of MAP1B expression (Figure 3C,D) were associated with worse DSS and MFS (all $p < 0.05$). Using multivariate analysis, we confirmed that advanced pathological tumor stage, an increased mitotic rate, and MAP1B expression remained significant in predicting reduced DSS and MFS (all $p < 0.05$) (Table 4).

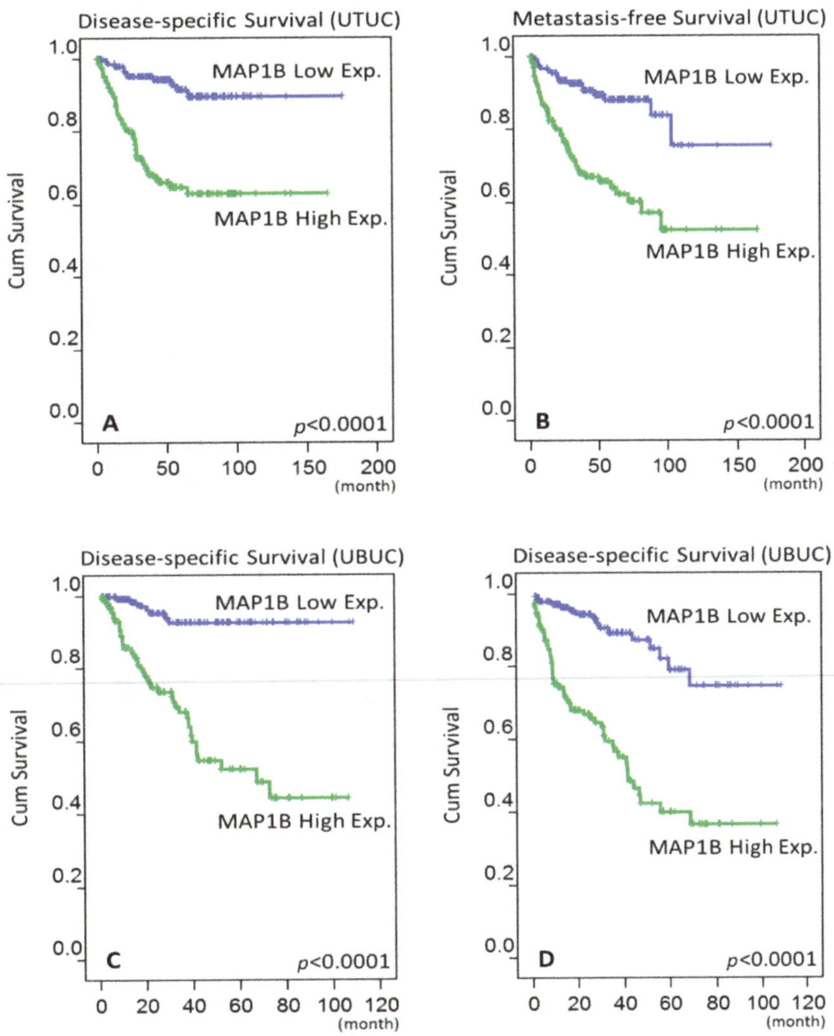

Figure 3. Kaplan–Meier survival analysis showing the prognostic significance of MAP1B expression for the DSS and MFS outcomes of UTUC (**A** and **B**) and UBUC (**C** and **D**).

Table 3. Univariate log-rank and multivariate analyses for DSS and MFS in UTUC.

Parameter	Category	Case No.	Disease-Specific Survival					Metastasis-Free Survival				
			Univariate Analysis		Multivariate Analysis			Univariate Analysis		Multivariate Analysis		
			No. of Event	*p*-value	R.R.	95% C.I.	*p*-value	No. of Event	*p*-value	R.R.	95% C.I.	*p*-value
Gender	Male	158	28	0.8730	-	-	-	32	0.8307	-	-	-
	Female	182	33		-	-	-	38		-	-	-
Age (years)	<65	138	26	0.9728	-	-	-	30	0.8667	-	-	-
	≥65	202	35		-	-	-	40		-	-	-
Tumor side	Right	177	34	0.7188	-	-	-	38	0.3903	-	-	-
	Left	154	26		-	-	-	32		-	-	-
	Bilateral	9	1		-	-	-	0		-	-	-
Tumor location	Renal pelvis	141	24	0.0100 *	1	-	0.562	31	0.0752	-	-	-
	Ureter	150	22		1.167	0.618–2.203		25		-	-	-
	Renal pelvis & ureter	49	15		1.261	0.345–4.615		14		-	-	
Multifocality	Single	273	48	0.0031 *	1	-	0.050 *	52	0.0144 *	1	-	0.001 *
	Multifocal	62	18		2.238	0.998–5.017		18		2.648	1.496–4.687	
Primary tumor (T)	Ta	89	2	<0.0001 *	1	-	0.008 *	4	<0.0001 *	1	-	0.036 *
	T1	92	9		2.641	0.561–12.419		15		2.643	0.563–12.410	
	T2–T4	159	50		5.667	1.250–25.699		51		5.538	1.236–24.817	
Nodal metastasis	Negative (N0)	312	42	<0.0001 *	1	-	<0.001 *	55	<0.0001 *	1	-	<0.001 *
	Positive (N1–N2)	28	19		4.188	2.244–7.819		15		4.421	2.415–8.094	
Histological grade	Low	56	4	0.0177 *	1	-	0.008 *	3	0.0022 *	1	-	0.008 *
	High	284	57		4.746	1.514–14.881		67		4.770	1.509–15.077	
Vascular invasion	Absent	234	24	<0.0001 *	1	-	0.139	26	<0.0001 *	1	-	0.147
	Present	106	37		1.571	0.863–2.859		44		1.565	0.855–2.868	
Perineural invasion	Absent	321	50	<0.0001 *	1	-	<0.001 *	61	<0.0001 *	1	-	<0.001 *
	Present	19	11		4.768	2.251–10.102	-	9		4.865	2.294–10.318	
Mitotic rate (per 10 high power fields)	<10	173	27	0.1442	-	-	-	30	0.0739	-	-	-
	≥10	167	34		-	-	-	40		-	-	-
MAP1B expression	Low	170	11	<0.0001 *	1	-	0.001 *	17	<0.0001 *	1	-	<0.001 *
	High	170	50		4.115	2.077–8.154		53		3.962	2.022–7.763	

* Statistically significant.

Table 4. Univariate log-rank and multivariate analyses for DSS and MFS in UBUC.

Parameter	Category	Case No.	Disease-Specific Survival					Metastasis-Free Survival				
			Univariate Analysis		Multivariate Analysis			Univariate Analysis		Multivariate Analysis		
			No. of Event	*p*-value	R.R.	95% C.I.	*p*-value	No. of Event	*p*-value	R.R.	95% C.I.	*p*-value
Gender	Male	216	41	0.4404	-	-	-	60	0.2786	-	-	-
	Female	79	11		-	-	-	16		-	-	-
Age (years)	<65	121	17	0.1010	-	-	-	31	0.6285	-	-	-
	≥65	174	35		-	-	-	45				
Primary tumor (T)	Ta	84	1	<0.0001 *	1	-	<0.001 *	4	<0.0001 *	1	-	<0.001 *
	T1	88	9		6.493	0.696–60.560		23		5.044	1.469–17.327	
	T2–T4	123	42		27.783	3.011–256.370		49		7.845	2.239–27.484	
Nodal metastasis	Negative (N0)	266	41	0.0001 *	1	-	0.729	61	<0.0001 *	1	-	0.100
	Positive (N1–N2)	29	11		1.132	0.560–2.288		15		1.685	0.905–3.137	
Histological grade	Low grade	56	2	0.0010 *	1	-	0.714	5	0.0005*	1	-	0.572
	High grade	239	50		0.744	0.153–3.610		71		0.729	0.244–2.179	
Vascular invasion	Absent	246	37	0.0017 *	1	-	0.174	54	0.0001 *	1	-	0.798
	Present	49	15		0.624	0.316–1.231		22		1.083	0.590–1.985	
Perineural invasion	Absent	275	44	<0.0001 *	1	-	0.099	66	0.0006 *	1	-	0.339
	Present	20	8		2.990	0.878–4.510		10		1.422	0.690–2.930	
Mitotic rate (per 10 high power fields)	<10	139	12	<0.0001 *	1	-	0.021 *	23	<0.0001 *	1	-	0.045 *
	≥10	156	40		2.184	1.124–4.246		53		1.697	1.012–2.846	
MAP1B expression	Low	147	7	<0.0001 *	1	-	<0.001 *	16	<0.0001 *	1	-	<0.001 *
	High	148	45		5.551	2.466–12.498		60		3.770	2.146–6.622	

* Statistically significant.

2.4. MAP1B Promotes the Cell Proliferation, Migration, and Invasion of UC Cell Lines

To investigate the biological effects of MAP1B, we first characterized endogenous MAP1B expression in eight UC cell lines and noticed RTCC1 and J82 cells had the most abundant MAP1B transcripts and protein expression (Figure 4A). We next successfully knocked down MAP1B in both the RTCC1 (Figure 4B, left) and J82 (Figure 4B, right) cell lines using short hairpin RNA (shRNA). We found significantly attenuated proliferation (viability) in stable MAP1B-silenced RTCC1 (Figure 4C1) and J82 (Figure 4C2) cells. Due to the positive relationship between MAP1B expression and the development of metastasis, we evaluated the effect of MAP1B in UC cell migration and invasion. MAP1B knockdown significantly decreased the migratory and invasive abilities of RTCC1 (Figure 4C3,C5) and J82 (Figure 4C4,C6) cells.

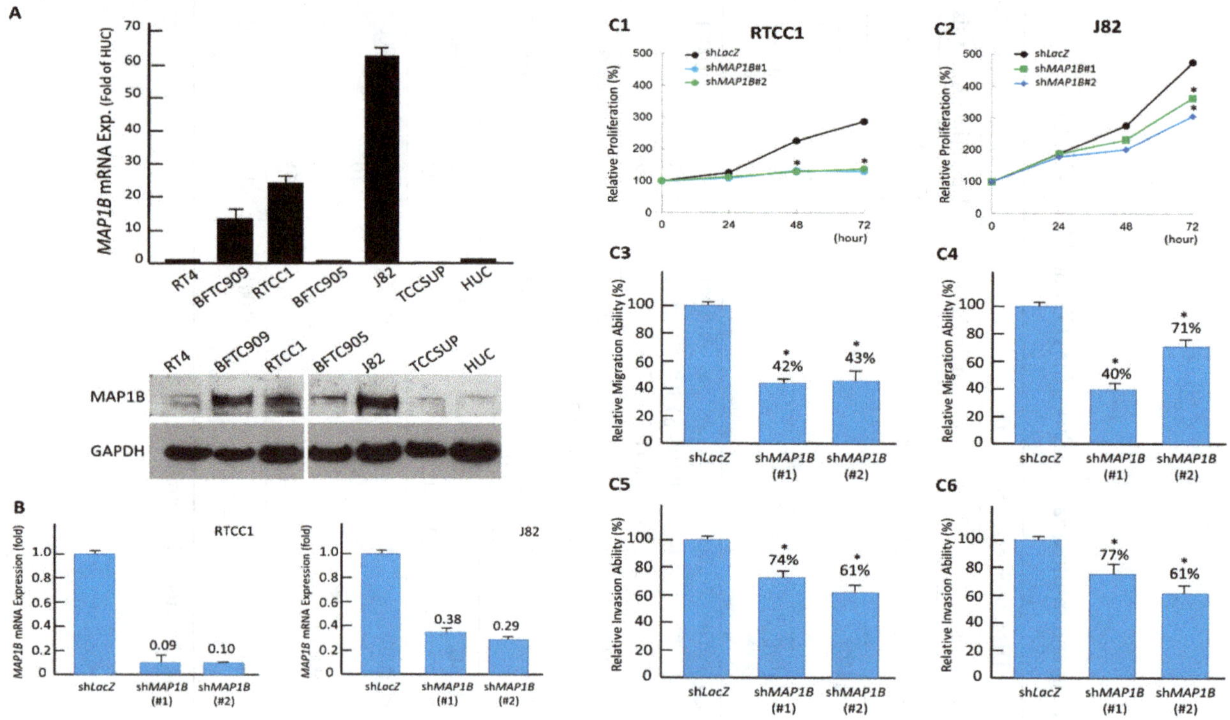

Figure 4. *MAP1B* expression promotes the growth of UC cells in vitro. (**A**) As compared with RT4 cells, endogenous *MAP1B* mRNA (upper) and protein (lower) expressions were increased in cells from the J82 and RTCC1 cell lines. (**B**) The two cell lines with high endogenous *MAP1B* expression were stably silenced against *MAP1B* expression by a lentiviral vector bearing one of the two clones of *MAP1B* shRNA with different sequences for both RTCC1 (left panel) and J82 (right panel) cells. Using an ELISA-based colorimetric assay to assess the rate of BrdU uptake, cell proliferation was significantly reduced in stable *MAP1B*-knockdown (**C1**) RTCC1 and (**C2**) J82 cell lines compared with that in the corresponding shLacZ controls. Similar trends were found for cell migration and invasion among cells from the (**C3** and **C5**) RTCC1 and (**C4** and **C6**) J82 cell lines. (* $p<0.05$). More details of western blot, please view at the supplementary materials.

2.5. MAP1B Expression Correlates with Chemoresistance In Vitro and In Vivo

Flow cytometric analysis of stable *MAP1B* knockdown RTCC1 and J82 cell lines showed stable *MAP1B* knockdown significantly increased the sub-G1 population, indicating induced cell apoptosis (Figures 5 and 6). Further analysis of vinblastine-treated RTCC1 and J82 cell lines also disclosed induced cell apoptosis (Figures 7 and 8). In other words, MAP1B expression might lead to a resistance to anti-mitotic chemotherapeutics. In the independent UBUC patient cohort receiving adjuvant chemotherapy, Kaplan–Meier survival analysis showed high MAP1B expression correlated with inferior DFS (Figure 9), further supporting the role of MAP1B in chemoresistance.

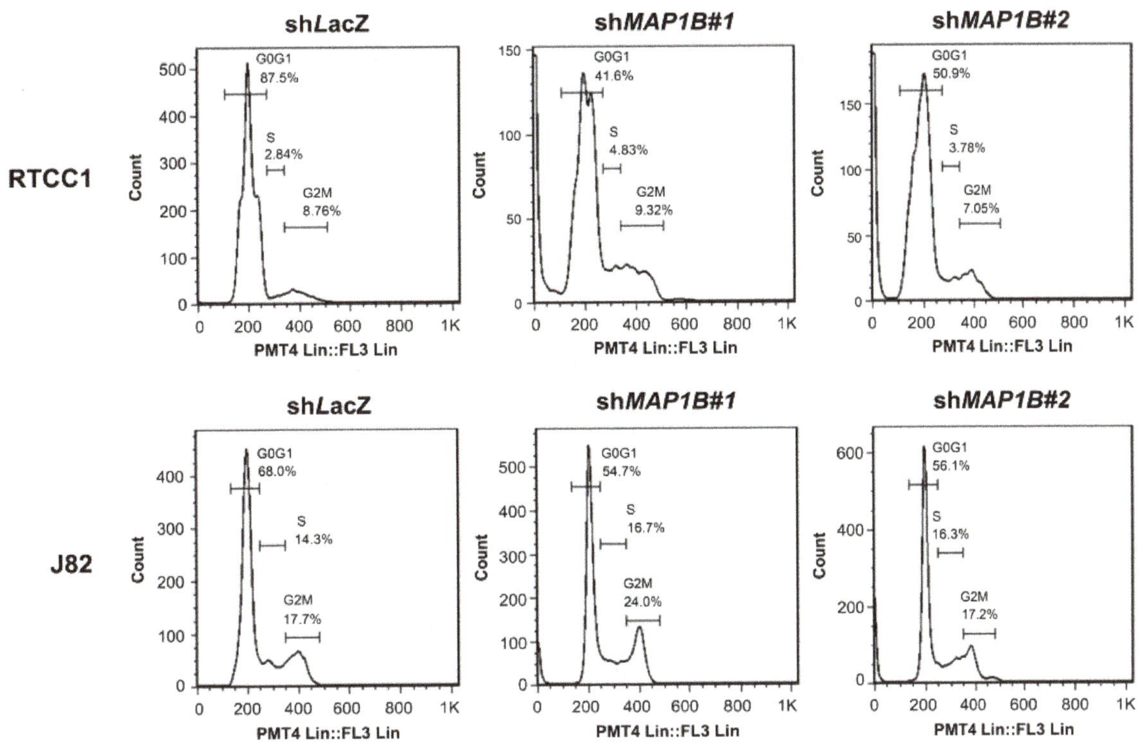

Figure 5. Stable *MAP1B* knockdown increases the sub-G1 population with significantly altered cell-cycle progression. Cell-cycle analysis as conducted by flow cytometry identified a remarkable increment of sub-G1 population indicating cell death in *MAP1B*-knockdown RTCC1 (upper panel) and J82 (lower panel) cells.

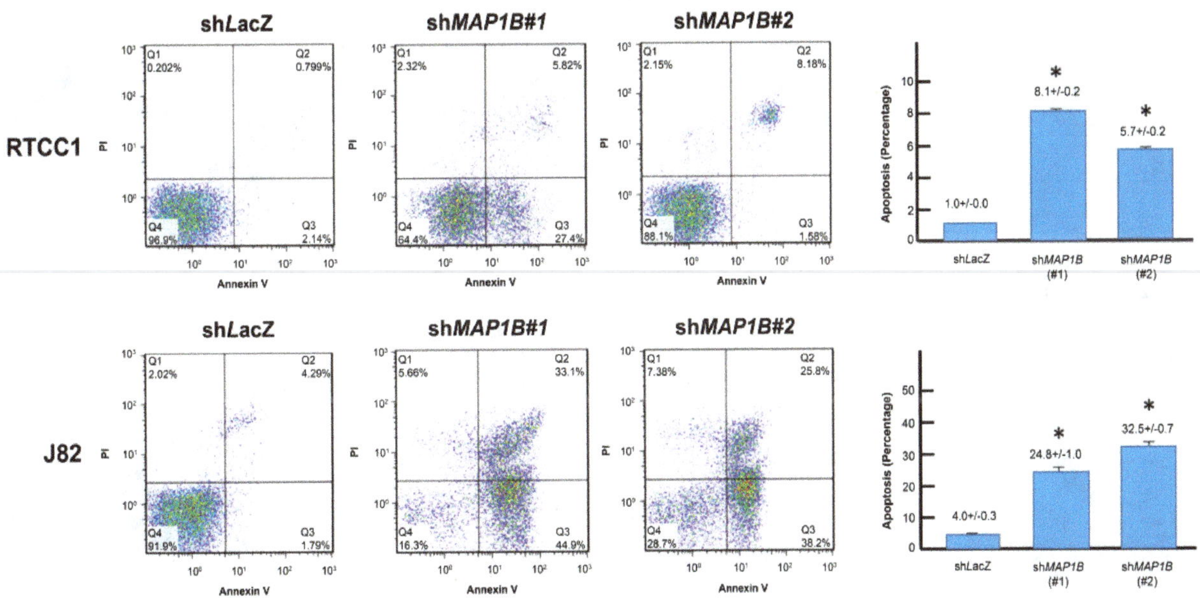

Figure 6. *MAP1B* knockdown induces apoptosis. Flow cytometric analysis of annexin V/propidium iodide-stained RTCC1 (upper panel) and J82 (lower panel) cell lines disclosed *MAP1B* knockdown significantly increased percentage of apoptosis. (* $p < 0.05$).

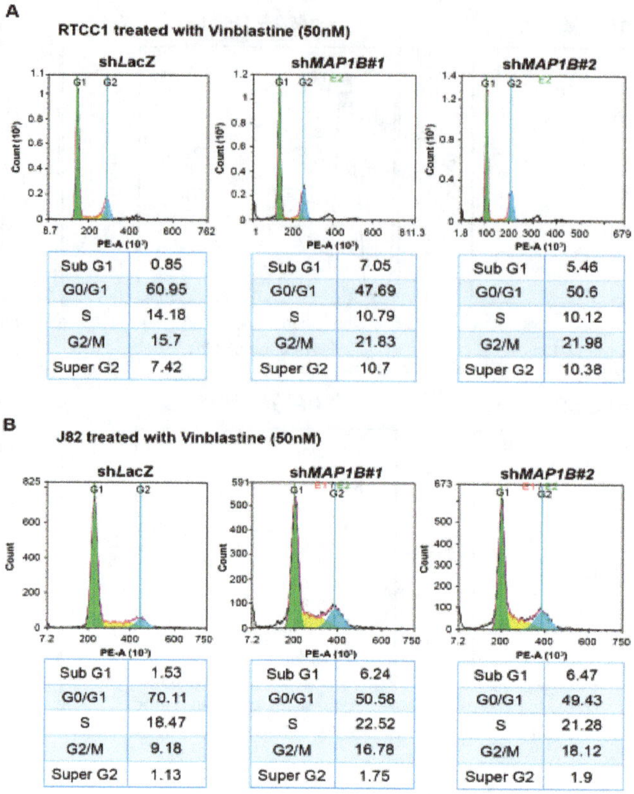

A — RTCC1 treated with Vinblastine (50nM)

	shLacZ	shMAP1B#1	shMAP1B#2
Sub G1	0.85	7.05	5.46
G0/G1	60.95	47.69	50.6
S	14.18	10.79	10.12
G2/M	15.7	21.83	21.98
Super G2	7.42	10.7	10.38

B — J82 treated with Vinblastine (50nM)

	shLacZ	shMAP1B#1	shMAP1B#2
Sub G1	1.53	6.24	6.47
G0/G1	70.11	50.58	49.43
S	18.47	22.52	21.28
G2/M	9.18	16.78	18.12
Super G2	1.13	1.75	1.9

Figure 7. Stable *MAP1B* knockdown increased vinblastine-induced apoptosis. Flow cytometric analysis of vinblastine-treated RTCC1 (upper panel) and J82 (lower panel) cell lines disclosed that *MAP1B* knockdown significantly increased the sub-G1 population, indicating induced cell apoptosis.

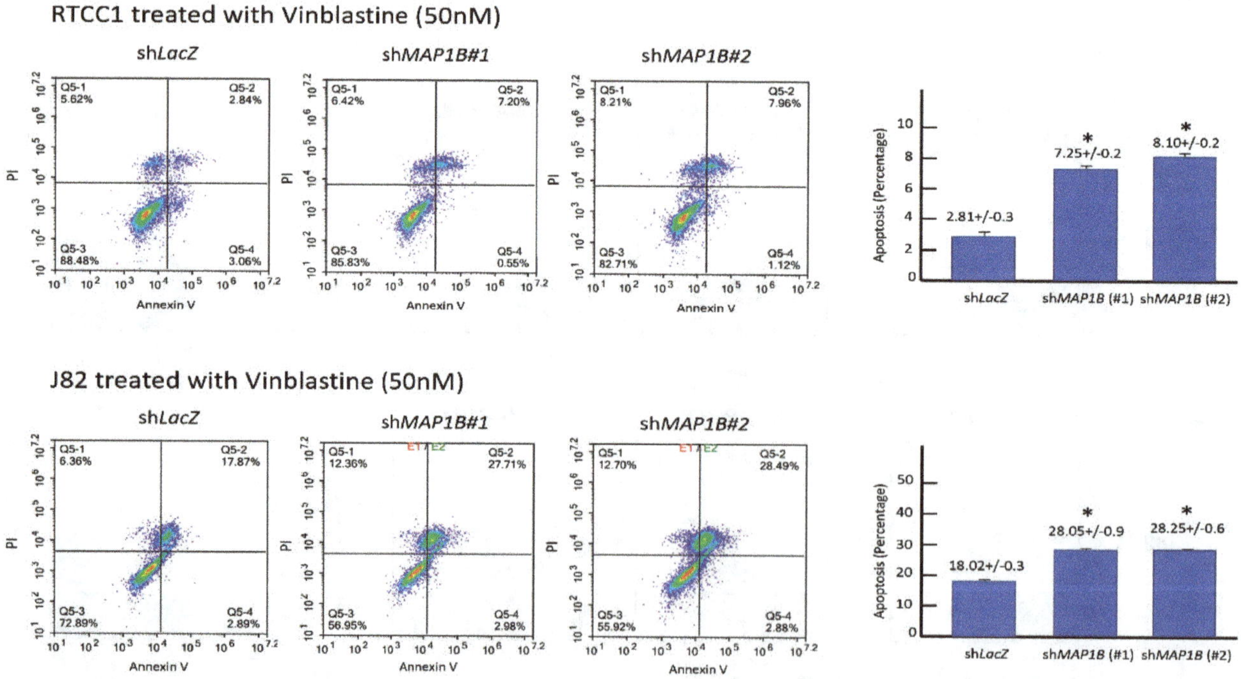

Figure 8. Stable *MAP1B* knockdown increase vinblastine-induced apoptosis. Flow cytometric analysis of annexin V/propidium iodide-stained RTCC1 (upper panel) and J82 (lower panel) cell lines demonstrated *MAP1B* knockdown significantly increased percentage of vinblastine-induced apoptosis. (* $p < 0.05$).

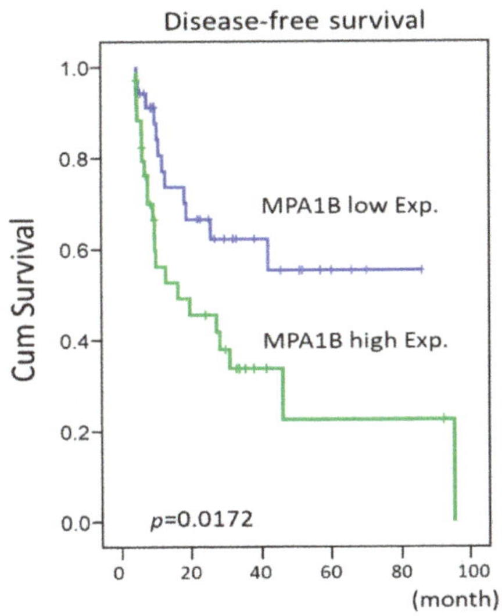

Figure 9. Kaplan–Meier survival analysis of *MAP1B* expression for the DFS of the UBUC patient cohort receiving adjuvant chemotherapy. Kaplan–Meier survival analysis showing the prognostic significance of *MAP1B* expression for the DFS of the UBUC patient cohort receiving adjuvant chemotherapy.

3. Discussion

It is estimated that one-third of patients with UBUC have advanced disease at presentation [16]. A similar poor prognosis was found among patients with advanced UTUC in that the DSS has not changed significantly during the last two decades [17]. Regardless of the high initial response, the therapeutic effects of current treatment were insufficient and resulted in recurrence and death. Currently, there are no effective salvage regimens for treating metastatic UC. Metastasis requires the inherent dynamic instability of microtubules for cell motility, and many changes in the microtubule network have been identified in various cancers [14]. There is accumulating evidence that MAPs are associated with changes in microtubule dynamics, that they can determine the effects of microtubule-targeting agents, and that they play a role in cancer resistance [14]. However, reliable tumor markers that predict the sensitivity to chemotherapy and resistance to tumor metastasis remain elusive.

MAPs contain products of oncogenes, tumor suppressors, and apoptosis regulators thought to be involved in microtubule assembly. On the other hand, vinblastine, listed in the World Health Organization's List of Essential Medicines, binds tubulin and inhibits the assembly of microtubules [18]. It causes M-phase–specific cell-cycle arrest by breaking microtubule assembly and proper formation of the mitotic spindle and the kinetochore, which were essential for the separation of chromosomes during the anaphase of mitosis. Due to the possibility of sharing a common function, the rational microtubule-targeting cancer therapeutic approaches should preferably include proteomic profiling of tumor MAPs before the administration of antimicrotubule agents preferentially in combination with agents that modulate the expression of relevant MAPs [14].

Histologically, MAPs were originally related to the development of the nervous system, based on their very early detection in neurons. However, the aberrant expression of primarily neuronal MAPs has since been detected in non-neural cancer tissues [14]. We also assessed MAP1B expression across various cancer types using Oncomine™ Platform (Thermo Fisher, Ann Arbor, MI). Data revealed a diverse expression of MAP1B in various cancers. Of these, CNS tumor has highest MAP1B expression; bladder tumor has moderate expression. In our present results and using a published transcriptome dataset (GSE31684), we first found that *MAP1B* was significantly upregulated in UC and associated with more advanced pT status and metastatic disease in UBUC. Next, we found using immunohistochemistry that *MAP1B* overexpression markedly correlated with disease status in affected patients. In patients with UTUC, *MAP1B* overexpression was positively associated with synchronous multiple tumors, advanced pathological tumor stage, positive lymph node metastasis, the presence of vascular invasion, and an increased mitotic rate. However, in patients with UBUC, *MAP1B* overexpression was associated with advanced pathological tumor stage, positive lymph node metastasis, high histological tumor grade, the presence of vascular invasion, and an increased mitotic rate. Furthermore, using survival analysis, we demonstrated an association between *MAP1B* and aggressive clinical progression, whereby *MAP1B* overexpression independently predicted poor DSS and MFS rates for all patients with UC. These findings indicate that standard clinical practices may benefit from evaluating the *MAP1B* status to improve the risk stratification of patients with UC.

Different *MAP1B* interactors can be grouped into seven different categories, including signaling, cytoskeleton, transmembrane proteins, RNA-binding proteins, apoptosis, neurodegeneration-linked proteins, and neurotransmitter receptors [19]. *MAP1B* is translated as a precursor polypeptide that undergoes proteolytic processing to cleave into an N-terminal heavy chain (*MAP1B* HC) and a C-terminal light chain (*MAP1B* LC1). *MAP1B* LC1 overexpression, which can generate protein aggregates, has been observed in endoplasmic reticulum-related stress-induced cell apoptosis. This effect is blocked by DJ-1, a Parkinson's disease–related protein that has been proposed to act like a molecular chaperone, and inhibits α-synuclein aggregation [20]. However, in contrast to the proapoptotic effects caused by LC1 overexpression, *MAP1B* overexpression is not related to cell death related to *p53*, a tumor-suppressor gene; in fact, *MAP1B* overexpression reduces *p53* transcriptional activity and inhibits doxorubicin-induced apoptosis [21]. In addition, we found that the percentages of cells in the early and late stages of apoptosis were significantly increased between shLacZ controls and shMAP1B-treated cells. Further in vivo studies are warranted to confirm our findings and to determine whether such results may lead to new therapeutic targets for UC.

Recent studies have found that changes in the expression of MAPs are associated with chemotherapy resistance and cancer progression [14,22]. For example, stathmin plays a role in regulating neuroblastoma cell migration and invasion [22]. Silencing stathmin expression using RNAi gene silencing significantly reduced lung metastasis in neuroblastoma in vivo. Similarly, we demonstrated using UC cell lines with high endogenous *MAP1B* expression that silencing by *MAP1B* shRNA significantly reduced cell proliferation, migration, and invasion ability. Based on these findings, we posit that *MAP1B* may be a clinically valuable diagnostic marker for early cancer detection and a promising prognostic marker.

Further, *MAP1B* interacts with several other proteins associated with cancer. For example, Ras-association domain family 1 isoform A (RASSF1A), a tumor suppressor whose inactivation is implicated in the development of many human cancers, interacts with *MAP1B* to influence microtubule dynamics in the cell cycle and is involved in the inhibition of cancer cell growth [23]. Through distinct bifunctional structural domains, C19ORF5, a sequence homolog of *MAP1B*, mediates the communication between the microtubular cytoskeleton and mitochondria in the control of cell death and defective genome destruction. In addition, it has been proposed that the accumulation of C19ORF5 results in microtubule hyperstability, which may be involved in the tumor suppression activity of RASSF1A [24]. In the mammary cancer susceptibility 1 (*Mcs1*) region in chromosome 2 (a region that expresses centromeric proteins), Laes et al. analyzed candidate genes in the region and found that *MAP1B* was expressed in the mammary glands of rats [25]. Interactions with other proteins not related to its role in stabilizing microtubules suggest that *MAP1B* may be part of a "signaling protein" that regulates molecular pathways [19]. We propose that *MAP1B* has multiple functions, and whether the main function of *MAP1B* is microtubule stabilization or whether it has many cellular functions warrants further investigation.

A recent study that focused on kidney glomerular development and function found that *MAP1B* was specifically expressed in podocytes in human and murine adult kidney tissues [26]. In a mouse model, *MAP1B* was not essential for glomerular filtration function but may play a role in the development and differentiation of the kidney tubular system. The authors hypothesize that *MAP1B* may be related to either stress maintenance or the aging process in the kidney. It is clear that the overall effects of *MAP1B* on UC are complex, with reports of associations between *MAP1B* and survival and metastasis. Research aimed at decoding the functional consequences of *MAP1B* and signaling cross-talk with other proteins in different cancers is needed in the future. However, due to a slight predominance toward females, it is unclear if the results can easily be transferred to the rest of the world.

4. Materials and Methods

4.1. Data Mining of GSE31684 to Identify Altered Gene Expression in UC

The transcriptome dataset GSE31684 (http://www.ncbi.nlm.nih.gov/geo/query/acc.cgi?acc=GSE31684), which includes 93 patients with UBUC who underwent radical cystectomy, was obtained from the Gene Expression Omnibus repository at the National Center for Biotechnology Information. Raw data were imported by Nexus Expression 3 (BioDiscovery, EI Segundo, CA, USA) to quantify the gene expression level. No pre-selection or filtering was conducted during the analysis of the data for all probes. Comparative analyses were performed to determine the significant differences in the expressed genes by comparing the primary tumor (pT) status (high-stage to low-stage) and the presence or absence of metastatic events.

4.2. Patients and Tumor Specimens

Between 1996 and 2004, 340 patients with UTUC and 295 with UBUC who underwent surgery with curative intent at the Chi Mei Medical Center were enrolled. This study was reviewed and approved by the institutional review board (105-01-005). Informed patient consent was obtained from all participants. Demographic characteristics and clinical information including pathological features, oncological follow-up, and cause of mortality were retrospectively collected. Patients who underwent neoadjuvant chemotherapy or radiotherapy; who had concurrent muscle-invasive bladder tumor, acute blood disorders, or bone marrow diseases; and those with incomplete clinical information were excluded from our study. The tumor stage was defined in accordance with the 2002 American Joint Committee Cancer (AJCC)'s Tumor, Node, Metastasis system. Two pathologists reviewed tumor tissues and reclassified then as low- or high-grade using the seventh edition of the AJCC staging system. As a rule, all patients were treated initially by surgery with curative intent. All UBUC patients with pT3 or pT4 diseases or with nodal involvement received cisplatin-based adjuvant chemotherapy. However, of the 106 UTUC patients with pT3 or pT4 and nodal positive diseases, only 29 received cisplatin-based adjuvant chemotherapy. One expert pathologist (CFL) re-evaluated the hematoxylin and eosin–stained sections of all cases. To determine the *MAP1B* transcript level, a pilot batch of 30 UTUC and 30 UBUC snap-frozen tissues with a high tumor percentage (> 70%) was retrieved. Each group included 10 tumor tissues of the pTa stage, 10 of the pT1 stage, and 10 that were muscle-invasive (pT2–pT4).

4.3. Immunohistochemical Staining

Immunohistochemistry was conducted to detect *MAP1B* protein expression in 340 UTUC and 295 UBUC cases. One representative slide of a tumor with most invasive area was evaluated by two pathologists manually. Tumor tissue slide preparation was performed as described in our previous study [27]. Slides were incubated with the primary antibody against *MAP1B* (1:100, clone AA6; Millipore, Beverly, MA, USA). We quantified *MAP1B* protein expression levels by combining the intensity and percentage of immunostaining in the cytoplasm of UC cells to generate an H score using the following equation: H score = $\Sigma Pi\ (i + 1)$, where Pi is the percentage of stained tumor cells (0–100%) and i represents the intensity of immunoreactivity (0–3+). The resulting scores ranged from 100 to 400 points, where a score of 100 points indicated that 100% of cancer cells were nonreactive and a score of 400 points meant that 100% of the cancer cells examined were strongly immunoreactive (3+).

4.4. Real-Time Reverse-Transcription Polymerase Chain Reaction (RT-PCR) to Assess the Transcription Levels of MAP1B in Cell Lines and UC Samples

We calculated the fold change in *MAP1B* gene expression of UC tumors relative to that of normal tissues as previously described [27]. We extracted total RNA from cell lines and a pilot batch of cases consisting of 30 UTUCs and 30 UBUCs to quantify the transcription level of *MAP1B* using real-time RT-PCR. Predesigned TaqMan assay reagents (Applied Biosystems, Waltham, MA, USA) were used to assess the mRNA abundance of *MAP1B* (Hs00195485_m1) using the ABI StepOnePlus™ system (Applied Biosystems, Waltham, MA, USA), for which *POLR2A* (Hs01108291_m1) was used as the internal control for normalization.

4.5. Cell Culture

The cell lines RT4, TCCSUP, J82, and HUC were purchased from the American Type Culture Collection (Manassas, VA, USA). The cell lines BFTC 909, and BFTC 905 were obtained from the Food Industry Research and Development Institute (Hsinchu, Taiwan). RTCC1 cells were kindly provided by Professor Lien-Chai Chiang at Kaohsiung Medical University [28]. Short-tandem repeat profiling cell authentication had been performed in all cell lines (Mission Biotech, Taipei, Taiwan).

4.6. RNA Interference

The lentiviral vectors pLKO.1-*shLacZ* (TRCN0000072223: 5′-TGTTCGCATTATCCGAACCAT-3′) and pLKO.1-*shMAP1B* (#1, TRCN0000116621: 5′-GCCTGGAATAAACAGCATGTT-3′; #2, TRCN0000290688: 5′- CCCTGACTTAGGAGTTGTATT-3′) were obtained from the Taiwan National RNAi Core Facility (Taipei, Taiwan) and used to establish stable *MAP1B*-silenced clones of RTCC1 and J82 cell lines using shRNAs against *MAP1B* (*shMAP1B*).Viruses were produced by transfecting HEK293 cells with the above three vectors using Lipofectamine 2000 (Thermo Fisher Scientific, Waltham, MA, USA) [29]. For viral infection, 3×10^6 RTCC1 and J82 cells were incubated with 8 mL of lentivirus in the presence of polybrene, followed by puromycin selection of the stable clones of lentivirus-transduced cells.

4.7. Western Blotting

Our previously published western blotting assay procedure was used to evaluate endogenous *MAP1B* expression and the *MAP1B*-knockdown efficiency in RTCC1 and J82 cell lines using primary antibodies against *MAP1B* (1:500, clone AA6; Millipore, Beverly, MA, USA) and glyceraldehyde 3-phosphate dehydrogenase (GADPH) (6C5, 1:10,000; Millipore, Beverly, MA, USA). Cell lysates with 25 μg of protein were separated using a 4% to 12% gradient NuPAGE gel (Invitrogen, Carlsbad, CA, USA), then transferred onto polyvinylidene difluoride membranes (Amersham Biosciences, Buckinghamshire, UK) for the immobilization of proteins. Membranes were incubated with tris-buffered saline containing Tween 20 (TBST) buffer and 5% skimmed milk at room temperature for one hour for blocking, followed by exposure to primary antibodies at 4 °C overnight against *MAP1B* (1:500, clone AA6; Millipore, Beverly, MA, USA) using GADPH as a loading control (6C5, 1:10,000; Millipore, Beverly, MA, USA). Membranes were incubated with the secondary antibody at room temperature for 1.5 h, and proteins were detected using a chemiluminescence system (Amersham Biosciences, Buckinghamshire, UK).

4.8. Bromodeoxyuridine (BrdU) Assay to Assess DNA Synthesis

DNA synthesis was measured using an enzyme-linked immunosorbent assay (ELISA)-based and colorimetric bromodeoxyuridine (BrdU) assay (Roche Holding AG, Basel, Switzerland). *MAP1B*-knockdown or *shLacA* control RTCC1 and J82 cell lines were plated into a 96-well plate at a density of 3000 cells per well. At 24, 48, and 72 h, we measured the amount of DNA synthesis. The labeling medium was removed after three hours of incubation with BrdU at 37 °C under 5% CO_2, followed by fixation and a final incubation with an anti-BrdU-POD solution. An ELISA reader

(Promega Corp., Madison, WI, USA) was used to measure the absorbance at 450 nm, and the reference was set at an absorbance of 690 nm.

4.9. Pharmacological Assays

The colorimetric 2,3-bis-(2-methoxy-4-nitro-5-sulfophenyl)-2H-tetrazolium-5-carboxanilide (XTT) assay (Sigma-Aldrich, St. Louis, MO, USA) was used to assess cell viability as previously described [30]. Vinblastine sulfate (Hospira UK Ltd., Maidenhead, UK) was obtained and suspended in normal saline. RTCC1 and J82 cells were seeded in 96-well plates at a density of 5×10^3 cells per well the day before treatment at the indicated time points with vehicle control (0.9% saline) or increasing concentrations of vinblastine sulfate. The length of treatment interval was 72 h. After incubation with XTT reaction mixture for three hours at 37 °C under 5% CO_2, the absorbance of the samples was determined using an ELISA reader (Promega Corp., Madison, WI, USA) at 450 nm, with the absorbance set at 630 nm as reference.

4.10. Migration and Invasion Assays

Cell migration assay was performed using Falcon HTS FluoroBlok 24-well inserts (BD Biosciences, Franklin Lakes, NJ, USA) and the cell invasion assay was performed using the 24-well Collagen-based Cell Invasion Assay (Millipore, Beverly, MA, USA). Briefly, we added serum-free medium to rehydrate each insert, then replaced it with a serum-free suspension with equal numbers of cells in the upper chamber, followed by a 12- to 24-h incubation period to allow cells to migrate toward (i.e., invade) the lower chamber, which contained medium with 10% fetal bovine serum. After removal of the noninvading cells in the upper chamber, cells that invaded through the inserts were stained, lysed in extraction buffer, and transferred to 96-well plates for colorimetric readings at 560 nm.

4.11. Flow Cytometry Analysis of Cell-Cycle Kinetics

Stable pools of *MAP1B* knockdown versus the corresponding *shLacZ* control of the RTCC1 and J82 cell lines were pelleted and fixed overnight in 75% cold ethanol at −20 °C. The cells were washed twice using cold phosphate-buffered saline with 10 mg/mL of DNase-free RNase. Next, the cells were labeled with 0.05 mg/mL of propidium iodide and analyzed using a NovoCyte flow cytometer (ACEA Biosciences, San Diego, CA, USA) to determine the different proportions of cells at each phase of the cell cycle. Our lower limit of the number of sorted cells after gating out fixation artifacts and cell debris was 10^4 cells for all experiments.

4.12. Flow Cytometry Analysis of Apoptosis

Cell apoptosis was evaluated by plating RTCC1 and J82 cells (10^5 cells each) with sh*LacZ* or sh*MAP1B* for 24 h, followed by 15 min of incubation using an Annexin V-FITC kit (BD Biosciences, Franklin Lakes, NJ, USA) that contained propidium iodide. The percentages of cells at late apoptosis were calculated from three independent experiments.

4.13. Mutation Analysis

To explore potential *MAP1B* mutation in UC, we randomly selected 15 UTUC and 15 UBUC cases (Table S1) with high protein expressions of *MAP1B* for mutation analysis. Mutation analyses were performed by using an ABI3100 sequencer targeting eight pathogenic point mutations occurring in other cancer types according to the database of COSMIC repository (https://cancer.sanger.ac.uk/cosmic/gene/analysis?ln=HSD11B1#variants). Validated *MAP1B* mutations and primers sets are shown in Table S2. The PCR amplification started with an initial denaturation step at 95 °C for 15 min, followed by 35 cycles of 95 °C for 30 s, 58 °C for 30 s, and 72 °C for 30 s, and a final extension step at 72 °C for 10 min. Then, these amplicons generated in individual PCR reactions were analyzed by direct sequencing.

4.14. Postoperative Adjuvant Chemotherapy in UBUC

To evaluate the role of *MAP1B* expression in the response to adjuvant chemotherapy in UBUC patients, an independent cohort containing 70 patients with pT3 or pT4 disease or with nodal involvement received cisplatin-based adjuvant chemotherapy combined with vinblastine and were enrolled for further survival analysis (Table S3).

4.15. Statistical Analyses

The Statistical Package for the Social Sciences version 12.0 software program (IBM Corp., Armonk, NY, USA) was used for all statistical analyses. Differences between categorical parameters were assessed using the chi-squared or Fisher's exact test. The median H scores of *MAP1B* immunoreactivity were used as cutoff values to separate UTUC and UBUC into two subgroups of high and low *MAP1B* expression. Pearson's chi-squared test was used to compare the association between *MAP1B* expression and clinicopathological parameters. The Kaplan–Meier method was applied to estimate the effect of *MAP1B* expression on DSS and MFS. The survival curves were compared using the log-rank test. We used a Cox proportional-hazards model to identify independent predictors for DSS and MFS. In all figure legend, continuous parameters (such as MAP1B transcript expression in Figure 1, mitotic activity in Figure 2, *MAP1B* mRNA expression, relative proliferation, migration and invasion in Figure 4, apoptosis rate in Figure 6) were assessed using a t-test or Mann–Whitney–Wilcoxon test. Survival analysis (DSS and MFS) were performed using Kaplan-Meier plots and compared by the log-rank test. Statistical significance was set at $p < 0.05$.

5. Conclusions

In summary, the present study demonstrated that MAP1B overexpression was not only an indicator of unfavorable clinicopathological parameters, but also an independent prognostic factor able to predict poor DSS and MFS rates in patients with UTUC or UBUC. Additional studies must be conducted to elucidate the details of the biological significance of MAP1B and its encoded protein in UC oncogenesis for exploring possible MAP1B-targeted therapy for both kinds of UC.

Author Contributions: Conceptualization, T.-M.C., S.K.-H.H., W.-J.W., C.-F.L.; Methodology, B.-W.Y.; Formal analysis, T.-C.C.; Data curation, T.-C.C., S.K.-H.H., W.-J.W., C.-F.L.; Writing—original draft preparation, T.-M.C.; Writing—review and editing, C.-N.H.; Supervision, W.-M.L., C.-C.L.; Project administration, C.-F.L. All authors have read and agreed to the published version of the manuscript.

Acknowledgments: The authors gratefully acknowledge the assistance of all the members in our group and the BioBank of Chi Mei Medical center. The authors would like to thank Enago (www.enago.tw) for the English language review.

References

1. Torre, L.A.; Bray, F.; Siegel, R.L.; Ferlay, J.; Lortet-Tieulent, J.; Jemal, A. Global cancer statistics, 2012. *CA Cancer J. Clin.* **2015**, *65*, 87–108. [CrossRef] [PubMed]
2. Lynch, C.F.; Davila, J.A.; Platz, C.E. Cancer of the urinary bladder. In *SEER Survival Monograph: Cancer Survival Among Adults: US SEER Program, 1988–2001, Patient and Tumor Characteristics, National*; Ries, Y.J., Keel, G.E., Eisner, M.P., Eds.; Cancer Institute, SEER Program: Bethesda, MD, USA, 2007; pp. 193–202.
3. Margulis, V.; Shariat, S.F.; Matin, S.F.; Kamat, A.M.; Zigeuner, R.; Kikuchi, E.; Lotan, Y.; Weizer, A.; Raman, J.D.; Wood, C.G. Outcomes of radical nephroureterectomy: A series from the Upper Tract Urothelial Carcinoma Collaboration. *Cancer* **2009**, *115*, 1224–1233. [CrossRef] [PubMed]
4. Lai, M.N.; Wang, S.M.; Chen, P.C.; Chen, Y.Y.; Wang, J.D. Population-based case-control study of Chinese herbal products containing aristolochic acid and urinary tract cancer risk. *J. Natl. Cancer Inst.* **2010**, *102*, 179–186. [CrossRef]
5. Li, C.C.; Chang, T.H.; Wu, W.J.; Ke, H.L.; Huang, S.P.; Tsai, P.C.; Chang, S.J.; Shen, J.T.; Chou, Y.H.; Huang, C.H. Significant predictive factors for prognosis of primary upper urinary tract cancer after radical nephroureterectomy in Taiwanese patients. *Eur. Urol.* **2008**, *54*, 1127–1134. [CrossRef] [PubMed]

6. Ploussard, G.; Xylinas, E.; Lotan, Y.; Novara, G.; Margulis, V.; Rouprêt, M.; Matsumoto, K.; Karakiewicz, P.I.; Montorsi, F.; Remzi, M.; et al. Conditional survival after radical nephroureterectomy for upper tract carcinoma. *Eur. Urol.* **2015**, *67*, 803–812. [CrossRef] [PubMed]
7. Raman, J.D.; Scherr, D.S. Management of patients with upper urinary tract transitional cell carcinoma. *Nat. Clin. Pract. Urol.* **2007**, *4*, 432–443. [CrossRef] [PubMed]
8. Knowles, M.A. What we could do now: Molecular pathology of bladder cancer. *Mol. Pathol.* **2001**, *54*, 215–221. [CrossRef] [PubMed]
9. McConkey, D.J.; Lee, S.; Choi, W.; Tran, M.; Majewski, T.; Lee, S.; Siefker-Radtke, A.; Dinney, C.; Czerniak, B. Molecular genetics of bladder cancer: Emerging mechanisms of tumor initiation and progression. *Urol. Oncol.* **2010**, *28*, 429–440. [CrossRef]
10. Amin, M.B. Histological variants of urothelial carcinoma: Diagnostic, therapeutic and prognostic implications. *Mod. Pathol.* **2009**, *22* (Suppl. 2), S96–S118. [CrossRef]
11. Zhang, Z.; Furge, K.A.; Yang, X.J.; Teh, B.T.; Hansel, D.E. Comparative gene expression profiling analysis of urothelial carcinoma of the renal pelvis and bladder. *BMC Med. Genom.* **2010**, *3*, 58. [CrossRef]
12. Halpain, S.; Dehmelt, L. The MAP1 family of microtubule-associated proteins. *Genome Biol.* **2006**, *76*, 224. [CrossRef] [PubMed]
13. Dehmelt, L.; Halpain, S. The MAP2/Tau family of microtubule-associated proteins. *Genome Biol.* **2005**, *6*, 204. [CrossRef] [PubMed]
14. Bhat, K.M.; Setaluri, V. Microtubule-associated proteins as targets in cancer chemotherapy. *Clin. Cancer Res.* **2007**, *13*, 2849–2854. [CrossRef] [PubMed]
15. Parker, A.L.; Kavallaris, M.; McCarroll, J.A. Microtubules and their role in cellular stress in cancer. *Front. Oncol.* **2014**, *4*, 153. [CrossRef] [PubMed]
16. Niegisch, G.; Lorch, A.; Droller, M.J.; Lavery, H.J.; Stensland, K.D.; Albers, P. Neoadjuvant chemotherapy in patients with muscle-invasive bladder cancer: Which patients benefit? *Eur. Urol.* **2013**, *64*, 355–357. [CrossRef] [PubMed]
17. Adibi, M.; Youssef, R.; Shariat, S.F.; Lotan, Y.; Wood, C.G.; Sagalowsky, A.I.; Zigeuner, R.; Montorsi, F.; Bolenz, C.; Margulis, V. Oncological outcomes after radical nephroureterectomy for upper tract urothelial carcinoma: Comparison over the three decades. *Int. J. Urol.* **2012**, *19*, 1060–1066. [CrossRef] [PubMed]
18. Altmann, K.H. Preclinical Pharmacology and Structure-Activity Studies of Epothilones. In *The Epothilones: An Outstanding Family of Anti-Tumor Agents. Fortschritte der Chemie Organischer Naturstoffe/Progress in the Chemistry of Organic Natural Products*; Springer: Vienna, Austria, 2009; Volume 90. [CrossRef]
19. Villarroel-Campos, D.; Gonzalez-Billault, C. The MAP1B case: An old MAP that is new again. *Dev. Neurobiol.* **2014**, *74*, 953–971. [CrossRef]
20. Wang, Z.; Zhang, Y.; Zhang, S.; Guo, Q.; Tan, Y.; Wang, X.; Xiong, R.; Ding, J.; Chen, S. DJ-1 can inhibit microtubule associated protein 1 B formed aggregates. *Mol. Neurodegener.* **2011**, *6*, 38. [CrossRef]
21. Lee, S.Y.; Kim, J.W.; Jeong, M.H.; An, J.H.; Jang, S.M.; Song, K.H.; Choi, K.H. Microtubule-associated protein 1B light chain (MAP1B-LC1) negatively regulates the activity of tumor suppressor p53 in neuroblastoma cells. *FEBS Lett.* **2008**, *582*, 2826–2832. [CrossRef]
22. Byrne, F.L.; Yang, L.; Phillips, P.A.; Hansford, L.M.; Fletcher, J.I.; Ormandy, C.J.; McCarroll, J.A.; Kavallaris, M. RNAi-mediated stathmin suppression reduces lung metastasis in an orthotopic neuroblastoma mouse model. *Oncogene* **2014**, *33*, 882–890. [CrossRef]
23. Dallol, A.; Agathanggelou, A.; Fenton, S.L.; Ahmed-Choudhury, J.; Hesson, L.; Vos, M.D.; Clark, G.J.; Downward, J.; Maher, E.R.; Latif, F. RASSF1A interacts with microtubule-associated proteins and modulates microtubule dynamics. *Cancer Res.* **2004**, *64*, 4112–4116. [CrossRef]
24. Liu, L.; Vo, A.; Liu, G.; McKeehan, W.L. Distinct Structural Domains within C19ORF5 Support Association with Stabilized Microtubules and Mitochondrial Aggregation and Genome Destruction. *Cancer Res.* **2005**, *65*, 4191–4201. [CrossRef] [PubMed]
25. Laes, J.F.; Quan, X.; Ravoet, M.; Stieber, D.; Van Vooren, P.; Van Reeth, T.; Szpirer, J.; Szpirer, C. Analysis of candidate genes included in the mammary cancer susceptibility 1 (Mcs1) region. *Mamm. Genome* **2001**, *12*, 199–206. [CrossRef] [PubMed]
26. Gödel, M.; Temerinac, D.; Grahammer, F.; Hartleben, B.; Kretz, O.; Riederer, B.M.; Propst, F.; Kohl, S.; Huber, T.B. Microtubule associated protein 1b (MAP1B) is a marker of the microtubular cytoskeleton in podocytes but is not essential for the function of the kidney filtration barrier in mice. *PLoS ONE* **2015**, *10*, e0140116. [CrossRef] [PubMed]

27. Fan, E.W.; Li, C.C.; Wu, W.J.; Huang, C.N.; Li, W.M.; Ke, H.L.; Yeh, H.C.; Wu, T.F.; Liang, P.I.; Ma, L.J.; et al. FGF7 Over expression is an independent prognosticator in patients with urothelial carcinoma of the upper urinary tract and bladder. *J. Urol.* **2015**, *194*, 223–229. [CrossRef] [PubMed]
28. Chiang, L.C.; Chiang, W.; Chang, L.L.; Wu, W.J.; Huang, C.H. Characterization of a new human transitional cell carcinoma cell line from the renal pelvis, RTCC-1/KMC. *Kaohsiung J. Med. Sci.* **1996**, *12*, 448–452. [PubMed]
29. Li, C.F.; Chen, L.T.; Lan, J.; Chou, F.F.; Lin, C.Y.; Chen, Y.Y.; Chen, T.J.; Li, S.H.; Yu, S.; Fang, F.M.; et al. AMACR amplification and overexpression in primary imatinib-naïve gastrointestinal stromal tumors: A driver of cell proliferation indicating adverse prognosis. *Oncotarget* **2014**, *5*, 11588–11630. [CrossRef]
30. Li, C.F.; Fang, F.M.; Chen, Y.Y.; Chen, Y.Y.; Liu, T.T.; Chan, T.C.; Yu, S.C.; Chen, L.T.; Huang, H.Y. Overexpressed fatty acid synthase in gastrointestinal stromal tumors: Targeting a progression-associated metabolic driver enhances the antitumor effect of imatinib. *Clin. Cancer Res.* **2017**, *23*, 4908–4918. [CrossRef]

8

Sex-Sparing Robot-Assisted Radical Cystectomy with Intracorporeal Padua Ileal Neobladder in Female: Surgical Technique, Perioperative, Oncologic and Functional Outcomes

Gabriele Tuderti [1,*], Riccardo Mastroianni [1,2], Simone Flammia [2], Mariaconsiglia Ferriero [1], Costantino Leonardo [2], Umberto Anceschi [1], Aldo Brassetti [1], Salvatore Guaglianone [1], Michele Gallucci [2] and Giuseppe Simone [1]

1 "Regina Elena" National Cancer Institute, Department of Urology, 00100 Rome, Italy; riccardomastroianniroma@gmail.com (R.M.); marilia.ferriero@gmail.com (M.F.); umberto.anceschi@gmail.com (U.A.); aldo.brassetti@gmail.com (A.B.); salvatore.guaglianone@ifo.gov.it (S.G.); puldet@gmail.com (G.S.)
2 "Sapienza" University of Rome, Department of Urology, 00100 Rome, Italy; roccosimone92@gmail.com (S.F.); costantino.leonardo@uniroma1.it (C.L.); michele.gallucci@ifo.gov.it (M.G.)
* Correspondence: gabriele.tuderti@gmail.com

Abstract: Our aim was to illustrate our technique of sex-sparing (SS)-robot-assisted radical cystectomy (RARC) in female patients receiving an intracorporeal neobladder (iN). From January 2013 to June 2018, 11 female patients underwent SS-RARC-iN at a single tertiary referral center. Inclusion criteria were a cT $\leq$ 2 N0 M0 bladder tumor at baseline imaging (CT or MRI) and an absence of tumors in the bladder neck, trigone and urethra at TURB. Baseline, perioperative, and outcomes at one year were reported. The median operative time was 255 min and the median hospital stay was seven days. Low-grade Clavien complications occurred in four patients (36.3%), while high-grade complications were not observed in any. Seven patients (63.7%) had an organ-confined disease at the pathologic specimen; nodal involvement and positive surgical margins were not detected in any of the cases. At a median follow-up of 28 months (IQR 14–51), no patients developed new onset of chronic kidney disease stage 3b. After one year, daytime and nighttime continence rates were 90.9% and 86.4% respectively. Quality of life as well as physical and emotional functioning improved significantly over time (all $p \leq 0.04$), while urinary symptoms and sexual function worsened at three months with a significant recovery taking place at one year (all $p \leq 0.04$). Overall, 8 out of 11 patients (72.7%) were sexually active at the 12-month evaluation. In select female patients, SS-RARC-iN is an oncologically sound procedure associated with favorable perioperative and functional outcomes.

Keywords: bladder cancer; female; intracorporeal neobladder; outcomes; radical cystectomy; robotic; sex-sparing

---

1. Introduction

Radical cystectomy (RC) with urinary diversion is the standard treatment for patients with muscle-invasive (MI) and high-risk non-muscle-invasive (NMI) urothelial carcinoma of the bladder and can offer an orthotopic neobladder (ON) diversion if technically and oncologically feasible [1].

Although bladder cancer (BCa) is more frequent among men, it remains the 17th most common cancer in women worldwide, with approximately 74,000 new diagnosed cases each year [2]. Moreover, women present an advanced stage at diagnosis more often, increasing the requirement of RC [3].

In female patients, the standard surgical procedure is represented by anterior pelvic exenteration including the removal of the bladder, ovaries, uterus, and anterior vaginal wall [1].

In this setting, when an ON is performed, the procedure can be associated with a considerable rate of voiding symptoms [4,5]. In addition, sexual dysfunction derived from such a highly demolitive surgical procedure is a key concern, especially in younger patients due to a significant impact on health-related quality of life (HRQoL) [6].

The improvement of imaging modalities, an increased knowledge of pelvic structure anatomy and function, and an advancement of surgical techniques have enabled less-destructive methods for treating high-risk BCa.

In this scenario, various types of pelvic-organ-preserving techniques, usually named "sex-sparing", have been proposed [5], aiming at the preservation of neurovascular bundles, vagina, and uterus, combining these techniques in order to optimize sexual and functional results without compromising oncological outcomes.

Functional outcomes of sex-sparing (sex) RC are essentially based on surgical dissection planes, with the sex-sparing approach being associated with the preservation of utero-vaginal hypogastric plexus, while during standard RC only rectal hypogastric plexus is preserved [7].

The Bern group were the first to describe the feasibility of nerve-sparing RC and ON replacement in female patients, highlighting the potential advantages which derive from preserving pelvic reproductive organs and their nervous structures both in terms of continence and urinary retention [7].

However, a recent systematic review aiming at the evaluation of the advantages and disadvantages of sexual-function-preserving RC and ON in female patients underlined the need for further and more robust comparisons between sex and standard RC as existing data are still immature [5].

Notwithstanding, for well-selected patients, sparing female reproductive organs during RC can be an oncologically safe procedure and can provide improved functional outcomes.

Accordingly, despite the widespread use of robot-assisted radical cystectomy (RARC), there is a paucity of data concerning outcomes of sex-RARC with intracorporeal ON (iON) performed in female patients.

In this paper we describe surgical steps of sex-RARC in female patients, highlighting differences with the standard technique and anatomical details of preservation of the inferior hypogastric plexus (IHP) and we report perioperative, pathologic, and functional outcomes.

2. Experimental Section

2.1. Patients

Our single-center Institutional-Review-Board-approved BCa database was queried for "Female", "RARC", "iON", and "Sex-sparing". Overall, 11 patients were treated between January 2013 and June 2018, with a minimum one year of follow-up. Inclusion criteria were a cT $\leq$ 2 N0 M0 bladder tumor at baseline imaging (CT or MRI) and an absence of tumors in the bladder neck, trigone, and urethra at transurethral resection of the bladder tumor (TURB). Exclusion criteria included any contraindication to ON. All subjects gave their written informed consent for inclusion before they participated in the study.

2.2. Surgical Technique

2.2.1. Sex-Sparing Robot-Assisted Radical Cystectomy

The patient was placed in a steep Trendelenburg position, and a six trocars access was performed as previously described [8].

Sex-RARC was performed replicating the principles of open technique described by Bhatta Dhar et al. [7]. After an incision of the posterior peritoneum up to the round ligament, the ureters were identified and meticulously isolated with a "no-touch" technique. The umbilical artery, uterine artery, superior and inferior vesical arteries, and vaginal branches were carefully prepared bilaterally.

Because the uterus was going to be spared, the peritoneum was incised at the level of the utero-vesical junction in order to deflect the uterus and develop a vesico-vaginal plane between the bladder and the anterior wall of the uterus. The vaginal wall dissection at the cervical level was performed in the anterior plane of the vagina at the 2 and 10 o'clock position in order to preserve the utero-vaginal and pararectal components of the IHP (highlighted in red and green colors respectively, in the video), while in the standard technique the dissection is usually performed dorsolaterally at the 4 and 8 o'clock position, preserving only the pararectal plexus and removing en bloc with the specimen and the utero-vaginal components of the IHP. The superior and inferior vesical arteries and veins were secured with Hem-o-lok clips (Teleflex, Wayne, PA, USA) and transected with LigaSure at their origin from the internal iliac vessels, while the uterine arteries and the vaginal branches directed to the paravaginal tissue were preserved. Both ureters were divided between Weck clips, and margins were sent for frozen sections. Next, the Retzius space was approached. Endopelvic fascia was incised very close to the bladder neck in order to reduce the risk of an accidental injury of neurovascular paraurethral structures, which is crucial for both sexual and continence functionality. The urethra was prepared and a sample was sent for frozen section. Bladder was secured in an endobag and extracted through a 3-cm prepubic incision.

2.2.2. Pelvic Lymph Node Dissection and Intracorporeal Orthotopic Neobladder

A meticulous separate package extending pelvic lymph node dissection (PLND) was performed, including obturator, internal, external, and common iliac nodes. Considering that superior hypogastric plexus (SHP) is usually located just below the aortic bifurcation, ventrally to the sacral promontory, presacral nodes are not removed. Moreover, lymphatic tissue medial to internal iliac arteries which is in close contact with uterine and vaginal vessels and with uterine and vaginal plexus is usually spared.

After RC and PLND, intracorporeal Padua ileal neobladder was performed as previously described [8].

2.3. Outcomes Evaluated

Collected demographic parameters were age, body mass index (BMI), gender, and American Society of Anesthesiologists (ASA) score. Clinical variables were preoperative eGFR, preoperative hemoglobin (Hgb), and neoadjuvant chemotherapy rate. Surgical outcomes reported consisted of operative time, Hgb at discharge, hospital stay, and complications according to the Clavien–Dindo system [9]. Pathological findings including pT stage, pN stage, histology, lymph node count, and the positive surgical margin status were analyzed. Functional outcomes assessed were the last eGFR, neobladder stones rate, the uretero-ileal strictures rate, and the need for intermittent self-catheterization. Daytime and nighttime continence recovery probabilities were assessed over time. EORTC QLQ-C30 and EORTC QLQ-BLM30 questionnaires were adopted to assess HRQoL and urinary symptoms respectively. Every item measured ranged in a score from 0 to 100. A Female Sexual Function Index (FSFI) questionnaire was adopted for sexual function assessment [10]. Each of the six sexual domains range in score from 0 to 6, with a maximum global score of 36. Questionnaires were administered at baseline, and at 3 and 12 month follow-up.

As supplementary data, we reported preoperative perioperative, pathologic and functional characteristics comparisons of sex-RARC and standard RARC cohorts.

2.4. Statistical Analysis

Descriptive analyses were used. Frequencies and proportions were reported for categorical variables. Medians and interquartile ranges (IQRs) were reported for continuously coded variables.

The Kaplan–Meier method was performed to report daytime and nighttime continence recovery probabilities. Continence rates were computed at 3, 6, 12 and 18 months after surgery.

Differences between questionnaires' domains scores evaluated at the baseline 3-month, and 1-year follow-up were assessed with the Friedman test.

In the supplementary outcomes, comparison, continuous, and categorical variables were compared with a Student's t-test and a chi-square test respectively. The Kaplan–Meier method was performed to compare daytime continence recovery probabilities between sex-RARC and standard RARC cohorts. Continence rates were computed at 3, 6, 12, and 18 months after surgery and the log-rank test was applied to assess any statistically significant differences between the two groups.

All p-values < 0.05 were considered statistically significant. Statistical analysis was performed using SPSS v24 (IBM Corp., Armonk, NY, USA).

3. Results

Baseline and clinical features were reported in Table 1. Median operative time was 255 min (IQR 250–399). The median hospital stay was 7 days (7–12). Low-grade Clavien complications occurred in four patients (36.3%) while high grade complications were not observed. Seven patients (63.7%) had an organ-confined disease at the pathologic specimen; nodal involvement and positive surgical margins were not detected in any case (Table 2).

All patients had a minimum follow-up period of one year. At a median follow-up of 28 months (IQR 14–51), no patient developed a new onset of chronic kidney disease stage 3b. One patient reported a neobladder stone formation, and one patient developed a ureteroileal anastomotic stricture and required robotic reimplantation 18 months following surgery (Table 2).

One-year daytime and nighttime continence recovery probability were 90.9% and 86.4%, respectively (Figure 1a,b). Three patients performed self-catheterization twice a day (early morning and before night rest).

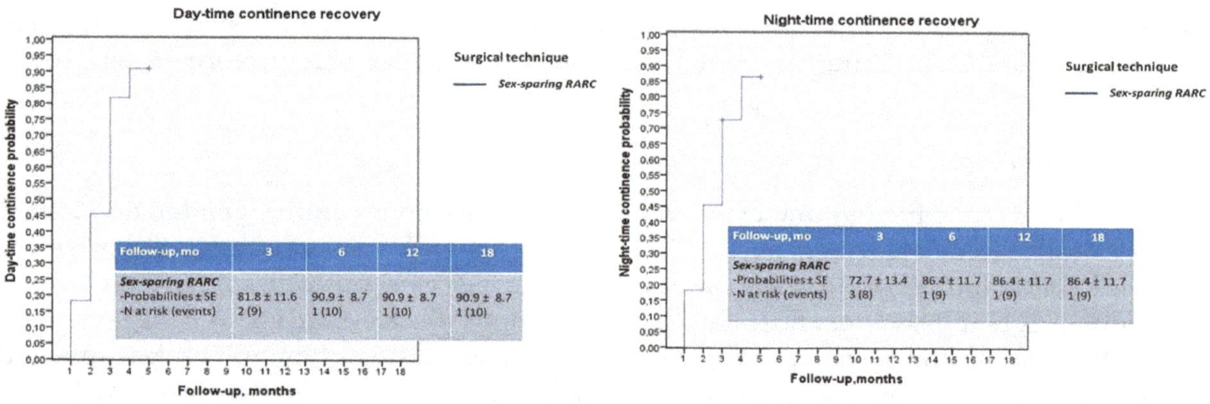

(a) (b)

Figure 1. (**a**,**b**) Kaplan–Meier analysis reporting daytime and nighttime continence recovery probabilities.

Table 1. Baseline and clinical characteristics.

Patients, n 11	Sex-Sparing RARC
Age, year, mean (±SD)	47.1 (13)
BMI, mean (±SD)	23.1 (3.3)
ASA score, n (%)	
1	4 (36.4)
2	6 (54.6)
3	1 (9)
4	-
Preoperative eGFR, mL/min, mean (±SD)	84 (26.8)
Preoperative Hgb, g/dL, mean (±SD)	12.6 (1.9)
Neoadjuvant Chemotherapy, n (%)	4 (36.3)

Table 2. Perioperative, pathologic, oncologic and functional outcomes.

Patients	*Sex-Sparing RARC (11)*
Operative time, min, median (IQR)	255 (250–399)
Hgb at discharge, g/dL, median (IQR)	10.8 (9.1–11.9)
Hospital stay, days, median (IQR)	7 (7–12)
Complications, *n* (%)	4 (36.3)
Clavien Low grade (1–2)	4 (36.3)
Clavien High grade (≥3)	0 (0)
pT stage, *n* (%)	
0, a, is	6 (54.6)
1	1 (9.1)
2	-
3	4 (36.3)
4	-
pN stage, *n* (%)	
0	11(100)
1	-
2	-
Lymph node count, mean (±SD)	26.2 (14.3)
Positive surgical margins, *n* (%)	0 (0)
Follow-up, months, median (IQR)	28 (14–51)
1-Year recurrence-free survival, *n* (%)	11 (100)
1-Year cancer-specific survival, *n* (%)	11 (100)
1-Year overall survival, *n* (%)	11 (100)
Last eGFR, mL/min, mean (±SD)	79.2 (23.7)
Ureteroileal strictures, pts (%)	1 (9)
Neobladder stones, *n* (%)	1 (9)
Need for intermittent self-catheterization, *n* (%)	3 (27.2)

Concerning the EORTC-QLQ-C30 questionnaire, global health status/quality of life, physical, and emotional functioning items improved significantly over time (all $p \leq 0.04$), while no differences were observed in any other items evaluated (all $p \geq 0.10$) (Supplementary Table S1, Figure 2).

According to the EORTC-QLQ-BLM30 questionnaire, specific for BCa, urinary symptoms worsened at three months with a significant recovery at one year ($p = 0.02$). Accordingly, when matching the baseline with 1-year scores, the values were comparable ($p = 0.08$) (Supplementary Table S2, Figure 2).

Finally, the FSFI global score and FSFI domains such as arousal, lubrication, orgasm, satisfaction, and pain worsened over the first three months with a subsequent improvement at one year (all $p \leq 0.04$). Moreover, comparing baseline vs. 1-year scores, arousal and orgasm domains experienced a complete recovery ($p = 0.10$ and $p = 0.10$, respectively), while lubrication, satisfaction, and pain domains, as well as FSFI global scores, experienced a satisfying improvement but were statistically significantly lower than baseline (all $p \leq 0.025$) (Supplementary Table S3, Figure 3). Overall, 8 out of 11 patients (72.7%) were sexually active at the 12-month evaluation.

As supplementary analysis, 36 standard RARC patients were compared with the sex-RARC cohort. The two cohorts were homogeneous for all baseline, clinical, and pathological features (all $p \geq 0.14$) except for age, with sex-sparing patients being significantly younger (47.1 vs. 61.7 years, $p < 0.001$) (Supplementary Tables S4 and S5).

Perioperative complications and hospital stay were comparable between groups ($p = 0.25$ and $p = 0.67$ respectively) (Supplementary Table S5).

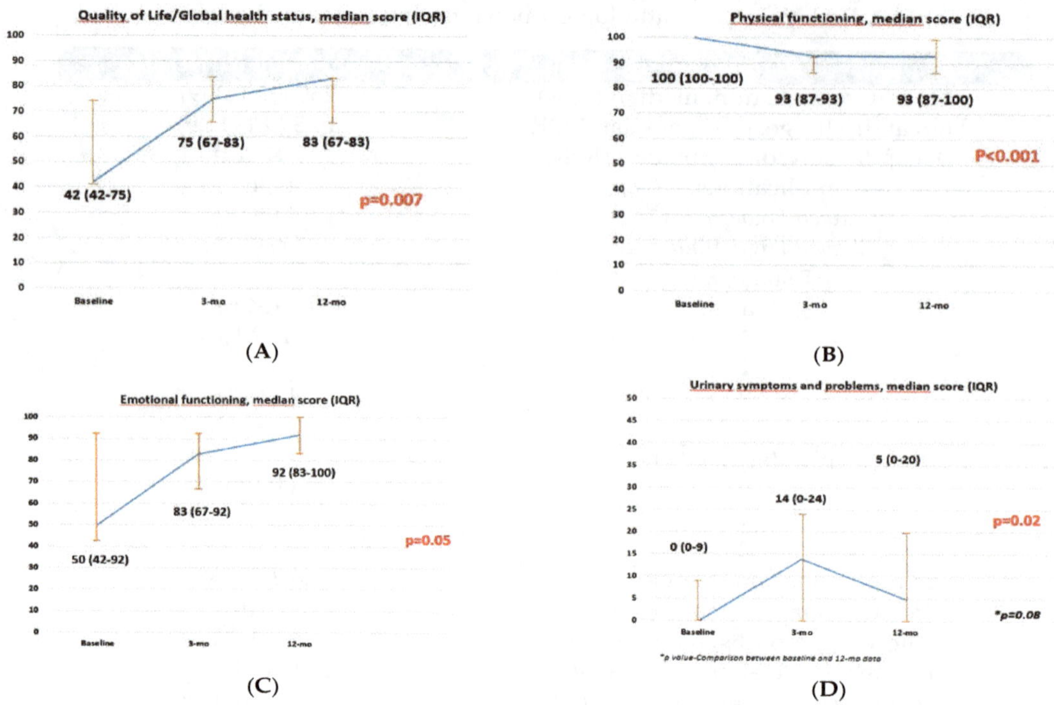

Figure 2. Graphs showing EORTC-QLQ-C30 and EORTC-QLQ-BLM30 questionnaire items displaying statistical significance according to the Friedman test. (**A**) Quality of Life/Global health status; (**B**) Emotional functioning; (**C**) Physical functioning; (**D**) Urinary symptoms and problems

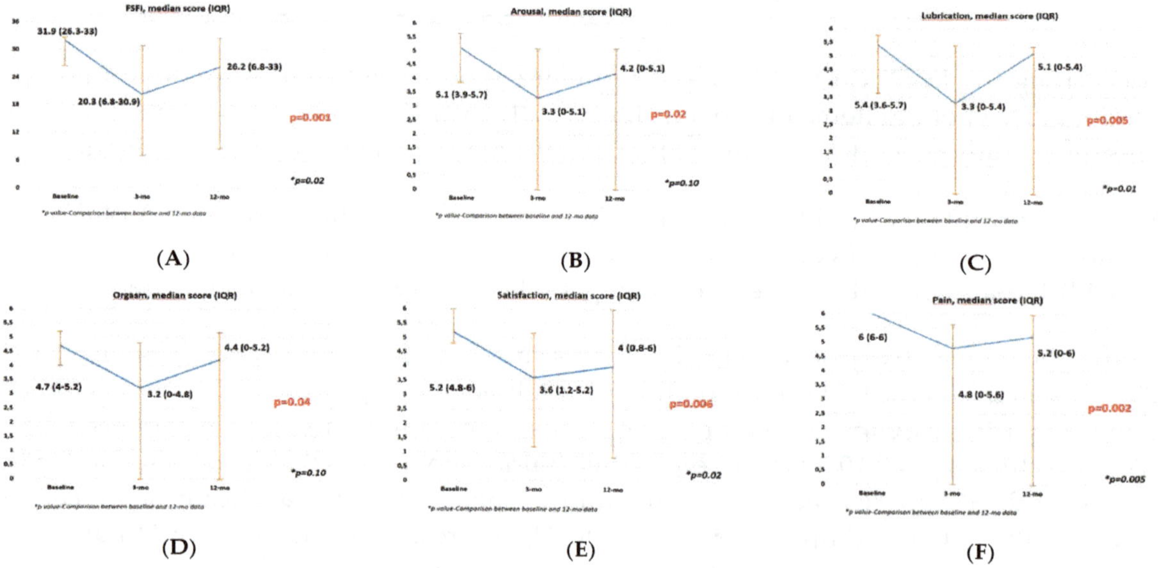

Figure 3. Graphs showing global Female Sexual Function Index (FSFI) and FSFI single domains questionnaire displaying statistical significance according to the Friedman test. (**A**) FSFI; (**B**) Arousal; (**C**) Lubrication; (**D**) Orgasm; (**E**) Satisfaction; (**F**) Pain.

With regard to functional outcomes, no significant differences were observed for the last estimated glomerular filtration rate ($p = 0.43$), neobladder stone formation rate ($p = 0.93$), and 1-year incidence of ureteroileal strictures ($p = 0.67$) (Supplementary Table S5). Daytime continence recovery probability was significantly higher in the sex-sparing cohort (1-year rate 90.9% vs. 74%, log-rank $p = 0.02$) (Supplementary Figure S1).

4. Discussion

Functional outcomes among women undergoing RC have been poorly addressed in the literature [11]. Urinary function is the most studied issue, although daytime and nighttime continence rates range significantly across studies due to a heterogeneity of definitions for continence, different inclusion criteria, and a lack of questionnaire adoption, as these are omitted in most studies [11]. In addition, Zahran et al. conducted a systematic review aiming to evaluate female sexual dysfunction post RC and urinary diversion, considering it an important predictor of HRQoL post RC. According to the 11 studies included, the most frequently detected sexual disorders were loss of sexual desire and orgasm disorders (49% and 39%, respectively) [12]. Notwithstanding, the authors called for the use of standardized tools in order to properly assess the outcomes of this technique from the patients' perspective and reported poor evidence from the available literature. Moreover, no data were available about RARC in females.

The concept of sex-RC in female patients was first introduced by the Bern team in 2007, when, in select female patients with an absence of invasive cancer at the level of the trigone or dorsolateral side walls of the bladder, they emphasized the functional advantages deriving from the preservation of the utero-vaginal hypogastric plexus, which is usually sacrificed in the standard procedure [7].

These results were corroborated by meticulous cadaveric studies elucidating topographic anatomic details of the nervous autonomic system in women, with their clinical nuances [13,14]. The SHP was identified as a single anatomical complex located below the aortic bifurcation, ventral to the sacral promontory. After the promontory, the SHP divides into right and left hypogastric nerves that more caudally plunge into the inferior pelvic IHP, composed by utero-vaginal, vesical, and rectal plexus.

As expected, preservation of these neural structures has an impact on recovery of urinary continence and on voiding function. Accordingly, data coming from gynecological studies report intrinsic sphincter deficiency resulting from hysterectomy as a consequence of urethral denervation after an extensive pelvic dissection [15,16]. Moreover, a pelvic autonomous nervous system affects all the domains of sexuality, such as sexual desire, arousal, lubrication, orgasm, satisfaction, and post-RC sexual dysfunction, often associated with pain disorders, such as dyspareunia, vulvodynia, and vaginismus, each being a consequence of autonomic and nociceptive nerve injuries, and a shortening or a narrowing of the vagina with an unavoidable negative impact on HRQoL [17].

In the literature, there are few existing series reporting sexual function results after sex-RC, all of them with an open approach and most of them with a small number of patients and without assessment of HRQoL through self-administered standardized questionnaires. Nandipati et al. focused on preservation of the lateral walls of the vagina, in which are embedded nervous fibers directed to the paraurethral tissue, involved in clitoral vascularization. In the small cohort of six women who underwent the sex-sparing approach, 12-month FSFI remained stable, while it declined in the standard RC group [18].

Furthermore, a significant improvement in all domains of the FSFI questionnaire has been reported in 13 sex-sparing RC patients evaluated at Mansoura Urology Department, with daytime and nighttime continence rates of 100% and 92%, respectively [19].

In this context, the EAU MIBCa Guideline Panel recently commissioned a systematic review aiming to assess the effect of sexual-function-preserving surgical techniques on outcomes in women receiving RC and ON substitution for BCa [5]. Sex-sparing approaches were found to be oncologically safe in well-selected patients, with sexual function appearing to be improved among those women undergoing gynecologic organ-preserving and nerve-sparing approaches. Nevertheless, most of the studies analyzed were retrospective and only contained a small number of patients [5]. Hence, according to EAU guidelines, data regarding sex RC in female patients are still considered immature and it is not yet considered a standard treatment, but an option to be taken into consideration for women highly motivated to preserve sexual function so long as strict oncologic inclusion criteria are met [1]. In addition, though the oncological equivalence of open and robotic RC has been extensively assessed, [20–22] and the robotic approach has been widely adopted in the male sex-sparing counterpart with excellent functional results [23], there are no reports on sex-RARC in female patients.

Hence, in this paper and in the accompanying video, we firstly described surgical steps of sex-RARC in female patients and reported perioperative and functional outcomes of our initial series with a minimum 1-year follow-up. In the video, we clearly highlight the differences with the standard technique with special attention paid to the preservation of the utero-vaginal component of the IHP. We strongly believe that robotic technology offers undebatable advantages in meticulously following and dissecting the appropriate surgical planes since IHP fibers are usually embedded in dense connective tissue, and consequently are not always easy to preserve. Despite the small cohort (11 patients), the excellent continence results (daytime 90.9% and nighttime 86.4% at one year) and the encouraging rate of sexually active patients (72.7% at one year) reflect the proper respect of the crucial anatomical structures and reinforce the efficacy of sex-RC in properly selected women. In addition, the oncological effectiveness with an absence of any recurrence corroborates our results.

Another important point of strength regarding the reliability of our results is our adoption of standardized questionnaires to assess the quality of life, urinary symptoms, and sexual activity (i.e., EORTC-C30, BLM30, and FSFI), which are rarely used in most studies. Moreover, the minimal invasiveness of the robotic approach represents a further issue to consider when considering young sexually and socially active women.

Furthermore, our technique may avoid devastating complications such as vaginal dehiscence and evisceration which have been reported after minimally invasive radical cystectomy [24,25].

Nevertheless, the present paper is not devoid of limitations. The small sample size, the strict inclusion criteria, and the need for advanced robotic surgical skills are significant limitations to a wide reproducibility of these outcomes in daily practice. Finally, BCa recurrence usually occurs within two years of radical cystectomy. In this respect, the follow-up duration might be inadequate.

5. Conclusions

In selected populations, sex-RARC-iN can be offered to female patients motivated to preserve sexual function as an oncologically safe procedure, associated with favorable functional outcomes. The meticulous anatomical preservation of utero-vaginal components of IHP represents the cornerstone of a quick and effective recovery of physiological functions in terms of urinary continence and sexual activity. A proper comparison of outcomes with the conventional RARC-iN technique requires properly designed prospective randomized trials.

Supplementary Materials
Table S1. Health-related quality of life assessment (EORTC QLQ-C30 questionnaire). Table S2. Bladder-cancer-specific quality of life EORTC QLQ-BLM30 questionnaire. Table S3. Female Sexual Function Index (FSFI) questionnaire. Table S4. Baseline and clinical characteristics of sex-sparing and standard RARC. Table S5. Perioperative, pathologic, and functional characteristics of sex-sparing and standard RARC. Figure S1. Kaplan–Meier analysis comparing day-time continence recovery probabilities between sex-sparing and standard RARC cohorts.

Author Contributions: Conceptualization, G.T, G.S.; methodology, G.T., R.M., G.S.; formal analysis, G.T.; data curation, R.M., S.F., M.F., C.L., U.A., A.B., S.G.; writing—original draft preparation, G.T., R.M.; writing—review and editing, G.T., G.S.; supervision, M.G., G.S. All authors have read and agreed to the published version of the manuscript.

References

1. Witjes, J.A.; Lebret, T.; Compérat, E.; Cowan, N.C.; De Santis, M.; Bruins, H.M.; Hernández, V.; Espinos, E.L.; Dunn, J.; Rouanne, M.; et al. Updated 2016 EAU Guidelines on Muscle-invasive and Metastatic Bladder Cancer. *Eur. Urol.* **2017**, *71*, 462–475. [CrossRef]
2. Burger, M.; Catto, J.; Dalbagni, G.; Grossman, H.B.; Herr, H.; Karakiewicz, P.; Kassouf, W.; Kiemeney, L.; La Vecchia, C.; Shariat, S.; et al. Epidemiology and risk factors of urothelial bladder cancer. *Eur. Urol.* **2013**, *63*, 234–241. [CrossRef] [PubMed]

3. Mungan, N.; Aben, K.K.; Schoenberg, M.P.; Visser, O.; Coebergh, J.-W.W.; Witjes, J.; Kiemeney, L. Gender differences in stage-adjusted bladder cancer survival. *Urology* **2000**, *55*, 876–880. [CrossRef]
4. Granberg, C.F.; Boorjian, S.A.; Crispen, P.L.; Tollefson, M.K.; Farmer, S.A.; Frank, I.; Blute, M.L. Functional and oncological outcomes after orthotopic neobladder reconstruction in women. *BJU Int.* **2008**, *102*, 1551–1555. [CrossRef] [PubMed]
5. Veskimäe, E.; Neuzillet, Y.; Rouanne, M.; MacLennan, S.; Lam, T.B.L.; Yuan, Y.; Compérat, E.; Cowan, N.C.; Gakis, G.; Van Der Heijden, A.G.; et al. Systematic review of the oncological and functional outcomes of pelvic organ preserving radical cystectomy (RC) compared with standard RC in women who undergo curative surgery and orthotopic neobladder substitution for bladder cancer. *BJU Int.* **2017**, *120*, 12–24. [CrossRef]
6. Zippe, C.D.; Raina, R.; Shah, A.D.; Massanyi, E.Z.; Agarwal, A.; Ulchaker, J.; Jones, S.; Klein, E. Female sexual dysfunction after radical cystectomy: A new outcome measure. *Urology* **2004**, *63*, 1153–1157. [CrossRef]
7. Dhar, N.B.; Kessler, T.M.; Mills, R.D.; Burkhard, F.; Studer, U.E. Nerve-sparing radical cystectomy and orthotopic bladder replacement in female patients. *Eur. Urol.* **2007**, *52*, 1006–1014. [CrossRef]
8. Simone, G.; Papalia, R.; Misuraca, L.; Tuderti, G.; Minisola, F.; Ferriero, M.; Vallati, G.E.; Guaglianone, S.; Gallucci, M. Robotic Intracorporeal Padua Ileal Bladder: Surgical Technique, Perioperative, Oncologic and Functional Outcomes. *Eur. Urol.* **2018**, *73*, 934–940. [CrossRef]
9. Mitropoulos, D.; Artibani, W.; Biyani, C.S.; Jensen, J.B.; Rouprêt, M.; Truss, M. Validation of the Clavien-Dindo grading system in urology by the European Association of Urology Guidelines Ad Hoc Panel. *Eur. Urol. Focus* **2018**, *4*, 608–613. [CrossRef]
10. Rosen, R.; Brown, C.; Heiman, J.; Leiblum, S.; Meston, C.; Shabsigh, R.; Ferguson, D.; D'Agostino, R., Jr. The Female Sexual Function Index (FSFI): A multidimensional self-report instrument for the assessment of female sexual function. *J. Sex Marital. Ther.* **2000**, *26*, 191–208. [CrossRef]
11. Smith, A.B.; Crowell, K.; Woods, M.E.; Wallen, E.M.; Pruthi, R.S.; Nielsen, M.E.; Lee, C.T. Functional Outcomes Following Radical Cystectomy in Women with Bladder Cancer: A Systematic Review. *Eur. Urol. Focus* **2017**, *3*, 136–143. [CrossRef] [PubMed]
12. Zahran, M.H.; Fahmy, O.; El-Hefnawy, A.S.; Ali-El-Dein, B. Female sexual dysfunction post radical cystectomy and urinary diversion. *Climateric* **2016**, *19*, 546–550. [CrossRef] [PubMed]
13. Ripperda, C.M.; Jackson, L.A.; Phelan, J.N.; Carrick, K.S.; Corton, M.M. Anatomic relationships of the pelvic autonomic nervous system in female cadavers: Clinical applications to pelvic surgery. *Am. J. Obstet. Gynecol.* **2017**, *216*, 388.e1–388.e7. [CrossRef] [PubMed]
14. Mauroy, B.; Demondion, X.; Bizet, B.; Claret, A.; Mestdagh, P.; Hurt, C. The female inferior hypogastric (= pelvic) plexus: Anatomical and radiological description of the plexus and its afferences—Applications to pelvic surgery. *Surg. Radiol. Anat.* **2007**, *29*, 55–66. [CrossRef] [PubMed]
15. Mundy, A.R. An anatomical explanation for bladder dysfunction following rectal and uterine surgery. *Br. J. Urol.* **1982**, *54*, 501–504. [CrossRef] [PubMed]
16. Morgan, J.L.; O'Connell, H.E.; McGuire, E.J. Is intrinsicsphincter deficiency a complication of simple hysterectomy? *J. Urol.* **2000**, *164*, 767–769. [CrossRef]
17. Pederzoli, F.; Campbell, J.D.; Matsui, H.; Sopko, N.; Bivalacqua, T.J. Surgical Factors Associated with Male and Female Sexual Dysfunction After Radical Cystectomy: What Do We Know and How Can We Improve Outcomes? *Sex Med. Rev.* **2018**, *6*, 469–481. [CrossRef]
18. Nandipati, C.; Bhat, A.; Zippe, C.D. Neurovascualr preservation in female orthotopic radical cystectomy significantly improves sexual function. *Urology* **2006**, *67*, 185–186. [CrossRef]
19. Ali-El-Dein, B.; Mosbah, A.; Osman, Y.; El-Tabey, N.; Abdel-Latif, M.; Eraky, I.; Shaaban, A.A. Preservation of the internal genital organs during radical cystectomy in selected women with bladder cancer: A report on 15 cases with long term follow-up B. *Eur. J. Surg. Oncol.* **2013**, *39*, 358–364. [CrossRef]
20. Bochner, B.H.; Dalbagni, G.; Sjoberg, D.D.; Silberstein, J.; Keren Paz, G.E.; Donat, S.M.; Coleman, J.A.; Mathew, S.; Vickers, A.; Schnorr, G.C.; et al. Comparing open radical cystectomy and robot-assisted laparoscopic radical cystectomy: A randomized clinical trial. *Eur. Urol.* **2015**, *67*, 1042–1050. [CrossRef]
21. Moschini, M.; Soria, F.; Mathieu, R.; Xylinas, E.; D'Andrea, D.; Tan, W.S.; Kelly, J.D.; Simone, G.; Tuderti, G.; Meraney, A.; et al. Propensity-score-matched comparison of soft tissue surgical margins status between open and robotic-assisted radical cystectomy. *Urol. Oncol.* **2019**, *37*, 179.e1–179.e7. [CrossRef] [PubMed]

22. Simone, G.; Tuderti, G.; Misuraca, L.; Anceschi, U.; Ferriero, M.; Minisola, F.; Guaglianone, S.; Gallucci, M. Perioperative and mid-term oncologic outcomes of robotic assisted radical cystectomy with totally intracorporeal neobladder: Results of a propensity score matched comparison with open cohort from a single-centre series. *Eur. J. Surg. Oncol.* **2018**, *44*, 1432–1438. [CrossRef] [PubMed]
23. Asimakopoulos, A.D.; Campagna, A.; Gakis, G.; Montes, V.E.C.; Piechaud, T.; Hoepffner, J.-L.; Mugnier, C.; Gaston, R.; Corona, M.V.E. Nerve sparing robot-assisted radical cystectomy with intracorporeal bladder substitution in the male. *J. Urol.* **2016**, *196*, 1549–1557. [CrossRef] [PubMed]
24. Lin, F.C.; Medendorp, A.; Van Kuiken, M.; Mills, S.A.; Tarnay, C.M. Vaginal Dehiscence and Evisceration after Robotic-Assisted Radical Cystectomy: A Case Series and Review of the Literature. *Urology* **2019**, *134*, 90–96. [CrossRef]
25. Kanno, T.; Ito, K.; Sawada, A.; Saito, R.; Kobayashi, T.; Yamada, H.; Inoue, T.; Ogawa, O. Complications and reoperations after laparoscopic radical cystectomy in a Japanese multicenter cohort. *Int. J. Urol.* **2019**, *26*, 493–498. [CrossRef]

9

Applications of Artificial Intelligence to Prostate Multiparametric MRI (mpMRI): Current and Emerging Trends

Michelle D. Bardis [1,*], Roozbeh Houshyar [1], Peter D. Chang [1], Alexander Ushinsky [2], Justin Glavis-Bloom [1], Chantal Chahine [1], Thanh-Lan Bui [1], Mark Rupasinghe [1], Christopher G. Filippi [3] and Daniel S. Chow [1]

1 Department of Radiology, University of California, Irvine, Orange, CA 92868-3201, USA; rhoushya@hs.uci.edu (R.H.); changp6@hs.uci.edu (P.D.C.); jglavisb@hs.uci.edu (J.G.-B.); cchahin1@hs.uci.edu (C.C.); thanhltb@hs.uci.edu (T.-L.B.); mrupasin@hs.uci.edu (M.R.); chowd3@hs.uci.edu (D.S.C.)

2 Mallinckrodt Institute of Radiology, Washington University Saint Louis, St. Louis, MO 63110, USA; aushinsky@wustl.edu

3 Department of Radiology, North Shore University Hospital, Manhasset, NY 11030, USA; sairaallapeikko@gmail.com

* Correspondence: mbardis@hs.uci.edu

Abstract: Prostate carcinoma is one of the most prevalent cancers worldwide. Multiparametric magnetic resonance imaging (mpMRI) is a non-invasive tool that can improve prostate lesion detection, classification, and volume quantification. Machine learning (ML), a branch of artificial intelligence, can rapidly and accurately analyze mpMRI images. ML could provide better standardization and consistency in identifying prostate lesions and enhance prostate carcinoma management. This review summarizes ML applications to prostate mpMRI and focuses on prostate organ segmentation, lesion detection and segmentation, and lesion characterization. A literature search was conducted to find studies that have applied ML methods to prostate mpMRI. To date, prostate organ segmentation and volume approximation have been well executed using various ML techniques. Prostate lesion detection and segmentation are much more challenging tasks for ML and were attempted in several studies. They largely remain unsolved problems due to data scarcity and the limitations of current ML algorithms. By contrast, prostate lesion characterization has been successfully completed in several studies because of better data availability. Overall, ML is well situated to become a tool that enhances radiologists' accuracy and speed.

Keywords: prostate carcinoma; prostate mpMRI; machine learning; artificial intelligence; deep learning; neural network

---

1. Introduction

Prostate carcinoma (PCa) is the most common cancer and the third leading cause of cancer-related death among men in the United States [1]. A major challenge for PCa management is the lack of non-invasive tools that can differentiate aggressive versus non-aggressive cancer types [2]. This limitation can result in overdiagnosis and overtreatment, as evidenced by the fact that only one death is prevented for every 48 patients treated for PCa [3]. This overdiagnosis and overtreatment can lead to unnecessary biopsies, surgeries, radiotherapy, chemotherapy, and patient anxiety [2]. Better diagnostic methods could mitigate these unwarranted procedures. To meet this need for more effective screening, multiparametric magnetic resonance imaging (mpMRI) could be implemented to examine the entire prostate.

MpMRI of the prostate has been increasingly used for PCa screening in recent years [4]. MpMRI's current utility in screening stems from a high negative predictive value for prostate cancer. However, the full potential of mpMRI has not yet been achieved [5]. PCa overdiagnosis could be reduced with an mpMRI analysis that accomplishes better lesion detection, lesion classification (benign versus malignant), and lesion volume quantification.

Accurate prostate segmentation and volume estimation can provide invaluable information for the diagnosis and clinical management of benign prostatic hyperplasia (BPH) and PCa. This can improve BPH treatment, surgical planning, and predictions of PCa prognosis [6–8]. Prostate segmentation is necessary for magnetic resonance imaging (MRI) transrectal ultrasound (TRUS) fusion biopsy, which is increasingly used to diagnose PCa. MRI/TRUS fusion biopsy yield depends on accurate prostate segmentation on magnetic resonance images because the prostate edges form the reference frames for fusion with the ultrasound data [8]. Therefore, any inaccuracy in tracing prostate boundaries may lead to biopsy errors [9]. In addition to segmentation, prostate volume estimation is also a useful metric, especially with regard to BPH treatment, surgical planning, and PCa prognosis. BPH is one of the most common diseases that affects elderly men and reaches a prevalence of 90% by the ninth decade of life [10]. Large prostate volumes in men with BPH indicate a higher likelihood of more severe lower urinary tract symptoms and urinary retention [11–13]. Furthermore, studies have shown that patients have differential responses to BPH-targeted medications, depending on prostate size [11]. Additionally, prostate volume is considered when determining a surgical approach, with each procedure having its own risk profile [14]. In addition to guiding BPH treatment, prostate volume is used in PCa prognosis. Prostate size alone is a valuable marker for PCa prognosis; PCa is more accurately detected in prostates under 50 cm^3 than in those over 50 cm^3 [6]. Prostate volume is also used to calculate prostate-specific antigen density, a figure that helps to differentiate BPH from PCa and can also be used to predict radical prostatectomy outcomes [15–17].

Accuracy of prostate lesion detection, segmentation, and volume estimation is important at different stages of PCa management. Lesion detection identifies regions for biopsy. Accurate segmentation is crucial for improved fusion biopsy yields. Additionally, segmentation improves radiotherapy delivery. Volume estimation predicts prognosis after prostatectomy [18–20]. Prostate lesion detection is crucial because the effective treatment of PCa directly depends on identifying cancer at its earliest stage [21–23]. Even though PCa most often follows an indolent course, it can show rapid progression in some cases. In these instances, lesion recognition on mpMRI is critical because it provides a region of high suspicion and a higher yield from targeted biopsy [24]. Without mpMRI lesion detection, random 12 core TRUS biopsies are performed, which may miss small or anteriorly located PCa [25].

While early prostate lesion detection improves timely PCa treatment, accurate lesion segmentation can improve radiotherapy [26]. Prostate lesion contouring is a major source of error when administering radiation therapy. This inexact segmentation can lead to the underdosage of the tumor as well as the overdosage of normal cells [20]. Although radiotherapy is an effective cancer treatment, its use is hampered by imprecise delineation. More precise contouring of a malignant lesion can improve lesion targeting and relative radiotherapeutic dosage, which can lead to lower recurrence rates [26,27].

Pre-operative prostate lesion volume estimation is a key metric for predicting the likelihood of positive surgical margins, biochemical prostate-specific antigen (PSA) recurrence, and cancer-specific survival post-prostatectomy [28–31]. This volume is a better indicator of surgical margins than other factors such as Gleason score and extracapsular extension [28]. Lesion volume also functions as an independent variable for PSA recurrence, an early sign of recurrent disease which may require salvage radiation therapy [32]. In addition, lesion volume predicts cancer-specific survival more accurately than variables such as lymphadenopathy, seminal vesical invasion, and Gleason score [29].

After prostate lesions have been detected on mpMRI, lesion characterization is important for selecting appropriate management options. Accurate prostate lesion classification on mpMRI could preclude biopsies in men with low-grade tumors, reduce the number of biopsy cores, and decrease the rate of overdiagnosis and false-negative biopsies [33]. Reduction in unnecessary biopsies is important, as potential TRUS biopsy complications include hematuria, lower urinary tract symptoms, and temporary erectile dysfunction [34]. Additionally, the number of biopsy cores obtained correlates with increased risk of complications, including rectal bleeding, hematospermia, bleeding complications, and acute urinary retention [34]. Furthermore, the overdetection of PCa exerts a major psychological toll on quality of life and increases the risk of overtreatment [2]. Overtreatment side effects that may occur after radical prostatectomy and radiotherapy include urinary incontinence, rectal bleeding and fistulae, and erectile dysfunction [2,35–37].

Artificial intelligence (AI) is a promising tool to improve prostate lesion detection, lesion characterization, and lesion volume quantification. AI can systematically evaluate mpMRI images [38]. Machine learning (ML), a branch of AI, and its sub-discipline, deep learning (DL), have become attractive techniques in medical imaging because of their ability to interpret large amounts of data [39]. By applying ML to prostate mpMRI data, imaging-based clinical decisions could be improved. The purpose of this review is to summarize ML applications for prostate mpMRI in regards to (1) prostate organ segmentation, (2) prostate lesion detection and segmentation, and (3) prostate lesion characterization.

2. Multiparametric Magnetic Resonance Imaging

Multiparametric magnetic resonance imaging (mpMRI) of the prostate is a form of advanced non-invasive imaging that combines standard anatomical sequences with functional imaging. It consists of T1-weighted images, T2-weighted images (T2W), and the following functional sequences: diffusion-weighted images (DWI) including the apparent diffusion coefficient maps (ADC) and dynamic contrast-enhanced images (DCE). Certain protocols also incorporate proton magnetic resonance spectroscopy imaging (MRSI) [40,41]. Typically, the functional techniques used are DWI and DCE. MRSI is more demanding than DWI and DCE because it requires more acquisition time, greater technical expertise, and intensive post-processing of the data. Therefore, it is not commonly used [42].

The advantages of seeing both the anatomy and functional ability of the prostate have made mpMRI an attractive imaging technique with many applications. It can accurately identify clinically relevant cancer. The combination of T2W, DWI, and DCE has high specificity, sensitivity, and negative predictive value in detecting PCa [43–45]. The use of all three functional sequences has been found to have a positive predictive value for PCa of 98% [46]. In addition to diagnosing PCa, mpMRI is also used in the management of the disease as the functional sequences aid in predicting tumor behavior. Prostate mpMRI has been used for active surveillance, tumor localization, staging, treatment planning, and monitoring of recurrence [40,41].

While mpMRI is a powerful imaging modality, it does have limitations. Differences in image acquisition techniques and protocols across institutions lead to heterogeneity in imaging quality and make it challenging to compare images [47]. Additionally, the learning curve for reading mpMRIs is steep, and there exists inter-observer variability [48–50]. The experience of radiologists reading these scans impacts the utility of prostate mpMRI images. In addition, the prostate gland is difficult to delineate, and various benign and pre-malignant processes can mimic PCa [51]. For example, the sensitivity for the detection of PCa in the transitional zone is limited by the heterogeneous nature of this zone in the setting of BPH, which can also exhibit increased cellularity further complicating the distinction. Furthermore, patient-related factors, including body habitus, prior procedures, and unconventional anatomy, can impact imaging. Artifacts, such as field inhomogeneity from rectal gas and metal implants, can substantially impede the interpretation and reporting of prostate mpMRI. Finally, it can be difficult to discriminate between post-treatment changes and local recurrence following treatment on mpMRI.

In an effort to assist in standardizing the acquisition, interpretation, and reporting of prostate mpMRI, the Prostate Imaging Reporting and Data System (PI-RADS) was developed by the European Society of Urogenital Radiology (ESUR) in 2012 [52]. The ESUR, in collaboration with the American

College of Radiology and the AdMeTech Foundation, released updated versions PI-RADS v2 in 2015 and PI-RADS v2.1 in 2019 [53,54]. All of the PI-RADS versions offer guidance for protocols and specifications for image acquisition. The scoring systems provide frameworks to evaluate individual sequences of T2W, DWI, and DCE and to integrate these findings into an overall risk assessment category from 1 to 5. These risk categories assist in the determination of biopsies and the management of clinically significant PCa.

3. Artificial Intelligence Paradigms: Machine Learning and Deep Learning

Although the terms AI, ML, and DL are commonly used interchangeably, each term has its own specific definition. AI is the broad, umbrella term that encompasses both ML and DL, with DL being a subset of ML (Figure 1). Marvin Minsky, an early AI developer, described AI as "the science of making machines do things that would require intelligence if done by men" [55]. AI is the ability of any tool to accept inputs of prior knowledge, experience, goals, and observations and then create an output that implements an action. This definition covers a wide range of tools varying from a simple thermostat to a self-driving car. AI research often falls under the domain of computer science because AI tools perform many computations to create appropriate outputs [56].

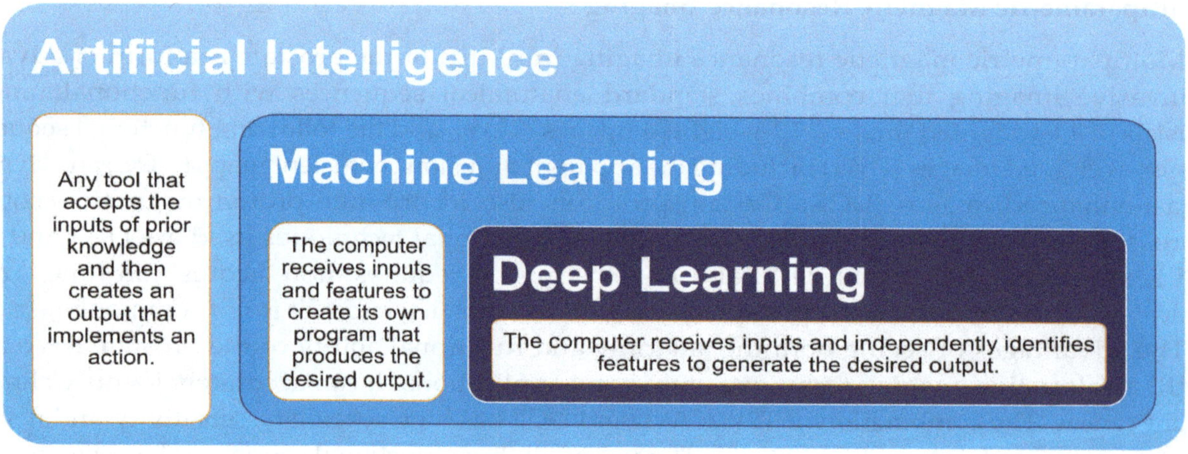

Figure 1. Relationship between artificial intelligence, machine learning, and deep learning. Artificial intelligence is an umbrella term that includes machine learning and deep learning. Deep learning is a hyponym of machine learning.

Whereas AI typically entails a fixed, rules-based computational method, ML dynamically improves upon computational methods as data is input and trained. In traditional programming, a computer receives data and a program as inputs and then produces the output in a one-to-one manner. All improvements to the results derive from alterations to the program rules. In ML, a computer receives data and labels as inputs and then creates a program to refine the outputs. The computer learns by comparing its own outputs, also known as predictions, to data that has already been defined and associated with a label. Over time, the ML algorithm will improve upon its ability to create a program that can match its own output to a label. The effectiveness of the program is highly dependent on the quality and size of data that the ML algorithm receives as input.

The data types that can be input into an ML algorithm vary widely, encompassing digitized handwriting, text from documents, DNA sequences, facial images, and more. A ML algorithm can utilize this data to train and make predictions. Two of the most common ML implementations are classification and regression [57]. In classification, ML receives data and then decides upon a category for each item in the data. For example, ML could look at images and decide whether the image is a plane, car, or boat. In regression, ML receives data and then predicts a numerical value for each item in the data. Examples include predicting tomorrow's ambient temperature or the price of a stock.

Within the ML discipline, DL has garnered significant attention because of the groundbreaking results that it achieved in the ImageNet Large Scale Visual Recognition Challenge competition, where competitors developed algorithms using a subset of a public dataset of images [58]. DL has flourished with the rise of big data and faster hardware [39]. In traditional ML, the algorithm has features that it will extract from the data before training begins [57] (Figure 2). These features are constant and are based upon established rules. For example, the algorithm can look for eyes when trying to recognize a face or search for wings when identifying an airplane. By contrast, a DL algorithm does not require feature selection before training. DL simply receives input and learns its salient features during training (Figure 2). DL architecture is also notable because it is formed by many tiered layers, which resemble a brain's neuronal network. These layers enable DL to extract features from progressively smaller sizes of input data and allow for increased feature complexity [59]. Although various DL architectures exist, convolutional neural networks (CNN) are considered well suited for medical imaging. The overall goal of these techniques is to allow the machine to determine and optimize features automatically for evaluating and classifying images.

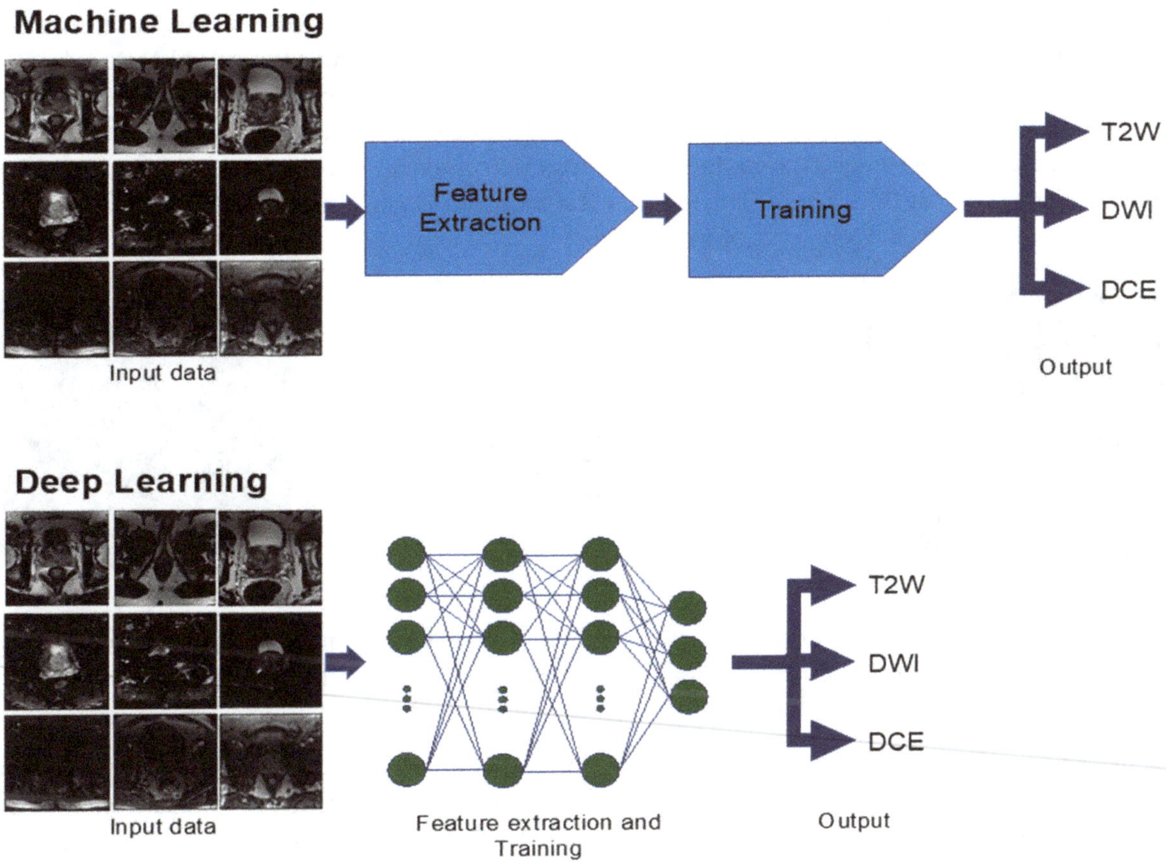

Figure 2. Machine learning versus deep learning used for multiparametric magnetic resonance imaging (mpMRI) sequence identification. In machine learning, the computer receives inputs of mpMRI images and goes through feature extraction specific to the different sequences of T2-weighted (T2W), diffusion-weighted imaging (DWI), and dynamic contrast-enhanced (DCE). Then, the computer is trained on additional images and is able to identify the correct sequence as an output. Deep learning differs from machine learning in that feature extraction and training can be done simultaneously to produce the output.

Medical imaging studies that use ML algorithms are frequently designed with three dataset types: training, validation, and test [60]. The study will first use training data as its input to develop an algorithm that produces the desired output. During this training period, the algorithm constantly uses validation data to provide correct feedback to modify itself. After the algorithm has finished development, final performance is then assessed with test data. Because test data was not used during the algorithm training, it is an objective method to assess performance.

4. Prostate Organ: Segmentation and Volume Estimation

Although prostate segmentation and volume approximation could greatly improve PCa and BPH management, existing techniques are limited. Currently, prostate segmentation is performed in a manual or semi-automated fashion and is limited by inter-observer variability [61]. According to a study by Rash et al. [62], the mean prostate organ volume among three radiation oncologists varied between 0.95 and 1.08. Currently, prostate volume is most often calculated during TRUS utilizing an ellipsoid estimate [63] or estimated during a prostate exam. Even though this volume approximation with TRUS is commonly used, it has significant intra-observer variation and is not as accurate as an approximation with mpMRI images [64,65]. Prostate volume approximation with software has been attempted with limited results. Medical students outperform the accuracy of a commercially available tool [66].

To meet this need for an automatic, accurate prostate segmentation and volume approximation tool, ML methods have been applied by various groups (Figure 3). A ML technique, fuzzy c-means clustering, categorizes data into groups via unsupervised learning and was used by Rundo et al. [67] to segment the prostate on T1-weighted and T2-weighted mpMRI images. Rundo et al. evaluated 21 patients to yield an average Dice score of 0.91 [67]. The Dice score is a standard statistic for assessing the spatial intersection between two images and ranges from 0 (no overlap) to 1 (perfect overlap) [68]. Therefore, a Dice score of 0.91 demonstrates that the technique was able to segment and estimate the volume of prostates with a high level of precision.

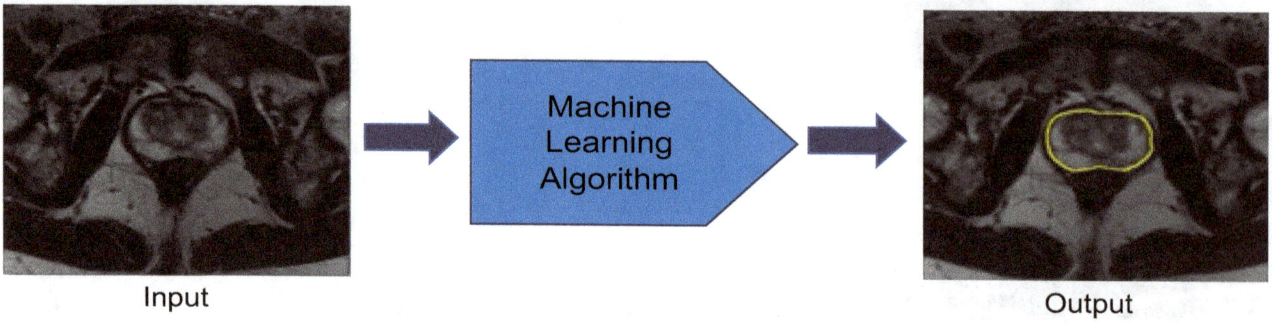

Figure 3. Prostate organ segmentation performed by machine learning methods. The computer takes multiparametric magnetic resonance imaging images as inputs and applies the developed machine learning algorithm to correctly identify the borders of the prostate.

Besides fuzzy c-means clustering, DL has been extensively used for complete prostate segmentation. In 2012, the release of the PROMISE12 challenge dataset, which contained 100 patients, prompted many studies on this topic [69,70]. Two groups led by Tian et al. [71] and Karimi et al. [70] both employed CNNs. Tian et al. [71] trained their CNN on T2-weighted mpMRI images from 140 patients and achieved a Dice score of 0.85. Karimi et al.'s [70] CNN was trained on a limited dataset of 49 T2-weighted mpMRI images supplemented by data augmentation. Their Dice score was 0.88. Both studies achieved high Dice scores and demonstrated that prostate segmentation could be achieved with commonly used technical designs.

Additionally, a uniquely designed DL network for biomedical images, U-Net, has also been proposed for complete prostate segmentation [72]. U-Net is an algorithm that successively compresses an image, derives features during these contractions, and classifies every pixel in the image [72]. Three studies used U-Net for prostate segmentation and obtained Dice scores of 0.89,

0.93, and 0.89 [73–75]. These three groups showed that U-Net could effectively segment the prostate with dataset sizes between 81 and 163 patients. The high Dice scores across multiple studies with comparable network architectures demonstrate substantial progress towards completely automated prostate segmentation and volume approximation. Table 1 lists the previously discussed studies along with several others that also segmented the prostate using various CNNs. To establish the ground truth label, which is used in establishing a Dice score, five studies used radiologists, two studies used clinicians of unstated specialties, one study used an expert, and one study used a radiologist for most of its data and an unnamed source for the rest of its data [67,70,71,73–78].

Table 1. Machine learning techniques applied to prostate organ segmentation.

Reference	Year	ML Algorithm	Patients	Dice	Modalities
Rundo et al. [67]	2017	Fuzzy C-means clustering. Features: T1 intensity, T2 intensity	21	0.91	T1W, T2W
Tian et al. [71]	2018	CNN: 7 layers	140	0.85	T2W
Karimi et al. [70]	2018	CNN: 3 layers	49	0.88	T2W
Clark et al. [73]	2017	CNN: U-Net	134	0.89	DWI
Zhu, Y. et al. [74]	2018	CNN: U-Net	163	0.93	DWI, T2W
Zhu, Q. et al. [75]	2017	CNN: U-Net	81	0.89	T2W
Milletari et al. [76]	2016	CNN: V-Net	80	0.87	T2W
Wang, B. et al. [77]	2019	CNN: 3D DSD-FCN	40	0.86	T2W
Cheng et al. [78]	2016	CNN and Active Appearance Model	120	0.93	T2W

5. Prostate Lesion: Detection, Segmentation, and Volume Estimation

Although prostate lesion detection, segmentation, and volume approximation could benefit PCa management, an effective tool that can automate these processes has not been created. For prostate lesion detection, satellite small lesions can be challenging to detect [19]. In a study by Steenbergen et al. [19], six different teams, each composed of one radiologist and one radiation oncologist, missed 66 out of 69 satellite lesions distributed across 20 patients. In addition to prostate lesion detection, segmentation is difficult because sparse tumors composed of benign glands and stroma are challenging to outline [79]. When segmentation across multiple institutions is compared, the contours reveal considerable differences [80]. As a result of inexact segmentation, volume approximation of prostate lesions is also challenging and often underestimates the histopathological volume [79]. This need for improved lesion metrics could be satisfied using ML algorithms that could learn to identify these features within mpMRI images.

For prostate lesion detection, ML approaches have been used to identify potential malignancies (Figure 4). Lay et al. [81] used a prostate computer-aided diagnosis (CAD) based on a random forest for prostate lesion detection (Table 2). This study's dataset used 224 patient cases across three sequences (T2-weighted, ADC, and DWI) for a total of 287 benign lesions and 123 lesions with a Gleason score of 6 or higher [81]. The Gleason scoring system describes PCa grades on a scale of 1 to 5 based on the pattern that the cancerous cells fall into, with 1 or 2 being low grade and 5 being high grade. It uses the combined grades of the most prominent and second most prominent patterns in a biopsy as the final score. A Gleason score of 6 or greater has malignant potential [82]. Lay et al.'s random forest technique yielded an area under the curve (AUC) score of 0.93 [81]; AUC is a measurement for binary classification and ranges from 0 to 1. Therefore, this study demonstrates that the ML model can detect lesions with high accuracy.

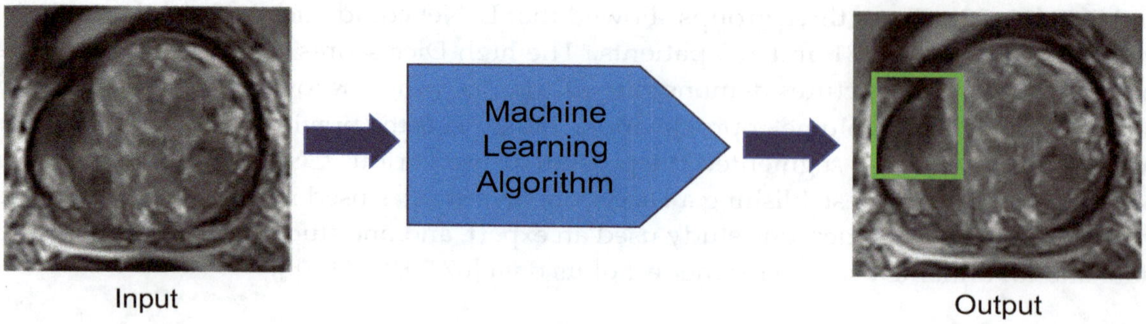

Figure 4. Prostate lesion detection using machine learning methods. The computer takes multiparametric magnetic resonance imaging images of the prostate as inputs and applies the developed machine learning algorithm to correctly localize lesions in the prostate.

Table 2. Machine learning techniques applied to prostate lesion detection.

Reference	Year	ML Algorithm	Patients	Lesions	AUC	Modalities
Lay et al. [81]	2017	Random Forest. Features: Intensity, Haralick texture	224	410	0.93	T2W, ADC, DWI
Sumathipala et al. [83]	2018	CNN: Holistically Nested Edge Detection	186	N/A	0.93	T2W, ADC, DWI
Xu et al. [84]	2019	CNN: ResNet	346	N/A	0.97	T2W, ADC, DWI
Tsehay et al. [85]	2017	CNN, 5 Layers	52	125	0.90	T2W, ADC, DWI

DL techniques have also been applied to prostate lesion detection (Table 2). Xu et al. [84] implemented a type of neural network with extensive layers, ResNet [86], to find lesions on T2-weighted, ADC, and DWI images. This study used images from the Cancer Imaging Archive data portal and included 346 patients. They achieved an AUC of 0.97 [84]. Tsehay et al. [85] also used a DL algorithm with a 5-layer CNN architecture that used an individual loss function for each layer. The CNN was trained and validated on a dataset of 39 benign lesions and 86 lesions with a Gleason 6 or higher [85]. Tsehay's group achieved an impressive AUC of 0.90 [85], which demonstrates high accuracy of prostate lesion detection. All four studies in Table 2 used radiologists for labeling the ground truth [81,83–85].

Although prostate lesion detection has been implemented with ML, automated prostate lesion segmentation and volume approximation remain largely unsolved (Figure 5). Few studies have attempted this task due to a dearth of well-curated data and its technical requirements. One obstacle for prostate lesion segmentation is a lack of guidelines across institutions for prostate lesion contours, which results in significant inter-observer variability [19,80]. Despite the lack of standardization, three studies have attempted prostate lesion segmentation (Table 3). A study by Liu et al. [87] used fuzzy Markov random fields to achieve a Dice score of 0.62 with 11 patients. Two other groups, Kohl et al. [88] and Dai et al. [89], both employed DL algorithms and used U-Net and Mask R-CNN, respectively. Kohl's group used a dataset of 152 patients and implemented U-Net combined with an adversarial network. Their architecture resulted in an average Dice score for prostate lesion segmentation of 0.41 [88]. Dai's group used a highly specialized DL algorithm, Mask R-CNN, and trained with 63 patients to achieve a prostate lesion Dice score of 0.46 [89]. To label the ground truth, Dai et al. [89] used a clinician, Kohl et al. [88] used a radiologist, and Liu et al. [87] used a pathologist. These studies' lower Dice scores demonstrate that the current techniques have limited precision. These studies show that prostate lesion segmentation and volume estimation remain challenging. A bigger dataset with more uniform labeling would permit the development of more ML models geared toward these tasks.

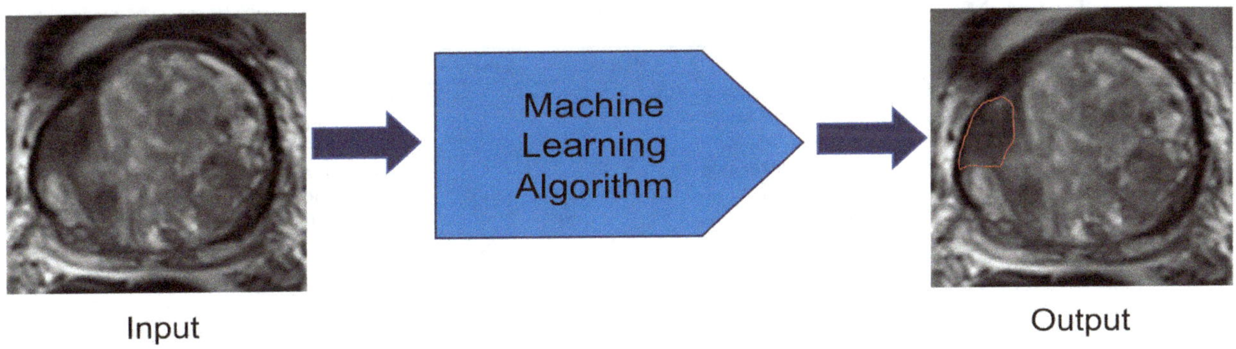

Figure 5. Prostate lesion segmentation using machine learning techniques. The computer takes multiparametric magnetic resonance imaging images of the prostate as inputs and applies the developed machine learning algorithm to correctly identify the borders of the lesion.

Table 3. Machine learning techniques applied to prostate lesion segmentation.

Reference	Year	ML Algorithm	Patients	Dice	Modalities
Dai et al. [89]	2019	CNN: Mask R-CNN	63	0.46	T2W, ADC
Kohl et al. [88]	2017	Adversarial Network and CNN: U-Net	152	0.41	T2W, ADC, DWI
Liu et al. [87]	2009	Fuzzy Markov Random Fields	11	0.62	T2W, quantitative T2, DWI, DCE

6. Prostate Lesion: Characterization

Although prostate lesions have been increasingly imaged with mpMRI since 2013 [4], their characterization has been hindered by the variability in classification conventions across different radiologists and institutions [4,47,90]. To establish better standardization, the PI-RADS scoring system was created in 2012, with an updated version PI-RADS v2 released in 2015, and the newest version PI-RADS v2.1 released in 2019 [53,54,91]. Since their conception, multiple studies have attempted to elucidate the clinical utility of PI-RADS, PI-RADS v2, and PI-RADS v2.1. Challenges to its broader acceptance include inter-reader agreement, radiologist experience, and the substantial interpretation time of images [4,47,90]. This need for more consistent lesion characterization makes ML an attractive method for accurate, quick classification.

ML algorithms can augment the PI-RADS scoring system as well as independently classify lesions (Table 4). Regarding PI-RADS, Litjens et al. [92] created a CAD system that applied a random forest for characterizing prostate lesions on a scale of suspicion for malignancy. After combining the ML generated scores and the radiologist provided PI-RADS scores on a dataset of 107 patients, the overall AUC was greater than either the ML generated scores or the PI-RADS scores [92]. Similarly, Wang, J. et al. [93], who used 54 patients in their dataset, also concluded that a support vector machine (SVM) algorithm enhanced the PI-RADS performance of radiologists. Song et al. [94] opted to use a DL algorithm based off of VGG-Net, a deep CNN, as a tool for improving PI-RADS scores assigned by radiologists. Song's group gathered data from 195 patients and also observed that their AUC improved when radiologists' decisions were combined with the VGG-Net [94].

Table 4. Machine-learning techniques applied to prostate lesion characterization.

Reference	Year	Algorithm	Patients	Lesions	AUC	Modalities
Litjens et al. [92]	2015	Random Forest. Features: Intensity, Position, Pharmacokinetic, Texture, Spatial Filter	107	141	Benign vs. Cancer; AUC increased from 0.81 to 0.88 with their ML tool Indolent vs. Aggressive; AUC increased from 0.78 to 0.88 with their ML tool	T2W, DCE, DWI
Wang, J. et al. [93]	2017	SVM. Features: Volumetric Radiomics	54	149	0.95	T2W, DWI
Song et al. [94]	2018	CNN: Deep CNN and Augmentation	195	547	0.94	T2W, ADC, DWI
Kwak et al. [95]	2015	SVM. Features: Texture	244	479	0.89	T2W, DWI
Wang, Z. et al. [96]	2018	CNN: Deep CNN	360	600	0.96	T2W, ADC
Seah et al. [97]	2017	CNN: Deep CNN	346	538	0.84	T2W, ADC, DCE
Liu et al. [98]	2017	CNN: XmasNet	341	538	0.84	T2W, ADC, DWI, Ktrans
Mehrtash et al. [99]	2017	CNN: 3D Implementation	344	538	0.80	ADC, DWI, DCE
Chen et al. [100]	2019	Two CNNs: Inception V3 and VGG-16	Training Data: 204 Test Data: N/A	538	Inception V3, 0.81 VGG-16, 0.83	T2W, DWI, DCE

In addition to bolstering lesion classification by radiologists, ML algorithms have been trained to characterize prostate lesions independently (Figure 6, Table 4). Many studies explored this task with the PROSTATEx challenge dataset that was released in 2017 [101]. The PROSTATEx dataset was gathered from 344 patients and contained segmented lesions along with their respective pathology-defined Gleason scores [101]. From this public database, Wang, Z. et al. [96] achieved an AUC of 0.96 by running two CNNs in parallel. Both Seah et al. [97] and Liu et al. [98] obtained an AUC of 0.84 by using deep layered CNNs. Mehrtash et al. [99] implemented a 3D CNN to reach an AUC of 0.80. One study by Kwak et al. [95] used its own proprietary dataset to implement an SVM that trained on T2-weighted and DWI images to characterize prostate lesions. In this study, 244 patients were used for a total of 333 benign and 146 malignant lesions [95]. The SVM method used discriminative features in training that resulted in an AUC score of 0.89 [95]. All of the studies listed in Table 4 used radiologists to determine their ground truth [77,92–95,97–100]. These studies highlight the ability of DL algorithms to predict the likelihood of a lesion's malignancy based upon Gleason scores.

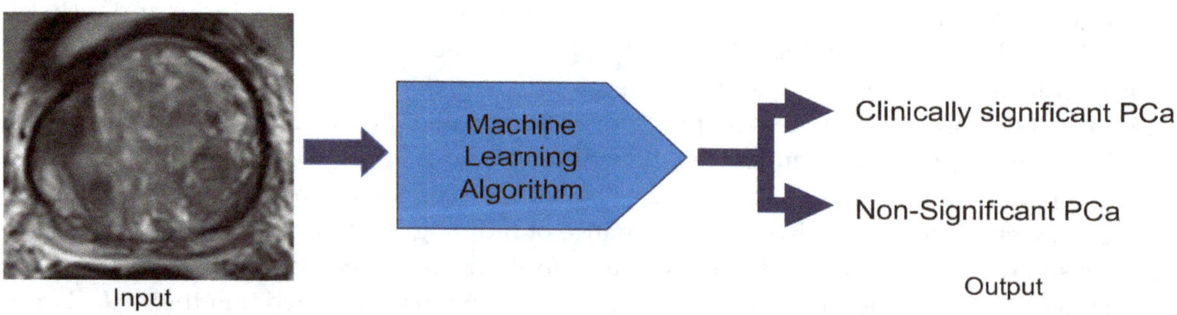

Figure 6. Prostate lesion characterization using machine-learning techniques. The computer receives multiparametric magnetic imaging images of prostate lesions and applies the developed machine learning algorithm to categorize the lesion as clinically significant prostate cancer or non-significant prostate cancer.

7. Future Work

The potential applications of ML to PCa surpass volume estimation, lesion detection, and lesion characterization. Further developments in prostate lesion classification may lead to a more practical clinical use, include training ML algorithms for tumor grade prediction. In addition to analyzing data solely from images, ML could augment the clinical management of PCa by incorporating demographic and biochemical data. ML could enable clinicians to make more assured decisions regarding the need for biopsy, medication dosing, and cancer recurrence. Biopsies that are performed for diagnosing PCa could be rendered unnecessary with a ML tool. Two studies by Hu et al. [102] and Chen et al. [103] used data such as age, digital rectal exam findings, PSA, and prostate volume for biopsy prediction. These studies made accurate PCa diagnoses and showed the potential for ML to eliminate the need for biopsy. In addition to diagnosis, ML could impact PCa medication dosing in PCa management. Radiation therapy requires accurate dosing, which is frequently operator dependent [104]. By minimizing operator dependency, ML could offer better standardization leading to more precise dosing. Nicola et al. [105] employed ML to predict prostate brachytherapy dosing by analyzing images and prior treatment plans from other patients. This study showed that ML implementation was comparable to brachytherapists and could be advanced by using a DL instead of a traditional ML algorithm. Along with diagnosis and dosing, ML could be used for predicting cancer recurrence after prostatectomy. Two studies by Wong et al. [106] and Cordon et al. [107] gathered data such as Gleason score, PSA, seminal vesical invasion, and surgical margins to predict recurrence after prostatectomy. The accuracy of these studies could be increased by adding postoperative imaging data for improved recurrence prediction.

8. Conclusions

AI applications in prostate mpMRI are promising tools for more effective and efficient image interpretation, leading to improved care. In pure image interpretation, ML has shown noteworthy progress in prostate organ segmentation and volume estimation. As better-curated data becomes available for prostate lesions, ML will likely become more successful at lesion detection, volume estimation, and characterization. As ML evolves, it will indisputably change radiologists' workflow by performing many of the simple tasks in image interpretation. However, ML will not replace the role of radiologists, who are critical to solving complex clinical problems [104]. AI is poised to enhance the decisions made by radiologists. It will enable radiologists to better care for their patients rather than supersede the need for radiologists.

Similarly, ML's ability to evaluate complex datasets across different domains suggests this technique may facilitate the bridging of advanced imaging, such as mpMRI, with emerging biomarker analysis or tumor genetics. Thus, ML may form the underpinnings of radiogenomics, allowing for the integration of imaging data, blood chemistry analysis, and pathologic evaluation in forming complex models that can predict treatment response. Enabled by larger datasets and more sophisticated mathematical techniques, ML could progress to creating completely automated tools that receive a patient's prostate mpMRI images and then delineate a range of desired features, as well as giving likelihood metrics for an array of pathologies.

References

1. Siegel, R.L.; Miller, K.D.; Jemal, A. Cancer statistics, 2017. *CA Cancer J. Clin.* **2017**, *67*, 7–30. [CrossRef] [PubMed]
2. Hugosson, J.; Carlsson, S. Overdetection in screening for prostate cancer. *Curr. Opin. Urol.* **2014**, *24*, 256–263. [CrossRef] [PubMed]
3. Schröder, F.H.; Hugosson, J.; Roobol, M.J.; Tammela, T.L.; Ciatto, S.; Nelen, V.; Kwiatkowski, M.; Lujan, M.; Lilja, H.; Zappa, M.; et al. Screening and prostate-cancer mortality in a randomized European study. *N. Engl. J. Med.* **2009**, *360*, 1320–1328. [CrossRef] [PubMed]

4. Oberlin, D.T.; Casalino, D.D.; Miller, F.H.; Meeks, J.J. Dramatic increase in the utilization of multiparametric magnetic resonance imaging for detection and management of prostate cancer. *Abdom. Radiol. (Ny)* **2017**, *42*, 1255–1258. [CrossRef] [PubMed]
5. Monni, F.; Fontanella, P.; Grasso, A.; Wiklund, P.; Ou, Y.C.; Randazzo, M.; Rocco, B.; Montanari, E.; Bianchi, G. Magnetic resonance imaging in prostate cancer detection and management: A systematic review. *Minerva. Urol. Nefrol.* **2017**, *69*, 567–578. [CrossRef] [PubMed]
6. Uzzo, R.G.; Wei, J.T.; Waldbaum, R.S.; Perlmutter, A.P.; Byrne, J.C.; Vaughan, D., Jr. The influence of prostate size on cancer detection. *Urology* **1995**, *46*, 831–836. [CrossRef]
7. Boyle, P.; Gould, A.L.; Roehrborn, C.G. Prostate volume predicts outcome of treatment of benign prostatic hyperplasia with finasteride: Meta-analysis of randomized clinical trials. *Urology* **1996**, *48*, 398–405. [CrossRef]
8. Sparks, R.; Bloch, B.N.; Feleppa, E.; Barratt, D.; Madabhushi, A. Fully automated prostate magnetic resonance imaging and transrectal ultrasound fusion via a probabilistic registration metric. *Proc. SPIE Int. Soc. Opt. Eng.* **2013**, *8671*. [CrossRef]
9. Tay, K.J.; Gupta, R.T.; Rastinehad, A.R.; Tsivian, E.; Freedland, S.J.; Moul, J.W.; Polascik, T.J. Navigating MRI-TRUS fusion biopsy: Optimizing the process and avoiding technical pitfalls. *Expert Rev. Anticancer Ther.* **2016**, *16*, 303–311. [CrossRef]
10. Lim, K.B. Epidemiology of clinical benign prostatic hyperplasia. *Asian J. Urol.* **2017**, *4*, 148–151. [CrossRef]
11. Garvey, B.; Türkbey, B.; Truong, H.; Bernardo, M.; Periaswamy, S.; Choyke, P.L. Clinical value of prostate segmentation and volume determination on MRI in benign prostatic hyperplasia. *Diagn. Interv. Radiol.* **2014**, *20*, 229. [CrossRef] [PubMed]
12. Kolman, C.; Girman, C.J.; Jacobsen, S.J.; Lieber, M.M. Distribution of post-void residual urine volume in randomly selected men. *J. Urol.* **1999**, *161*, 122–127. [CrossRef]
13. Girman, C.J.; Jacobsen, S.J.; Guess, H.A.; Oesterling, J.E.; Chute, C.G.; Panser, L.A.; Lieber, M.M. Natural history of prostatism: Relationship among symptoms, prostate volume and peak urinary flow rate. *J. Urol.* **1995**, *153*, 1510–1515. [CrossRef]
14. Oelke, M.; Bachmann, A.; Descazeaud, A.; Emberton, M.; Gravas, S.; Michel, M.C.; N'dow, J.; Nordling, J.; Jean, J. EAU guidelines on the treatment and follow-up of non-neurogenic male lower urinary tract symptoms including benign prostatic obstruction. *Eur. Urol.* **2013**, *64*, 118–140. [CrossRef] [PubMed]
15. Bretton, P.R.; Evans, W.P.; Borden, J.D.; Castellanos, R.D. The use of prostate specific antigen density to improve the sensitivity of prostate specific antigen in detecting prostate carcinoma. *Cancer Interdiscip. Int. J. Am. Cancer Soc.* **1994**, *74*, 2991–2995. [CrossRef]
16. Benson, M.C.; Seong Whang, I.; Pantuck, A.; Ring, K.; Kaplan, S.A.; Olsson, C.A.; Cooner, W.H. Prostate specific antigen density: A means of distinguishing benign prostatic hypertrophy and prostate cancer. *J. Urol.* **1992**, *147*, 815–816. [CrossRef]
17. Sfoungaristos, S.; Perimenis, P. PSA density is superior than PSA and Gleason score for adverse pathologic features prediction in patients with clinically localized prostate cancer. *Can. Urol. Assoc. J.* **2012**, *6*, 46. [CrossRef]
18. May, M.; Siegsmund, M.; Hammermann, F.; Loy, V.; Gunia, S. Visual estimation of the tumor volume in prostate cancer: A useful means for predicting biochemical-free survival after radical prostatectomy? *Prostate Cancer Prostatic Dis.* **2007**, *10*, 66. [CrossRef]
19. Steenbergen, P.; Haustermans, K.; Lerut, E.; Oyen, R.; De Wever, L.; Van den Bergh, L.; Kerkmeijer, L.G.; Pameijer, F.A.; Veldhuis, W.B.; Pos, F.J. Prostate tumor delineation using multiparametric magnetic resonance imaging: Inter-observer variability and pathology validation. *Radiother. Oncol.* **2015**, *115*, 186–190. [CrossRef]
20. Njeh, C. Tumor delineation: The weakest link in the search for accuracy in radiotherapy. *J. Med. Phys./Assoc. Med. Phys. India* **2008**, *33*, 136. [CrossRef]
21. Denis, L.J.; Murphy, G.P.; Schroder, F.H. Report of the consensus workshop on screening and global strategy for prostate cancer. *Cancer* **1995**, *75*, 1187–1207. [CrossRef]
22. Edwards, B.K.; Ward, E.; Kohler, B.A.; Eheman, C.; Zauber, A.G.; Anderson, R.N.; Jemal, A.; Schymura, M.J.; Lansdorp-Vogelaar, I.; Seeff, L.C.; et al. Annual report to the nation on the status of cancer, 1975-2006, featuring colorectal cancer trends and impact of interventions (risk factors, screening, and treatment) to reduce future rates. *Cancer* **2010**, *116*, 544–573. [CrossRef] [PubMed]

23. Etzioni, R.; Tsodikov, A.; Mariotto, A.; Szabo, A.; Falcon, S.; Wegelin, J.; DiTommaso, D.; Karnofski, K.; Gulati, R.; Penson, D.F.; et al. Quantifying the role of PSA screening in the US prostate cancer mortality decline. *Cancer Causes Control.* **2008**, *19*, 175–181. [CrossRef] [PubMed]
24. Lahdensuo, K.; Erickson, A.; Saarinen, I.; Seikkula, H.; Lundin, J.; Lundin, M.; Nordling, S.; Bützow, A.; Vasarainen, H.; Bostrom, P.J.; et al. Loss of PTEN expression in ERG-negative prostate cancer predicts secondary therapies and leads to shorter disease-specific survival time after radical prostatectomy. *Mod. Pathol.* **2016**, *29*, 1565–1574. [CrossRef]
25. Rothwax, J.T.; George, A.K.; Wood, B.J.; Pinto, P.A. Multiparametric MRI in biopsy guidance for prostate cancer: Fusion-guided. *Biomed. Res. Int.* **2014**, *2014*, 439171. [CrossRef]
26. Lips, I.M.; van der Heide, U.A.; Haustermans, K.; van Lin, E.N.; Pos, F.; Franken, S.P.; Kotte, A.N.; van Gils, C.H.; van Vulpen, M. Single blind randomized phase III trial to investigate the benefit of a focal lesion ablative microboost in prostate cancer (FLAME-trial): Study protocol for a randomized controlled trial. *Trials* **2011**, *12*, 255. [CrossRef]
27. Cellini, N.; Morganti, A.G.; Mattiucci, G.C.; Valentini, V.; Leone, M.; Luzi, S.; Manfredi, R.; Dinapoli, N.; Digesu', C.; Smaniotto, D. Analysis of intraprostatic failures in patients treated with hormonal therapy and radiotherapy: Implications for conformal therapy planning. *Int. J. Radiat. Oncol. Biol. Phys.* **2002**, *53*, 595–599. [CrossRef]
28. Chun, F.K.-H.; Briganti, A.; Jeldres, C.; Gallina, A.; Erbersdobler, A.; Schlomm, T.; Walz, J.; Eichelberg, C.; Salomon, G.; Haese, A. Tumour volume and high grade tumour volume are the best predictors of pathologic stage and biochemical recurrence after radical prostatectomy. *Eur. J. Cancer* **2007**, *43*, 536–543. [CrossRef]
29. Chung, B.I.; Tarin, T.V.; Ferrari, M.; Brooks, J.D. Comparison of prostate cancer tumor volume and percent cancer in prediction of biochemical recurrence and cancer specific survival. *Urol. Oncol.* **2011**, *29*, 314–318. [CrossRef]
30. Nelson, B.A.; Shappell, S.B.; Chang, S.S.; Wells, N.; Farnham, S.B.; Smith, J.A., Jr.; Cookson, M.S. Tumour volume is an independent predictor of prostate-specific antigen recurrence in patients undergoing radical prostatectomy for clinically localized prostate cancer. *BJU Int.* **2006**, *97*, 1169–1172. [CrossRef]
31. Fukuhara, H.; Kume, H.; Suzuki, M.; Fujimura, T.; Enomoto, Y.; Nishimatsu, H.; Ishikawa, A.; Homma, Y. Maximum tumor diameter: A simple independent predictor for biochemical recurrence after radical prostatectomy. *Prostate Cancer Prostatic Dis.* **2010**, *13*, 244. [CrossRef] [PubMed]
32. Stephenson, A.J.; Scardino, P.T.; Kattan, M.W.; Pisansky, T.M.; Slawin, K.M.; Klein, E.A.; Anscher, M.S.; Michalski, J.M.; Sandler, H.M.; Lin, D.W. Predicting the outcome of salvage radiation therapy for recurrent prostate cancer after radical prostatectomy. *J. Clin. Oncol. Off. J. Am. Soc. Clin. Oncol.* **2007**, *25*, 2035. [CrossRef] [PubMed]
33. Bjurlin, M.A.; Taneja, S.S. Standards for prostate biopsy. *Curr. Opin. Urol.* **2014**, *24*, 155–161. [CrossRef] [PubMed]
34. Borghesi, M.; Ahmed, H.; Nam, R.; Schaeffer, E.; Schiavina, R.; Taneja, S.; Weidner, W.; Loeb, S. Complications After Systematic, Random, and Image-guided Prostate Biopsy. *Eur. Urol.* **2017**, *71*, 353–365. [CrossRef] [PubMed]
35. Walsh, P.C.; Marschke, P.; Ricker, D.; Burnett, A.L. Patient-reported urinary continence and sexual function after anatomic radical prostatectomy. *Urology* **2000**, *55*, 58–61. [CrossRef]
36. Hu, K.; Wallner, K. Clinical course of rectal bleeding following I-125 prostate brachytherapy. *Int. J. Radiat. Oncol. Biol. Phys.* **1998**, *41*, 263–265. [CrossRef]
37. Theodorescu, D.; Gillenwater, J.Y.; Koutrouvelis, P.G. Prostatourethral-rectal fistula after prostate brachytherapy: Incidence and risk factors. *Cancer Interdiscip. Int. J. Am. Cancer Soc.* **2000**, *89*, 2085–2091. [CrossRef]
38. Shaver, M.M.; Kohanteb, P.A.; Chiou, C.; Bardis, M.D.; Chantaduly, C.; Bota, D.; Filippi, C.G.; Weinberg, B.; Grinband, J.; Chow, D.S. Optimizing neuro-oncology imaging: A review of deep learning approaches for glioma imaging. *Cancers* **2019**, *11*, 829. [CrossRef]
39. Jordan, M.I.; Mitchell, T.M. Machine learning: Trends, perspectives, and prospects. *Science* **2015**, *349*, 255–260. [CrossRef]
40. Johnson, L.M.; Turkbey, B.; Figg, W.D.; Choyke, P.L. Multiparametric MRI in prostate cancer management. *Nat. Rev. Clin. Oncol.* **2014**, *11*, 346–353. [CrossRef]

41. Stabile, A.; Giganti, F.; Rosenkrantz, A.B.; Taneja, S.S.; Villeirs, G.; Gill, I.S.; Allen, C.; Emberton, M.; Moore, C.M.; Kasivisvanathan, V. Multiparametric MRI for prostate cancer diagnosis: Current status and future directions. *Nat. Rev. Urol.* **2020**, *17*, 41–61. [CrossRef] [PubMed]
42. Dickinson, L.; Ahmed, H.U.; Allen, C.; Barentsz, J.O.; Carey, B.; Futterer, J.J.; Heijmink, S.W.; Hoskin, P.J.; Kirkham, A.; Padhani, A.R.; et al. Magnetic resonance imaging for the detection, localisation, and characterisation of prostate cancer: Recommendations from a European consensus meeting. *Eur. Urol.* **2011**, *59*, 477–494. [CrossRef] [PubMed]
43. De Rooij, M.; Hamoen, E.H.; Futterer, J.J.; Barentsz, J.O.; Rovers, M.M. Accuracy of multiparametric MRI for prostate cancer detection: A meta-analysis. *AJR Am. J. Roentgenol.* **2014**, *202*, 343–351. [CrossRef] [PubMed]
44. Fütterer, J.J.; Briganti, A.; De Visschere, P.; Emberton, M.; Giannarini, G.; Kirkham, A.; Taneja, S.S.; Thoeny, H.; Villeirs, G.; Villers, A. Can clinically significant prostate cancer be detected with multiparametric magnetic resonance imaging? A systematic review of the literature. *Eur. Urol.* **2015**, *68*, 1045–1053. [CrossRef] [PubMed]
45. Daun, M.; Fardin, S.; Ushinsky, A.; Batra, S.; Nguyentat, M.; Lee, T.; Uchio, E.; Lall, C.; Houshyar, R. PI-RADS version 2 is an excellent screening tool for clinically significant prostate cancer as designated by the validated international society of urological pathology criteria: A retrospective analysis. *Curr. Probl. Diagn. Radiol.* **2019**. [CrossRef]
46. Turkbey, B.; Mani, H.; Shah, V.; Rastinehad, A.R.; Bernardo, M.; Pohida, T.; Pang, Y.; Daar, D.; Benjamin, C.; McKinney, Y.L.; et al. Multiparametric 3T prostate magnetic resonance imaging to detect cancer: Histopathological correlation using prostatectomy specimens processed in customized magnetic resonance imaging based molds. *J. Urol.* **2011**, *186*, 1818–1824. [CrossRef]
47. Leake, J.L.; Hardman, R.; Ojili, V.; Thompson, I.; Shanbhogue, A.; Hernandez, J.; Barentsz, J. Prostate MRI: Access to and current practice of prostate MRI in the United States. *J. Am. Coll. Radiol.* **2014**, *11*, 156–160. [CrossRef]
48. Latchamsetty, K.C.; Borden, L.S., Jr.; Porter, C.R.; Lacrampe, M.; Vaughan, M.; Lin, E.; Conti, N.; Wright, J.L.; Corman, J.M. Experience improves staging accuracy of endorectal magnetic resonance imaging in prostate cancer: What is the learning curve? *Can. J. Urol.* **2007**, *14*, 3429–3434.
49. Gaziev, G.; Wadhwa, K.; Barrett, T.; Koo, B.C.; Gallagher, F.A.; Serrao, E.; Frey, J.; Seidenader, J.; Carmona, L.; Warren, A.; et al. Defining the learning curve for multiparametric magnetic resonance imaging (MRI) of the prostate using MRI-transrectal ultrasonography (TRUS) fusion-guided transperineal prostate biopsies as a validation tool. *BJU Int.* **2016**, *117*, 80–86. [CrossRef]
50. Rosenkrantz, A.B.; Babb, J.S.; Taneja, S.S.; Ream, J.M. Proposed adjustments to PI-RADS Version 2 decision rules: Impact on prostate cancer detection. *Radiology* **2017**, *283*, 119–129. [CrossRef]
51. De Visschere, P.J.; Vral, A.; Perletti, G.; Pattyn, E.; Praet, M.; Magri, V.; Villeirs, G.M. Multiparametric magnetic resonance imaging characteristics of normal, benign and malignant conditions in the prostate. *Eur. Radiol.* **2017**, *27*, 2095–2109. [CrossRef] [PubMed]
52. Barentsz, J.O.; Richenberg, J.; Clements, R.; Choyke, P.; Verma, S.; Villeirs, G.; Rouviere, O.; Logager, V.; Futterer, J.J.; European Society of Urogenital, R. ESUR prostate MR guidelines 2012. *Eur. Radiol.* **2012**, *22*, 746–757. [CrossRef] [PubMed]
53. Weinreb, J.C.; Barentsz, J.O.; Choyke, P.L.; Cornud, F.; Haider, M.A.; Macura, K.J.; Margolis, D.; Schnall, M.D.; Shtern, F.; Tempany, C.M.; et al. PI-RADS Prostate imaging—Reporting and data system: 2015, version 2. *Eur. Urol.* **2016**, *69*, 16–40. [CrossRef] [PubMed]
54. Turkbey, B.; Rosenkrantz, A.B.; Haider, M.A.; Padhani, A.R.; Villeirs, G.; Macura, K.J.; Tempany, C.M.; Choyke, P.L.; Cornud, F.; Margolis, D.J.; et al. Prostate imaging reporting and data system version 2.1: 2019 update of prostate imaging reporting and data system version 2. *Eur. Urol.* **2019**, *76*, 340–351. [CrossRef] [PubMed]
55. Stonier, T. The evolution of machine intelligence. In *Beyond Information: The Natural History of Intelligence*; Springer: London, UK, 1992; pp. 107–133. [CrossRef]
56. Poole, D.; Mackworth, A.; Goebel, R. *Computational Intelligence*; Oxford University Press: Oxford, UK, 1998; Volume 1.
57. Goodfellow, I.; Bengio, Y.; Courville, A. *Deep Learning*; MIT Press: Cambridge, MA, USA, 2016.
58. Krizhevsky, A.; Sutskever, I.; Hinton, G.E. Imagenet classification with deep convolutional neural networks. In Proceedings of the Advances in Neural information Processing Systems, Lake Tahoe, NV, USA, 3–6 December 2012; pp. 1097–1105.

59. LeCun, Y.; Bengio, Y.; Hinton, G. Deep learning. *Nature* **2015**, *521*, 436. [CrossRef] [PubMed]
60. Ueda, D.; Shimazaki, A.; Miki, Y. Technical and clinical overview of deep learning in radiology. *Jpn. J. Radiol.* **2019**, *37*, 15–33. [CrossRef] [PubMed]
61. Ghose, S.; Oliver, A.; Martí, R.; Lladó, X.; Vilanova, J.C.; Freixenet, J.; Mitra, J.; Sidibé, D.; Meriaudeau, F. A survey of prostate segmentation methodologies in ultrasound, magnetic resonance and computed tomography images. *Comput. Methods Prog. Biomed.* **2012**, *108*, 262–287. [CrossRef] [PubMed]
62. Rasch, C.; Barillot, I.; Remeijer, P.; Touw, A.; van Herk, M.; Lebesque, J.V. Definition of the prostate in CT and MRI: A multi-observer study. *Int. J. Radiat. Oncol. Biol. Phys.* **1999**, *43*, 57–66. [CrossRef]
63. Kachouie, N.N.; Fieguth, P.; Rahnamayan, S. An elliptical level set method for automatic TRUS prostate image segmentation. In Proceedings of the 2006 IEEE International Symposium on Signal Processing and Information Technology, Vancouver, BC, Canada, 27–30 August 2006; pp. 191–196.
64. Ko, J.S.; Landis, P.; Carter, H.B.; Partin, A.W. Effect of intra-observer variation in prostate volume measurement on prostate-specific antigen density calculations among prostate cancer active surveillance participants. *BJU Int.* **2011**, *108*, 1739–1742. [CrossRef]
65. Dianat, S.S.; Ruiz, R.M.R.; Bonekamp, D.; Carter, H.B.; Macura, K.J. Prostate volumetric assessment by magnetic resonance imaging and transrectal ultrasound: Impact of variation in calculated prostate-specific antigen density on patient eligibility for active surveillance program. *J. Comput. Assist. Tomogr.* **2013**, *37*, 589–595. [CrossRef]
66. Bezinque, A.; Moriarity, A.; Farrell, C.; Peabody, H.; Noyes, S.L.; Lane, B.R. Determination of prostate volume: A comparison of contemporary methods. *Acad. Radiol.* **2018**, *25*, 1582–1587. [CrossRef] [PubMed]
67. Rundo, L.; Militello, C.; Russo, G.; Garufi, A.; Vitabile, S.; Gilardi, M.C.; Mauri, G. Automated prostate gland segmentation based on an unsupervised fuzzy C-means clustering technique using multispectral T1w and T2w MR imaging. *Information* **2017**, *8*, 49. [CrossRef]
68. Zou, K.H.; Warfield, S.K.; Bharatha, A.; Tempany, C.M.; Kaus, M.R.; Haker, S.J.; Wells III, W.M.; Jolesz, F.A.; Kikinis, R. Statistical validation of image segmentation quality based on a spatial overlap index1: Scientific reports. *Acad. Radiol.* **2004**, *11*, 178–189. [CrossRef]
69. Litjens, G.; Toth, R.; van de Ven, W.; Hoeks, C.; Kerkstra, S.; van Ginneken, B.; Vincent, G.; Guillard, G.; Birbeck, N.; Zhang, J.; et al. Evaluation of prostate segmentation algorithms for MRI: The PROMISE12 challenge. *Med. Image Anal.* **2014**, *18*, 359–373. [CrossRef] [PubMed]
70. Karimi, D.; Samei, G.; Kesch, C.; Nir, G.; Salcudean, S.E. Prostate segmentation in MRI using a convolutional neural network architecture and training strategy based on statistical shape models. *Int. J. Comput. Assist. Radiol. Surg.* **2018**. [CrossRef] [PubMed]
71. Tian, Z.; Liu, L.; Zhang, Z.; Fei, B. PSNet: Prostate segmentation on MRI based on a convolutional neural network. *J. Med. Imaging* **2018**, *5*, 021208. [CrossRef]
72. Ronneberger, O.; Fischer, P.; Brox, T. U-net: Convolutional networks for biomedical image segmentation. In Proceedings of the 2015 International Conference on Medical Image Computing and Computer-Assisted Intervention, Munich, Germany, 5–9 October 2015; pp. 234–241.
73. Clark, T.; Wong, A.; Haider, M.A.; Khalvati, F. *Fully Deep Convolutional Neural Networks for Segmentation of the Prostate Gland in Diffusion-Weighted MR Images*; Springer: Cham, Switzerland, 2017; pp. 97–104.
74. Zhu, Y.; Wei, R.; Gao, G.; Ding, L.; Zhang, X.; Wang, X.; Zhang, J. Fully automatic segmentation on prostate MR images based on cascaded fully convolution network. *J. Magn. Reson. Imaging* **2018**, *49*, 1149–1156. [CrossRef]
75. Zhu, Q.; Du, B.; Turkbey, B.; Choyke, P.L.; Yan, P. Deeply-supervised CNN for prostate segmentation. In Proceedings of the 2017 International Joint Conference on Neural Networks (IJCNN), Anchorage, AK, USA, 14–19 May 2017; pp. 178–184.
76. Milletari, F.; Navab, N.; Ahmadi, S.-A. V-net: Fully convolutional neural networks for volumetric medical image segmentation. In Proceedings of the 2016 Fourth International Conference on 3D Vision (3DV), Stanford, CA, USA, 25–28 October 2016; pp. 565–571.
77. Wang, B.; Lei, Y.; Tian, S.; Wang, T.; Liu, Y.; Patel, P.; Jani, A.B.; Mao, H.; Curran, W.J.; Liu, T.; et al. Deeply supervised 3D fully convolutional networks with group dilated convolution for automatic MRI prostate segmentation. *Med. Phys.* **2019**, *46*, 1707–1718. [CrossRef]

78. Cheng, R.; Roth, H.R.; Lu, L.; Wang, S.; Turkbey, B.; Gandler, W.; McCreedy, E.S.; Agarwal, H.K.; Choyke, P.; Summers, R.M. Active appearance model and deep learning for more accurate prostate segmentation on MRI. In Proceedings of the Medical Imaging 2016: Image Processing, San Diego, CA, USA, 27 February–3 March 2016; p. 97842I.
79. Le Nobin, J.; Orczyk, C.; Deng, F.M.; Melamed, J.; Rusinek, H.; Taneja, S.S.; Rosenkrantz, A.B. Prostate tumour volumes: Evaluation of the agreement between magnetic resonance imaging and histology using novel co-registration software. *BJU Int.* **2014**, *114*, E105–E112. [CrossRef]
80. Van Schie, M.A.; Dinh, C.V.; van Houdt, P.J.; Pos, F.J.; Heijmink, S.W.; Kerkmeijer, L.G.; Kotte, A.N.; Oyen, R.; Haustermans, K.; van der Heide, U.A. Contouring of prostate tumors on multiparametric MRI: Evaluation of clinical delineations in a multicenter radiotherapy trial. *Radiother. Oncol.* **2018**, *128*, 321–326. [CrossRef]
81. Lay, N.; Tsehay, Y.; Greer, M.D.; Turkbey, B.; Kwak, J.T.; Choyke, P.L.; Pinto, P.; Wood, B.J.; Summers, R.M. Detection of prostate cancer in multiparametric MRI using random forest with instance weighting. *J. Med. Imaging (Bellingham)* **2017**, *4*, 024506. [CrossRef] [PubMed]
82. Epstein, J.I.; Zelefsky, M.J.; Sjoberg, D.D.; Nelson, J.B.; Egevad, L.; Magi-Galluzzi, C.; Vickers, A.J.; Parwani, A.V.; Reuter, V.E.; Fine, S.W. A contemporary prostate cancer grading system: A validated alternative to the Gleason score. *Eur. Urol.* **2016**, *69*, 428–435. [CrossRef] [PubMed]
83. Sumathipala, Y.; Lay, N.; Turkbey, B.; Smith, C.; Choyke, P.L.; Summers, R.M. Prostate cancer detection from multi-institution multiparametric MRIs using deep convolutional neural networks. *J. Med. Imaging* **2018**, *5*, 044507. [CrossRef] [PubMed]
84. Xu, H.; Baxter, J.S.; Akin, O.; Cantor-Rivera, D. Prostate cancer detection using residual networks. *Int. J. Comput. Assist. Radiol. Surg.* **2019**, *14*, 1647–1650. [CrossRef]
85. Tsehay, Y.K.; Lay, N.S.; Roth, H.R.; Wang, X.; Kwak, J.T.; Turkbey, B.I.; Pinto, P.A.; Wood, B.J.; Summers, R.M. Convolutional neural network based deep-learning architecture for prostate cancer detection on multiparametric magnetic resonance images. In *Medical Imaging 2017: Computer-Aided Diagnosis*; SPIE: Bellingham, WA, USA, 2017; p. 1013405. [CrossRef]
86. He, K.; Zhang, X.; Ren, S.; Sun, J. Deep residual learning for image recognition. In Proceedings of the 2016 IEEE Conference on Computer Vision and Pattern Recognition, Las vegas, NV, USA, 26 June–1 July 2016; pp. 770–778.
87. Liu, X.; Langer, D.L.; Haider, M.A.; Yang, Y.; Wernick, M.N.; Yetik, I.S. Prostate cancer segmentation with simultaneous estimation of Markov random field parameters and class. *IEEE Trans. Med. Imaging* **2009**, *28*, 906–915. [CrossRef]
88. Kohl, S.; Bonekamp, D.; Schlemmer, H.-P.; Yaqubi, K.; Hohenfellner, M.; Hadaschik, B.; Radtke, J.-P.; Maier-Hein, K. Adversarial networks for the detection of aggressive prostate cancer. *ArXiv* **2017**, arXiv:1702.08014.
89. Dai, Z.; Carver, E.; Liu, C.; Lee, J.; Feldman, A.; Zong, W.; Pantelic, M.; Elshaikh, M.; Wen, N. Segmentation of the Prostatic Gland and the Intraprostatic Lesions on Multiparametic MRI Using Mask-RCNN. *ArXiv* **2019**, arXiv:1904.02575.
90. Dickinson, L.; Ahmed, H.U.; Allen, C.; Barentsz, J.O.; Carey, B.; Futterer, J.J.; Heijmink, S.W.; Hoskin, P.; Kirkham, A.P.; Padhani, A.R. Scoring systems used for the interpretation and reporting of multiparametric MRI for prostate cancer detection, localization, and characterization: Could standardization lead to improved utilization of imaging within the diagnostic pathway? *J. Magn. Reson. Imaging* **2013**, *37*, 48–58. [CrossRef]
91. Nguyentat, M.; Ushinsky, A.; Miranda-Aguirre, A.; Uchio, E.; Lall, C.; Shirkhoda, L.; Lee, T.; Green, C.; Houshyar, R. Validation of Prostate Imaging-Reporting and Data System Version 2: A Retrospective Analysis. *Curr. Probl. Diagn. Radiol.* **2018**, *47*, 404–409. [CrossRef]
92. Litjens, G.J.; Barentsz, J.O.; Karssemeijer, N.; Huisman, H.J. Clinical evaluation of a computer-aided diagnosis system for determining cancer aggressiveness in prostate MRI. *Eur. Radiol.* **2015**, *25*, 3187–3199. [CrossRef]
93. Wang, J.; Wu, C.-J.; Bao, M.-L.; Zhang, J.; Wang, X.-N.; Zhang, Y.-D. Machine learning-based analysis of MR radiomics can help to improve the diagnostic performance of PI-RADS v2 in clinically relevant prostate cancer. *Eur. Radiol.* **2017**, *27*, 4082–4090. [CrossRef] [PubMed]
94. Song, Y.; Zhang, Y.D.; Yan, X.; Liu, H.; Zhou, M.; Hu, B.; Yang, G. Computer-aided diagnosis of prostate cancer using a deep convolutional neural network from multiparametric MRI. *J. Magn. Reson. Imaging* **2018**, *48*, 1570–1577. [CrossRef] [PubMed]

95. Kwak, J.T.; Xu, S.; Wood, B.J.; Turkbey, B.; Choyke, P.L.; Pinto, P.A.; Wang, S.; Summers, R.M. Automated prostate cancer detection using T2-weighted and high-b-value diffusion-weighted magnetic resonance imaging. *Med. Phys.* **2015**, *42*, 2368–2378. [CrossRef] [PubMed]
96. Wang, Z.; Liu, C.; Cheng, D.; Wang, L.; Yang, X.; Cheng, K.-T. Automated detection of clinically significant prostate cancer in mp-MRI images based on an end-to-end deep neural network. *IEEE Trans. Med. Imaging* **2018**, *37*, 1127–1139. [CrossRef]
97. Seah, J.C.; Tang, J.S.; Kitchen, A. Detection of prostate cancer on multiparametric MRI. In Proceedings of the Medical Imaging 2017: Computer-Aided Diagnosis, Orlando, FL, USA, 13–16 February 2017; p. 1013429.
98. Liu, S.; Zheng, H.; Feng, Y.; Li, W. Prostate cancer diagnosis using deep learning with 3D multiparametric MRI. In Proceedings of the Medical Imaging 2017: Computer-Aided Diagnosis, Orlando, FL, USA, 13–16 February 2017; p. 1013428.
99. Mehrtash, A.; Sedghi, A.; Ghafoorian, M.; Taghipour, M.; Tempany, C.M.; Wells, W.M., III; Kapur, T.; Mousavi, P.; Abolmaesumi, P.; Fedorov, A. Classification of clinical significance of MRI prostate findings using 3D convolutional neural networks. *Proc. Spie Int. Soc. Opt. Eng.* **2017**, *10134*. [CrossRef]
100. Chen, Q.; Hu, S.; Long, P.; Lu, F.; Shi, Y.; Li, Y. A transfer learning approach for malignant prostate lesion detection on multiparametric MRI. *Technol. Cancer Res. Treat.* **2019**, *18*. [CrossRef]
101. Armato, S.G.; Huisman, H.; Drukker, K.; Hadjiiski, L.; Kirby, J.S.; Petrick, N.; Redmond, G.; Giger, M.L.; Cha, K.; Mamonov, A. PROSTATEx Challenges for computerized classification of prostate lesions from multiparametric magnetic resonance images. *J. Med. Imaging* **2018**, *5*, 044501. [CrossRef]
102. Hu, X.; Cammann, H.; Meyer, H.-A.; Miller, K.; Jung, K.; Stephan, C. Artificial neural networks and prostate cancer—Tools for diagnosis and management. *Nat. Rev. Urol.* **2013**, *10*, 174. [CrossRef]
103. Chen, T.; Li, M.; Gu, Y.; Zhang, Y.; Yang, S.; Wei, C.; Wu, J.; Li, X.; Zhao, W.; Shen, J. Prostate cancer differentiation and aggressiveness: Assessment with a radiomic-based model vs. PI-RADS v2. *J. Magn. Reson. Imaging* **2019**, *49*, 875–884. [CrossRef]
104. European Society of Radiology. What the radiologist should know about artificial intelligence—An ESR white paper. *Insights Imaging* **2019**, *10*, 44. [CrossRef]
105. Nicolae, A.; Morton, G.; Chung, H.; Loblaw, A.; Jain, S.; Mitchell, D.; Lu, L.; Helou, J.; Al-Hanaqta, M.; Heath, E.; et al. Evaluation of a machine-learning algorithm for treatment planning in prostate low-dose-rate brachytherapy. *Int. J. Radiat. Oncol. Biol. Phys.* **2017**, *97*, 822–829. [CrossRef]
106. Wong, N.C.; Lam, C.; Patterson, L.; Shayegan, B. Use of machine learning to predict early biochemical recurrence after robot-assisted prostatectomy. *BJU Int.* **2019**, *123*, 51–57. [CrossRef] [PubMed]
107. Cordon-Cardo, C.; Kotsianti, A.; Verbel, D.A.; Teverovskiy, M.; Capodieci, P.; Hamann, S.; Jeffers, Y.; Clayton, M.; Elkhettabi, F.; Khan, F.M.; et al. Improved prediction of prostate cancer recurrence through systems pathology. *J. Clin. Invest.* **2007**, *117*, 1876–1883. [CrossRef] [PubMed]

10

FOXA1 Gene Expression for Defining Molecular Subtypes of Muscle-Invasive Bladder Cancer after Radical Cystectomy

Danijel Sikic [1,*], Markus Eckstein [2], Ralph M. Wirtz [3], Jonas Jarczyk [4], Thomas S. Worst [4], Stefan Porubsky [5], Bastian Keck [1], Frank Kunath [1], Veronika Weyerer [2], Johannes Breyer [6], Wolfgang Otto [6], Sebastien Rinaldetti [7], Christian Bolenz [8], Arndt Hartmann [2], Bernd Wullich [1] and Philipp Erben [4] on behalf of the BRIDGE Consortium e.V., Germany

1. Department of Urology and Pediatric Urology, University Hospital Erlangen, Friedrich-Alexander University Erlangen-Nuremberg, 91054 Erlangen, Germany; bastian.keck@web.de (B.K.); frank.kunath@uk-erlangen.de (F.K.); bernd.wullich@uk-erlangen.de (B.W.)
2. Institute of Pathology, University Hospital Erlangen, Friedrich-Alexander University Erlangen-Nuremberg, 91054 Erlangen, Germany; markus.eckstein@uk-erlangen.de (M.E.); veronika.weyerer@uk-erlangen.de (V.W.); arndt.hartmann@uk-erlangen.de (A.H.)
3. STRATIFYER Molecular Pathology GmbH, 50935 Cologne, Germany; ralph.wirtz@STRATIFYER.de
4. Department of Urology, University Medical Centre Mannheim, Medical Faculty Mannheim, University of Heidelberg, 68167 Mannheim, Germany; jonas.jarczyk@umm.de (J.J.); thomas.worst@umm.de (T.S.W.); philipp.erben@medma.uni-heidelberg.de (P.E.)
5. Institute of Pathology, University Medical Centre Mannheim, Medical Faculty Mannheim, University of Heidelberg, 68167 Mannheim, Germany; stefan.porubsky@umm.de
6. Department of Urology, University of Regensburg, 93053 Regensburg, Germany; johannes.breyer@ukr.de (J.B.); wolfgang.otto@ukr.de (W.O.)
7. Department of Hematology and Oncology, University Medical Centre Mannheim, Medical Faculty Mannheim, University of Heidelberg, 68167 Mannheim, Germany; sebastien.rinaldetti@medma.uni-heidelberg.de
8. Department of Urology and Pediatric Urology, University Hospital Ulm, 89081 Ulm, Germany; christian.bolenz@uniklinik-ulm.de

* Correspondence: danijel.sikic@uk-erlangen.de

Abstract: It remains unclear how to implement the recently revealed basal and luminal subtypes of muscle-invasive bladder cancer (MIBC) into daily clinical routine and whether molecular marker panels can be reduced. The mRNA expression of basal (KRT5) and luminal (FOXA1, GATA3, KRT20) markers was measured by reverse transcription quantitative real-time polymerase chain reaction (RT-qPCR) and correlated to clinicopathological features, recurrence-free survival (RFS), disease-free survival (DFS), and overall survival (OS) in 80 patients with MIBC who underwent radical cystectomy. Additionally, the correlation of single markers with the basal and non-basal subtypes defined by a 36-gene panel was examined and then validated in the TCGA (The Cancer Genome Atlas) cohort. High expression of FOXA1 (p = 0.0048) and KRT20 (p = 0.0317) was associated with reduced RFS. In the multivariable analysis, only FOXA1 remained an independent prognostic marker for DFS (p = 0.0333) and RFS (p = 0.0310). FOXA1 expression (AUC = 0.79; p = 0.0007) was closest to the combined marker expression (AUC = 0.79; p = 0.0015) in resembling the non-basal subtype defined by the 36-gene panel. FOXA1 in combination with KRT5 may be used to distinguish the basal and non-basal subtypes of MIBC.

Keywords: FOXA1; GATA3; KRT20; molecular markers; mRNA; muscle-invasive bladder cancer; PCR; urothelial carcinoma

---

1. Introduction

Urothelial carcinoma of the bladder (UCB) is the 10th most common cancer worldwide, with an estimated 549,000 new cases and 200,000 deaths per year [1]. While the majority of patients have non-muscle-invasive bladder cancer (NMIBC), approximately 25% of patients with UCB have muscle-invasive bladder cancer (MIBC) or metastases at the time of diagnosis [2]. While radical cystectomy and platin-based chemotherapy have remained the therapeutic standard for MIBC and metastatic disease in the last few decades, the treatment and follow-up of MIBC continues to be very challenging [3,4]. Radical cystectomy is associated with high rates of perioperative morbidity and mortality [5], and approximately 50% of patients experience distant disease recurrence after cystectomy, mostly within the first two years, although later recurrences have also been reported [6–8]. The median survival of patients treated with cisplatin-based chemotherapy for metastatic disease ranges between nine and 26 months [3]. The need for lifelong surveillance as well as high treatment costs result in UCB being the most expensive cancer per patient from diagnosis to death in the US [9–11]. Given the high costs and poor outcome of patients with UCB, there is a high demand for novel molecular markers to improve diagnostics and serve as targets for new therapies.

In recent years, several independent groups have demonstrated the existence of distinct molecular subtypes in UCB comparable to the molecular subtypes in breast cancer [12–16]. It was also shown that these molecular subtypes were associated with different outcomes and responses to chemotherapy [15, 17]. While these findings bear great potential to improve the diagnostics and treatment of UCB in the future, there are still many uncertainties. Based on genetic expression patterns, most groups defined the basal and luminal subtypes of UCB by measuring the expression of hundreds of genes, which is not conveyable into daily clinical practice because of the high cost and effort [12–16]. The identification of relevant surrogate markers is necessary for the easy and feasible implementation of the molecular subtyping of UCB into daily clinical routine, as is the case in breast cancer [18].

Moreover, the exact number and definition of clinically relevant subtypes remain unclear. A recent consensus meeting agreed on the structure and features of a basal-squamous-like subtype, which is characterized by the high expression of the keratins KRT5/6 and KRT14 as well as the low expression of the transcription factors FOXA1 and GATA3 [19], which are suggested to drive luminal cell biology in bladder cancer [20]. However, to date, there has been no agreement on the definition of other non-basal subtypes or the markers necessary to define them.

Recently, using a 36-gene panel quantified by NanoString nCounter (NanoString Technologies Germany GmbH, Hamburg, Germany) in patients with MIBC treated with radical cystectomy, we were able to discriminate three prognostically distinct molecular subtypes (basal, luminal, and infiltrated) [21]. In an attempt to further reduce the required marker panel, we previously analyzed the prognostic relevance of the mRNA expression of KRT5 and KRT20 as surrogate markers for the basal and luminal subtypes of UCB, respectively [22,23]. However, it remains unclear if such a reduced marker panel adequately mirrors subtypes defined by larger marker panels.

In the present study, we investigated the association of the mRNA expression of suggested surrogate markers for the basal (KRT5) and luminal (FOXA1, GATA3, KRT20, androgen receptor (AR)) subtypes of MIBC with clinical and pathological characteristics and survival. Furthermore, the association of the surrogate markers with the subtypes defined by the previously established 36-gene panel was examined with the intent to reduce marker panels for the non-basal subtypes [21].

2. Materials and Methods

2.1. Patient Population and Histological Assessment

In this study, we retrospectively analyzed tissue samples and clinical data from 80 patients with MIBC (stage pT2–pT4) who were treated between 1998 and 2006 with radical cystectomy and bilateral lymphadenectomy at the Department of Urology of the Medical Faculty Mannheim (Mannheim, Germany). Only patients who were treated with curative intention were included. All patients with metastases (n = 7) or unresectable (n = 1) tumors at the time of diagnosis were excluded, leaving a total of 73 patients to be included in this analysis. None of the patients received neoadjuvant or adjuvant therapy. The median follow-up time was 24 months (range: 1–184 months). All patients gave written informed consent. The study was approved by the relevant institutional review board at the Medical Faculty Mannheim under numbers 2013-517N-MA and 2016-814R-MA. Hematoxylin-eosin stained sections of the tumor samples were evaluated for pathological stage according to the 2010 TNM classification and were graded according to the common grading systems (WHO 1973, WHO 2016) by an experienced uropathologist (AH).

Expression data and clinicopathological information from the publicly available cancer genome atlas network (TCGA) cohort were used for validation (n = 406) [14]. Only patients with MIBC (T2–T4) were included, while all patients with no documented T or N stage and patients who received neoadjuvant therapy were excluded, leaving a total of 365 patients to be included in the analysis. Based on gene expression, the samples were clustered into five molecular subtypes (basal-squamous, luminal, luminal-papillary, luminal-infiltrated, and neuronal) [24].

2.2. Assessment of mRNA Expression by RT-qPCR

A reverse transcription quantitative real-time polymerase chain reaction (RT-qPCR)-based assessment was used for the objective quantification of FOXA1, GATA3, and AR mRNA expression, as previously described and performed with KRT5 and KRT20 [22,25]. In brief, RNA was extracted from a single 10-µm section of formalin-fixed paraffin embedded (FFPE) routine tissue using a commercially available bead-based extraction method (Xtract® kit; STRATIFYER Molecular Pathology GmbH, Cologne, Germany). After a lysation and purification process, the nucleic acids were eluted and treated with DNase I. After the DNA was digested, the RNA eluates were stored at −80 °C until use.

One-step RT-qPCR was applied for the relative quantification of the mRNA expression of the genes of interest (FOXA1, GATA3 and AR) as well as the reference gene (Calmodulin 2 (CALM2)) by gene-specific TaqMan®-based assays using the SuperScript III PLATINUM One-Step, quantitative RT-PCR System (Invitrogen, Karlsruhe, Germany) on a Stratagene Mx3005p system (Agilent Technologies, Böblingen, Germany) with 30 minutes at 50 °C, two minutes at 95 °C, followed by 40 cycles of 15 seconds at 95 °C and 30 seconds at 60 °C as described previously [22,25].

Forty amplification cycles were applied, and the cycle threshold (Ct) values of the genes of interest and CALM2 for each sample were estimated as the mean value of the duplicate measurements. Ct values were then normalized against the mean expression levels of CALM2 using the 40-ΔCt method to ensure that normalized gene expression obtained by the test was proportional to the corresponding mRNA expression levels.

A set of 36 genes was previously quantified in 28 patients of this cohort using standard nCounter chemistry as previously described [21]. The nCounter assay was normalized using the geometric mean of six reference genes (CALM2, RPL37A, B2M, TUBB, GAPDH, and G6PD) and six internal positive controls, while negative background subtraction was conducted by eight negative internal controls, as previously described. Based on gene expression, urothelial carcinomas were assigned to one of three subtypes (basal, luminal, or infiltrated) [21]. Because of the small cohort size of 28 patients with available data on expression of the 36-gene panel, the subtypes were dichotomized into basal and non-basal subtypes.

The datasets for the TCGA cohort were downloaded as processed data from the open access cBioPortal database (http://www.cbioportal.org/study?id=blca_tcga#clinical) provided by the Memorial Sloan Kettering Cancer Center (New York, NY, USA). Gene expression analyses were based on paired-end RNA-Seq analysis on an Illumina HiSeq. All RSEM (RNA-Seq by Expectation Maximization) values were log2 transformed [24].

2.3. Statistical Methods

Correlation between variables was investigated by Spearman's rank correlation coefficient, Wilcoxon/Kruskal–Wallis test, or Fisher's exact test, whichever was appropriate. In addition, the cohort was stratified into patients with high or low marker expression using the median mRNA expression of KRT5, KRT20, FOXA1, GATA3, and AR as objective cut-offs. Recurrence-free survival (RFS), disease-free survival (DFS), and overall survival (OS) were analyzed by the Kaplan–Meier method and log-rank test. Univariable and multivariable analyses were performed by a Cox proportional hazards regression model. Receiver operating characteristic (ROC) curve analyses were used to measure the correlation between the markers and molecular subtypes.

Statistical analysis was performed with JMP SAS 13.0 (SAS Institute, Cary, NC, USA) or Graph Pad Prism 5 (GraphPad Software Inc., La Jolla, CA, USA). All p-values were two-sided, and a p-value <0.05 was considered to be significant.

3. Results

3.1. Association of the Surrogate Markers with Clinicopathological Features

The characteristics of the included patients are summarized in Table 1. The median mRNA expression of all analyzed markers is shown in Figure 1.

Table 1. Patient characteristics of the Mannheim cohort.

Patient Characteristic	*n* (%)
Tumor stage	
T2	18 (24.7)
T3	43 (58.9)
T4	12 (16.4)
Nodal status	
N0	44 (60.3)
N positive	29 (39.7)
Sex	
male	54 (74.0)
female	19 (26.0)
Grade (WHO 1973)	
G2	15 (20.5)
G3	58 (79.5)
Age	
<70	47 (64.4)
≥70	26 (35.6)
Histology	
Pure urothelial carcinoma	43 (58.9)
Histologic variants	30 (41.1)
Squamous cell	10 (13.7)
Sarcomatoid	7 (9.6)
Micropapillary	5 (6.9)
Small cell	3 (4.1)
Adenocarcinoma	2 (2.7)
Neuroendocrine	1 (1.4)
Nested	1 (1.4)
Plasmacytoid	1 (1.4)

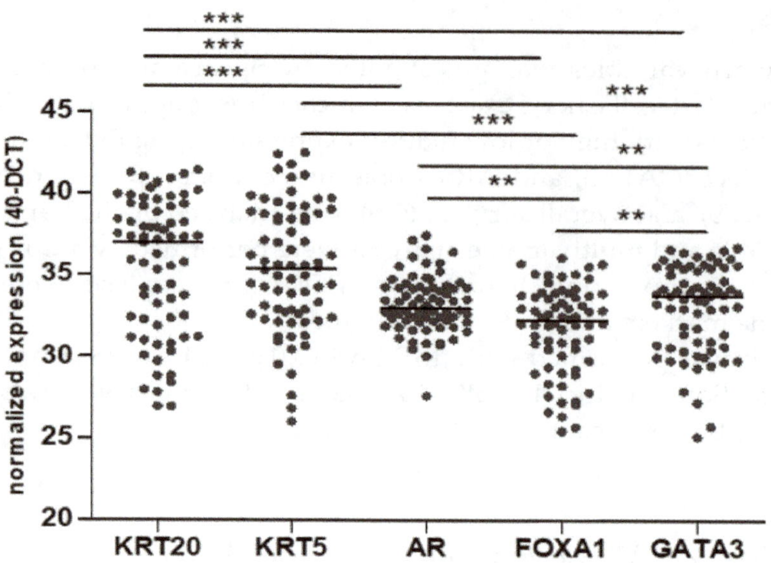

Figure 1. Distribution of normalized mRNA expression of KRT5, KRT20, FOXA1, GATA3, and androgen receptor (AR) in the Mannheim cohort (** $p < 0.01$; *** $p < 0.001$).

Spearman correlation demonstrated a significant positive association of FOXA1 and GATA3 with the luminal marker KRT20 (Figure 2). All three luminal markers showed a significantly negative association with the basal marker KRT5. Moreover, AR also showed a significantly positive association with all luminal markers, while the association between AR and KRT5 was negative.

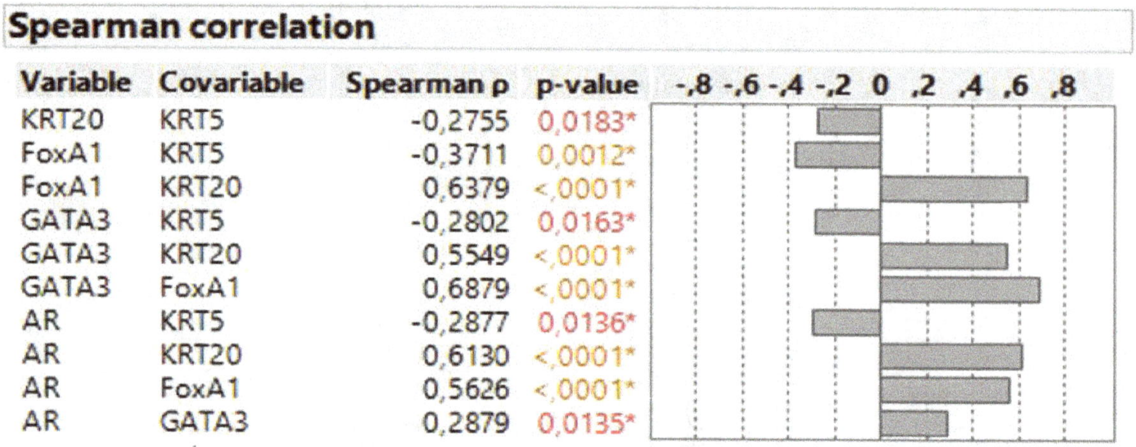

Spearman correlation

Variable	Covariable	Spearman ρ	p-value
KRT20	KRT5	-0,2755	0,0183*
FoxA1	KRT5	-0,3711	0,0012*
FoxA1	KRT20	0,6379	<,0001*
GATA3	KRT5	-0,2802	0,0163*
GATA3	KRT20	0,5549	<,0001*
GATA3	FoxA1	0,6879	<,0001*
AR	KRT5	-0,2877	0,0136*
AR	KRT20	0,6130	<,0001*
AR	FoxA1	0,5626	<,0001*
AR	GATA3	0,2879	0,0135*

Figure 2. Spearman correlation of all measured markers (* $p < 0.05$).

The Wilcoxon/Kruskal–Wallis test showed significant positive associations between grade and both KRT5 (0.0388) and GATA3 ($p = 0.0133$). There were no significant associations with tumor stage, nodal status, sex, or age.

3.2. Association of the Surrogate Markers with Survival

For survival analysis, the median mRNA expression levels of each marker were used as an objective cut-off to stratify patients with high and low marker expression. Kaplan–Meier analysis indicated that high KRT20 ($p = 0.0317$) and FOXA1 ($p = 0.0048$) expression was associated with significantly reduced RFS. GATA3 ($p = 0.0629$) and KRT5 ($p = 0.0513$) were not significantly associated with RFS. When analyzing the association with DFS and OS, only FOXA1 was significantly associated with reduced DFS ($p = 0.0186$) (Figure 3), while KRT5, KRT20, and GATA3 showed no associations with OS or DFS. AR mRNA expression showed no relevant associations with RFS, DFS, or OS.

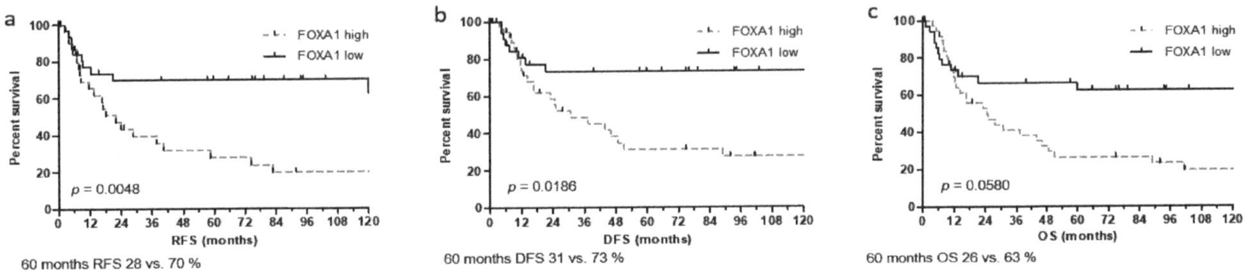

Figure 3. Kaplan Meier analysis for recurrence-free survival (RFS) (**a**), disease-free survival (DFS) (**b**) and overall survival (OS) (**c**) based on FOXA1 mRNA expression within the Mannheim cohort.

In univariable Cox regression analysis, positive nodal status, tumor stage, and expression of FOXA1 and KRT20 were associated with worse outcome (Tables 2–4). In the multivariable analysis, of all examined markers, only FOXA1 remained an independent prognostic marker for DFS ($p = 0.0333$) and RFS ($p = 0.0310$) (Tables 2–4). When analyzing patients with pure urothelial carcinomas ($n = 43$) and patients with histologic variants ($n = 30$) separately, we found an improved survival for patients with low FOXA1 expression and pure urothelial carcinomas but not histologic variants, which might be attributed to the low number of 30 patients and high heterogeneity of the histologic variants (Figure S1).

Table 2. Univariable and multivariable Cox regression analyses for RFS (Recurrence-free survival), accounting for all five analyzed markers and clinicopathological features.

Parameter	Univariable		Multivariable	
	Hazard Ratio	*p*-Value	Hazard Ratio	*p*-Value
Tumor stage T3/4 vs. T2	1.6203	0.2156		
Nodal status N+ vs. N0	2.8737	**0.0027**	2.4330	**0.0146**
Sex male vs. female	1.0155	0.9698		
Grade (WHO 1973) G2 vs. G3	0.4709	0.8186		
Age <70 vs. ≥70	0.8428	0.6454		
KRT5 >median vs. <median	0.5081	0.0513		
KRT20 >median vs. <median	2.1233	**0.0317**	1.2927	0.5083
FOXA1 >median vs. <median	2.7209	**0.0048**	2.2670	**0.0310**
GATA3 >median vs. <median	1.9211	0.0629		
AR >median vs. <median	1.6121	0.1670		

Multivariable analysis was performed only for significant parameters in univariable analysis (significant values in bold).

Table 3. Univariable and multivariable Cox regression analyses for DFS (Disease-free survival), accounting for all five analyzed markers and clinicopathological features.

Parameter	Univariable		Multivariable	
	Hazard Ratio	*p*-Value	Hazard Ratio	*p*-Value
Tumor stage T3/4 vs. T2	2.0330	0.0926		
Nodal status N+ vs. N0	2.7727	**0.0044**	2.6057	**0.0077**
Sex male vs. female	1.5435	0.2715		
Grade (WHO 1973) G2 G3	1.1484	0.7558		
Age <70 ≥70	0.8833	0.7404		
KRT5 >median vs. <median	0.6999	0.3072		
KRT20 >median vs. <median	1.3249	0.4235		
FOXA1 >median vs. <median	2.3617	**0.0186**	2.1946	**0.0333**
GATA3 >median vs. <median	1.2429	0.5359		
AR >median vs. <median	1.3717	0.3670		

Multivariable analysis was performed only for significant parameters in univariable analysis (significant values in bold).

There was no association between FOXA1 expression and DFS in the TCGA cohort (Figure S2).

3.3. Correlation of Surrogate Markers with Molecular Subtypes Defined by Multigene Panels

In the Mannheim cohort, a total of 28 patients were clustered into three molecular subtypes (basal, luminal, and infiltrated) according to the expression of a 36-gene panel previously quantified with nCounter [21]. Because of the small cohort with available data on molecular subtypes, we dichotomized the subtypes into basal and non-basal subtypes in the present study. The Mann–Whitney test showed that FOXA1 ($p = 0.0028$) and KRT20 ($p = 0.011$) expression was significantly higher in the non-basal subtype (Figure 4). The expression of KRT5 ($p = 0.083$) and GATA3 ($p = 0.11$) was not significantly different between the two subtypes in the Mannheim cohort. In the TCGA cohort, all three luminal markers had significantly higher expression in the non-basal subtype, while KRT5 was significantly higher in the basal subtype (each $p < 0.0001$).

Table 4. Univariable and multivariable Cox regression analyses for OS (Overall survival), accounting for all five analyzed markers and clinicopathological features.

Parameter	Univariable		Multivariable	
	Hazard Ratio	*p*-Value	Hazard Ratio	*p*-Value
Tumor stage T3/4 vs. T2	2.0601	**0.0048**	1.7819	0.1251
Nodal status N+ vs. N0	2.2720	**0.0086**	2.0806	**0.0206**
Sex male vs. female	1.3586	0.3820		
Grade (WHO 1973) G2 vs. G3	0.7678	0.4590		
Age <70 vs. ≥70	0.8253	0.5544		
KRT5 >median vs. <median	0.7012	0.2408		
KRT20 >median vs. <median	1.1560	0.6334		
FOXA1 >median vs. <median	1.7986	0.0580		
GATA3 >median vs. <median	1.0844	0.7800		
AR >median vs. <median	1.3104	0.3728		

Multivariable analysis was performed only for significant parameters in univariable analysis (significant values in bold).

Using the median marker expression as the cut-off, ROC analyses showed a high but not significant correlation of KRT5 with the basal subtype (AUC = 0.65; $p = 0.097$) in the Mannheim cohort. FOXA1 (AUC = 0.79; $p = 0.0007$) and KRT20 (AUC = 0.75; $p = 0.0066$) correlated significantly with the non-basal subtype, unlike GATA3 (AUC = 0.65; $p = 0.097$). The use of all three luminal markers combined showed no relevantly improved approximation to the non-basal subtype (AUC = 0.79; $p = 0.0015$) over the use of KRT20 or especially FOXA1 alone. Validation in the TCGA cohort showed that the use of FOXA1 alone (AUC = 0.77; $p < 0.0001$) achieved a high approximation to the non-basal subtype, similar to the use of all three markers combined (AUC = 0.79; $p < 0.0001$), while KRT5 achieved a close approximation to the basal subtype (AUC = 0.75; $p < 0.0001$). To exclude the possibility that the high association of KRT5 and FOXA1 with the basal and non-basal subtypes is mainly based on the central role of KRT5 and FOXA1 in the classification of subtypes using the 36-gene panel and the TCGA classification, we applied the BASE47 signature, which does not include KRT5 and FOXA1 for defining subtypes, on the TCGA cohort for validation [16]. This way, KRT5 and FOXA1 still showed a significantly higher distribution in the basal and luminal subtype, respectively (Figure S3). Furthermore, there was still a high association between the basal subtype and KRT5 (AUC = 0.72; $p < 0.0001$) and the luminal subtype and FOXA1 (AUC = 0.77; $p < 0.0001$).

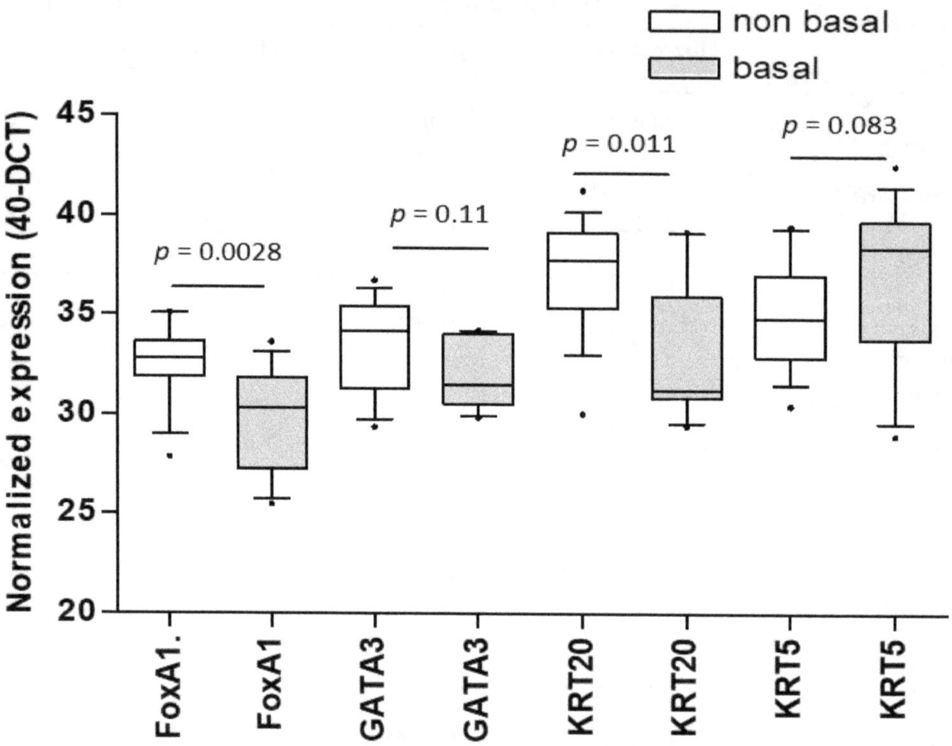

Figure 4. Distribution of FOXA1, GATA3, KRT20, and KRT5 within the basal and non-basal subtypes defined by a 36-gene panel within the Mannheim cohort showing significantly higher expression of FOXA1 and KRT20 in the non-basal subtype.

4. Discussion

With the advent of molecular subtyping in UCB, researchers and clinicians are faced with several problems, as was the case with molecular subtyping in breast cancer 15 years ago. First, apart from a basal squamous-like subtype, no consensus on the number and essential characteristics of other molecular subtypes has yet been reached [19]. As most groups have defined various numbers of luminal-like subtypes, these differences in labeling, subclassification and marker expression have hindered the general acceptance of these non-basal subtypes so far [12,14,16,21].

Second, it is necessary that subtypes are either prognostically or therapeutically relevant; otherwise, they are useless for daily clinical routine. For instance, analogous to breast cancer, a claudin-low subset of basal UCB was previously defined which demonstrated a similar outcome as regular basal UCB [16], therefore being of no interest for clinical routine.

Third, the analysis of hundreds of genes per patient currently used by most groups for the definition of their subtypes is too time-consuming and cost-intensive for easy transfer into a routine clinical setting, which is why a small set of surrogate markers per subtype has to be determined. In breast cancer, it was shown that the analysis of only four markers (estrogen receptor, progesterone receptor, HER2, and Ki-67) is enough to make a valid therapeutically relevant molecular classification [18,26]. In addition, a recent study in prostate cancer showed that the status of the PTEN gene alone matched a multigene panel to predict the risk of metastasis in patients treated with radical prostatectomy, allowing for more cost-saving diagnostics [27].

By analogy to previous findings in breast and prostate cancer, the goal of the present study was to identify surrogate markers for molecular subtypes with regard to their prognostic relevance and concordance with subtypes defined by multigene panels. Given that there is consensus about the basal subtype, we focused on non-basal subtypes. Therefore, we decided to analyze the mRNA expression of the two prominent luminal markers, FOXA1 and GATA3, together with the previously measured luminal marker KRT20 and the basal marker KRT5 [22], alongside AR as a potential target associated with the luminal subtype of MIBC [28].

Regarding the expression pattern, our results are in concordance with previous findings, as FOXA1 and GATA3 are strongly associated with KRT20 expression and show a negative association with KRT5 [12,16]. As before, we found AR to be associated with the luminal subtype in MIBC [28].

When comparing single-marker analysis to the subtypes defined by the 36-gene panel, FOXA1 and KRT20 expression was significantly higher in the non-basal subtype than in the basal subtype. Moreover, the analysis of only FOXA1 or KRT20 showed a similar high correlation with the 36-gene panel when compared to the analysis of FOXA1, GATA3 and KRT20 combined. The use of FOXA1 alone showed an almost identical AUC in the Mannheim (0.79) and TCGA (0.77) cohorts when compared to the use of all three luminal markers together (Mannheim 0.79; TCGA 0.76). FOXA1 is known to play a central role in urothelial differentiation. In addition, the low expression or loss of FOXA1 in basal tumors was described in the development of squamous cell carcinoma in preclinical models of bladder cancer, which is in concordance with the subtype association in the current study [29]. The nonsignificant correlation of GATA3 with the non-basal subtype and KRT5 with the basal subtype in the Mannheim cohort might be attributed to the small sample size of only 28 patients for whom the 36-gene panel results were available. The correlation of all markers with their respective subtype was confirmed in the TCGA cohort. The current results indicate that the measurement of one of the luminal markers, could be enough to determine a non-basal subtype, potentially allowing for more cost-saving diagnostics in daily clinical routine.

When analyzing the prognostic relevance, high KRT5 showed a non-significant trend for prolonged RFS, while FOXA1 was the only luminal marker that remained an independent prognostic marker for reduced RFS when all markers were accounted for, which suggests that a combined analysis of all three luminal markers does not provide any additional prognostically relevant information. These results are in contrast to several previous studies that found the basal subtype to be associated with worse outcome [15,17]. With regard to FOXA1 in particular, Yuk and colleagues reported higher FOXA1 expression to be associated with a positive prognostic outcome using immunohistochemistry on tissue microarray slides [30]. One possible reason for this discrepancy might be the high percentage (41%) of histologic variants within the analyzed Mannheim cohort, which are often associated with poorer prognosis than pure urothelial carcinomas and demonstrate a higher expression of luminal markers such as FOXA1 [20,31]. Furthermore, some studies show an association between the high expression of luminal markers such as KRT20 and high tumor stage, grade and micrometastasis, which are known to be associated with worse survival, which further indicates a luminal patient group with impaired survival [32,33]. On the other hand, no prognostic relevance for any of the luminal markers could be shown in the TCGA cohort. Tumor heterogeneity, which was not accounted for in the current study, might also be a factor for these contradictory results [34]. Further studies are necessary to clarify the prognostic role of molecular markers in MIBC.

Moreover, while the analysis of only one basal and one luminal marker seems to be enough to make a valid distinction between the basal and non-basal subtypes, additional markers still might be necessary for subclassification. In a comprehensive molecular analysis of MIBC within the TCGA cohort, Robertson et al. were able to identify three distinct luminal subclasses, with the luminal and luminal-infiltrated subtypes being associated with reduced survival compared to the luminal-papillary subtype [24]. All three luminal subtypes showed comparable expression patterns of FOXA1, GATA3, and KRT20 but differed with regard to FGFR3 mutations, lymphocytic infiltration, smooth muscle gene signatures, and uroplakin expression. Differences in luminal subclasses were not accounted for in our current study. The analysis of one or two additional markers (for instance, the epithelial–mesenchymal transition (EMT) markers TWIST1 or SNAI1) might be enough to draw clinically relevant conclusions. Moreover, a rare neuronal/neuroendocrine-like subtype associated with poor survival has previously been described in approximately 5% of patients with MIBC [24,35]. These tumors are mainly characterized by the upregulation of genes of neuroendocrine origin, such as TUBB2B but can also express FOXA1 and GATA3. Markers to distinguish these neuronal/neuroendocrine-like subtypes from luminal subtypes still have to be defined.

As previously mentioned, with a total of 73 included patients, our cohort is relatively small compared to other multicentric studies. On the other hand, given that this is a single center study, we have exact information on treatment modalities, which is necessary to interpret the prognostic relevance of markers, although some data on salvage therapies is missing due to the retrospective nature of the study. However, this is also the case in the TCGA cohort, where no precise information on the treatment modality is provided, rendering statements about prognosis even more difficult.

5. Conclusions

In conclusion, we were able to demonstrate that the measurement of only one of the prominent luminal markers alongside KRT5 as the basal marker is enough to make a valid distinction between the basal and non-basal subtypes and potentially draw prognostically relevant conclusions. Given the closest concordance with subtypes defined by multigene panels as well as strongest prognostic relevance, FOXA1 seems to be the marker best suited as a surrogate marker to distinguish the non-basal subtypes from the basal subtypes. The measurement of FOXA1, GATA3, and KRT20 combined does not provide any additional relevant information. However, additional studies are necessary to further clarify the prognostic role of molecular markers in MIBC. Moreover, surrogate markers for the further subclassification of the luminal subtype still have to be defined.

Author Contributions: Conceptualization: D.S., R.M.W., B.K., C.B., B.W., and P.E.; Methodology, D.S., M.E, R.M.W., J.J., S.P., V.W., S.R., A.H., and P.E.; Validation: M.E., T.S.W., F.K., V.W., J.B., W.O., S.R., C.B., and B.W.; Formal Analysis: D.S., R.M.W., A.H., and P.E.; Investigation, D.S., R.M.W., J.B., and P.E.; Data Curation: D.S., J.J., T.S.W., S.P., and P.E.; Writing—Original Draft Preparation: D.S., B.K., J.B., B.W., and P.E.; Writing—Review and Editing: D.S., M.E., J.J., T.S.W., F.K., V.W., J.B., W.O., S.R., C.B., A.H., and P.E.; Visualization: D.S., R.M.W., and P.E.; Supervision: T.S.W., S.P., B.K., F.K., W.O., S.R., C.B., A.H., and B.W.; Project Administration: D.S. and P.E. All authors have read and agreed to the published version of the manuscript.

Acknowledgments: D.S. is supported by a Ferdinand Eisenberger grant from the German Society of Urology (Deutsche Gesellschaft für Urologie), grant ID SiD1/FE-16.

References

1. Bray, F.; Ferlay, J.; Soerjomataram, I.; Siegel, R.L.; Torre, L.A.; Jemal, A. Global cancer statistics 2018: GLOBOCAN estimates of incidence and mortality worldwide for 36 cancers in 185 countries. *CA A Cancer J. Clin.* **2018**, *68*, 394–424. [CrossRef] [PubMed]
2. Burger, M.; Catto, J.W.; Dalbagni, G.; Grossman, H.B.; Herr, H.; Karakiewicz, P.; Kassouf, W.; Kiemeney, L.A.; La Vecchia, C.; Shariat, S.; et al. Epidemiology and risk factors of urothelial bladder cancer. *Eur. Urol.* **2013**, *63*, 234–241. [CrossRef] [PubMed]
3. Alfred Witjes, J.; Lebret, T.; Comperat, E.M.; Cowan, N.C.; De Santis, M.; Bruins, H.M.; Hernandez, V.; Espinos, E.L.; Dunn, J.; Rouanne, M.; et al. Updated 2016 EAU Guidelines on Muscle-invasive and Metastatic Bladder Cancer. *Eur. Urol.* **2017**, *71*, 462–475. [CrossRef] [PubMed]
4. Babjuk, M.; Bohle, A.; Burger, M.; Capoun, O.; Cohen, D.; Comperat, E.M.; Hernandez, V.; Kaasinen, E.; Palou, J.; Roupret, M.; et al. EAU Guidelines on Non-Muscle-invasive Urothelial Carcinoma of the Bladder: Update 2016. *Eur. Urol.* **2017**, *71*, 447–461. [CrossRef] [PubMed]
5. Aziz, A.; Gierth, M.; Rink, M.; Schmid, M.; Chun, F.K.; Dahlem, R.; Roghmann, F.; Palisaar, R.J.; Noldus, J.; Ellinger, J.; et al. Optimizing outcome reporting after radical cystectomy for organ-confined urothelial carcinoma of the bladder using oncological trifecta and pentafecta. *World J. Urol.* **2015**, *33*, 1945–1950. [CrossRef] [PubMed]
6. Donat, S.M. Staged based directed surveillance of invasive bladder cancer following radical cystectomy: Valuable and effective? *World J. Urol.* **2006**, *24*, 557–564. [CrossRef] [PubMed]
7. Hassan, J.M.; Cookson, M.S.; Smith, J.A., Jr.; Chang, S.S. Patterns of initial transitional cell recurrence in patients after cystectomy. *J. Urol.* **2006**, *175*, 2054–2057. [CrossRef]
8. Yoo, S.H.; Kim, H.; Kwak, C.; Kim, H.H.; Jung, J.H.; Ku, J.H. Late Recurrence of Bladder Cancer following Radical Cystectomy: Characteristics and Outcomes. *Urol. Int.* **2019**, *103*, 1–6. [CrossRef]

9. Svatek, R.S.; Hollenbeck, B.K.; Holmang, S.; Lee, R.; Kim, S.P.; Stenzl, A.; Lotan, Y. The economics of bladder cancer: Costs and considerations of caring for this disease. *Eur. Urol.* **2014**, *66*, 253–262. [CrossRef]
10. Botteman, M.F.; Pashos, C.L.; Redaelli, A.; Laskin, B.; Hauser, R. The health economics of bladder cancer: A comprehensive review of the published literature. *PharmacoEconomics* **2003**, *21*, 1315–1330. [CrossRef]
11. Gore, J.L.; Gilbert, S.M. Improving bladder cancer patient care: A pharmacoeconomic perspective. *Expert Rev. Anticancer. Ther.* **2013**, *13*, 661–668. [CrossRef]
12. Choi, W.; Porten, S.; Kim, S.; Willis, D.; Plimack, E.R.; Hoffman-Censits, J.; Roth, B.; Cheng, T.; Tran, M.; Lee, I.-L.; et al. Identification of distinct basal and luminal subtypes of muscle-invasive bladder cancer with different sensitivities to frontline chemotherapy. *Cancer Cell* **2014**, *25*, 152–165. [CrossRef] [PubMed]
13. Sjödahl, G.; Lauss, M.; Lövgren, K.; Chebil, G.; Gudjonsson, S.; Veerla, S.; Patschan, O.; Aine, M.; Fernö, M.; Ringnér, M.; et al. A molecular taxonomy for urothelial carcinoma. *Clin. Cancer Res.* **2012**, *18*, 3377–3386. [CrossRef] [PubMed]
14. Network, C.G.A.R. Comprehensive molecular characterization of urothelial bladder carcinoma. *Nature* **2014**, *507*, 315–322. [CrossRef]
15. Choi, W.; Czerniak, B.; Ochoa, A.; Su, X.; Siefker-Radtke, A.; Dinney, C.; McConkey, D.J. Intrinsic basal and luminal subtypes of muscle-invasive bladder cancer. *Nat. Rev. Urol.* **2014**, *11*, 400–410. [CrossRef]
16. Damrauer, J.S.; Hoadley, K.A.; Chism, D.D.; Fan, C.; Tiganelli, C.J.; Wobker, S.E.; Yeh, J.J.; Milowsky, M.I.; Iyer, G.; Parker, J.S.; et al. Intrinsic subtypes of high-grade bladder cancer reflect the hallmarks of breast cancer biology. *Proc. Natl. Acad. Sci. USA* **2014**, *111*, 3110–3115. [CrossRef]
17. Seiler, R.; Ashab, H.A.D.; Erho, N.; van Rhijn, B.W.G.; Winters, B.; Douglas, J.; Van Kessel, K.E.; Fransen van de Putte, E.E.; Sommerlad, M.; Wang, N.Q.; et al. Impact of Molecular Subtypes in Muscle-invasive Bladder Cancer on Predicting Response and Survival after Neoadjuvant Chemotherapy. *Eur. Urol.* **2017**, *72*, 544–554. [CrossRef]
18. Goldhirsch, A.; Wood, W.C.; Coates, A.S.; Gelber, R.D.; Thurlimann, B.; Senn, H.J.; Panel, M. Strategies for subtypes–dealing with the diversity of breast cancer: Highlights of the St. Gallen International Expert Consensus on the Primary Therapy of Early Breast Cancer 2011. *Ann. Oncol.* **2011**, *22*, 1736–1747. [CrossRef]
19. Lerner, S.P.; McConkey, D.J.; Hoadley, K.A.; Chan, K.S.; Kim, W.Y.; Radvanyi, F.; Hoglund, M.; Real, F.X. Bladder Cancer Molecular Taxonomy: Summary from a Consensus Meeting. *Bladder Cancer* **2016**, *2*, 37–47. [CrossRef]
20. Warrick, J.I.; Kaag, M.; Raman, J.D.; Chan, W.; Tran, T.; Kunchala, S.; Shuman, L.; DeGraff, D.; Chen, G. FOXA1 and CK14 as markers of luminal and basal subtypes in histologic variants of bladder cancer and their associated conventional urothelial carcinoma. *Virchows Arch. Int. J. Pathol.* **2017**, *471*, 337–345. [CrossRef]
21. Rinaldetti, S.; Rempel, E.; Worst, T.S.; Eckstein, M.; Steidler, A.; Weiss, C.A.; Bolenz, C.; Hartmann, A.; Erben, P. Subclassification, survival prediction and drug target analyses of chemotherapy-naive muscle-invasive bladder cancer with a molecular screening. *Oncotarget* **2018**, *9*, 25935–25945. [CrossRef] [PubMed]
22. Eckstein, M.; Wirtz, R.M.; Gross-Weege, M.; Breyer, J.; Otto, W.; Stoehr, R.; Sikic, D.; Keck, B.; Eidt, S.; Burger, M.; et al. mRNA-Expression of KRT5 and KRT20 Defines Distinct Prognostic Subgroups of Muscle-Invasive Urothelial Bladder Cancer Correlating with Histological Variants. *Int. J. Mol. Sci.* **2018**, *19*, 3396. [CrossRef] [PubMed]
23. Breyer, J.; Wirtz, R.M.; Otto, W.; Erben, P.; Kriegmair, M.C.; Stoehr, R.; Eckstein, M.; Eidt, S.; Denzinger, S.; Burger, M.; et al. In stage pT1 non-muscle-invasive bladder cancer (NMIBC), high KRT20 and low KRT5 mRNA expression identify the luminal subtype and predict recurrence and survival. *Virchows Arch. Int. J. Pathol.* **2017**, *470*, 267–274. [CrossRef]
24. Robertson, A.G.; Kim, J.; Al-Ahmadie, H.; Bellmunt, J.; Guo, G.; Cherniack, A.D.; Hinoue, T.; Laird, P.W.; Hoadley, K.A.; Akbani, R.; et al. Comprehensive Molecular Characterization of Muscle-Invasive Bladder Cancer. *Cell* **2017**, *171*, 540–556.e55. [CrossRef] [PubMed]
25. Breyer, J.; Otto, W.; Wirtz, R.M.; Wullich, B.; Keck, B.; Erben, P.; Kriegmair, M.C.; Stoehr, R.; Eckstein, M.; Laible, M.; et al. ERBB2 Expression as Potential Risk-Stratification for Early Cystectomy in Patients with pT1 Bladder Cancer and Concomitant Carcinoma in situ. *Urol. Int.* **2016**. [CrossRef] [PubMed]
26. Perou, C.M.; Sorlie, T.; Eisen, M.B.; van de Rijn, M.; Jeffrey, S.S.; Rees, C.A.; Pollack, J.R.; Ross, D.T.; Johnsen, H.; Akslen, L.A.; et al. Molecular portraits of human breast tumours. *Nature* **2000**, *406*, 747–752. [CrossRef] [PubMed]

27. Leapman, M.S.; Nguyen, H.G.; Cowan, J.E.; Xue, L.; Stohr, B.; Simko, J.; Cooperberg, M.R.; Carroll, P.R. Comparing Prognostic Utility of a Single-marker Immunohistochemistry Approach with Commercial Gene Expression Profiling Following Radical Prostatectomy. *Eur. Urol.* **2018**, *74*, 668–675. [CrossRef]
28. Sikic, D.; Wirtz, R.M.; Wach, S.; Dyrskjot, L.; Erben, P.; Bolenz, C.; Breyer, J.; Otto, W.; Hoadley, K.A.; Lerner, S.P.; et al. Androgen Receptor mRNA Expression in Urothelial Carcinoma of the Bladder: A Retrospective Analysis of Two Independent Cohorts. *Transl. Oncol.* **2019**, *12*, 661–668. [CrossRef]
29. DeGraff, D.J.; Clark, P.E.; Cates, J.M.; Yamashita, H.; Robinson, V.L.; Yu, X.; Smolkin, M.E.; Chang, S.S.; Cookson, M.S.; Herrick, M.K.; et al. Loss of the urothelial differentiation marker FOXA1 is associated with high grade, late stage bladder cancer and increased tumor proliferation. *PLoS ONE* **2012**, *7*, e36669. [CrossRef]
30. Yuk, H.D.; Jeong, C.W.; Kwak, C.; Kim, H.H.; Moon, K.C.; Ku, J.H. Clinical outcomes of muscle invasive bladder Cancer according to the BASQ classification. *BMC Cancer* **2019**, *19*, 897. [CrossRef]
31. Lopez-Beltran, A.; Henriques, V.; Montironi, R. Variants and new entities of bladder cancer. *Histopathology* **2019**, *74*, 77–96. [CrossRef] [PubMed]
32. Christoph, F.; Muller, M.; Schostak, M.; Soong, R.; Tabiti, K.; Miller, K. Quantitative detection of cytokeratin 20 mRNA expression in bladder carcinoma by real-time reverse transcriptase-polymerase chain reaction. *Urology* **2004**, *64*, 157–161. [CrossRef] [PubMed]
33. Gazquez, C.; Ribal, M.J.; Marin-Aguilera, M.; Kayed, H.; Fernandez, P.L.; Mengual, L.; Alcaraz, A. Biomarkers vs conventional histological analysis to detect lymph node micrometastases in bladder cancer: A real improvement? *BJU Int.* **2012**, *110*, 1310–1316. [CrossRef] [PubMed]
34. Thomsen, M.B.H.; Nordentoft, I.; Lamy, P.; Vang, S.; Reinert, L.; Mapendano, C.K.; Hoyer, S. Comprehensive multiregional analysis of molecular heterogeneity in bladder cancer. *Sci. Rep.* **2017**, *7*, 11702. [CrossRef] [PubMed]
35. Sjodahl, G.; Eriksson, P.; Liedberg, F.; Hoglund, M. Molecular classification of urothelial carcinoma: Global mRNA classification versus tumour-cell phenotype classification. *J. Pathol.* **2017**, *242*, 113–125. [CrossRef]

11

The Impact of Whole Genome Data on Therapeutic Decision-Making in Metastatic Prostate Cancer: A Retrospective Analysis

Megan Crumbaker [1,2,3,†], Eva K. F. Chan [1,2,†], Tingting Gong [1,4], Niall Corcoran [5,6,7], Weerachai Jaratlerdsiri [1], Ruth J. Lyons [1], Anne-Maree Haynes [1], Anna A. Kulidjian [8,9], Anton M. F. Kalsbeek [1], Desiree C. Petersen [10], Phillip D. Stricker [11], Christina A. M. Jamieson [12], Peter I. Croucher [1,13], Christopher M. Hovens [5,6,*], Anthony M. Joshua [1,2,3,*] and Vanessa M. Hayes [1,2,4,*]

1 Garvan Institute of Medical Research, Darlinghurst, NSW 2010, Australia; m.crumbaker@garvan.org.au (M.C.); e.chan@garvan.org.au (E.K.F.C.); t.gong@garvan.org.au (T.G.); w.Jaratlerdsiri@garvan.org.au (W.J.); R.Lyons@garvan.org.au (R.J.L.); a.Haynes@garvan.org.au (A.-M.H.); amfkalsbeek@gmail.com (A.M.F.K.); p.croucher@garvan.org.au (P.I.C.)

2 St. Vincent's Clinical School, University of New South Wales, Sydney, Randwick, NSW 2031, Australia

3 Kinghorn Cancer Centre, Department of Medical Oncology, St. Vincent's Hospital, Darlinghurst, NSW 2010, Australia

4 Central Clinical School, University of Sydney, Sydney, Camperdown, NSW 2050, Australia

5 Australian Prostate Cancer Research Centre Epworth, Richmond, VIC 3121, Australia; niallmcorcoran@gmail.com

6 Department of Surgery, University of Melbourne, Melbourne, VIC 3010, Australia

7 Division of Urology, Royal Melbourne Hospital, Melbourne, VIC 3050, Australia

8 Department of Orthopedic Surgery, Scripps Clinic, La Jolla, CA 92037, USA.; Kulidjian.Anna@scrippshealth.org

9 Orthopedic Oncology Program, Scripps MD Anderson Cancer Center, La Jolla, CA 92037, USA

10 The Centre for Proteomic and Genomic Research, Cape Town 7925, South Africa; desiree.petersen@cpgr.org.za

11 Department of Urology, St. Vincent's Hospital, Darlinghurst, NSW 2010, Australia; phillip@stricker.com.au

12 Department of Urology, Moores Cancer Center, University of California, San Diego, La Jolla, CA 92037, USA; camjamieson@health.ucsd.edu

13 School of Biotechnology and Biomolecular Sciences, University of New South Wales, Sydney, Randwick, NSW 2031, Australia

* Correspondence: cbhovens@gmail.com (C.M.H.); anthony.joshua@svha.org.au (A.M.J.); v.hayes@garvan.org.au (V.M.H)

† These authors contributed equally to this work.

Abstract: *Background*: While critical insights have been gained from evaluating the genomic landscape of metastatic prostate cancer, utilizing this information to inform personalized treatment is in its infancy. We performed a retrospective pilot study to assess the current impact of precision medicine for locally advanced and metastatic prostate adenocarcinoma and evaluate how genomic data could be harnessed to individualize treatment. *Methods*: Deep whole genome-sequencing was performed on 16 tumour-blood pairs from 13 prostate cancer patients; whole genome optical mapping was performed in a subset of 9 patients to further identify large structural variants. Tumour samples were derived from prostate, lymph nodes, bone and brain. *Results*: Most samples had acquired genomic alterations in multiple therapeutically relevant pathways, including DNA damage response (11/13 cases), PI3K (7/13), MAPK (10/13) and Wnt (9/13). Five patients had somatic copy number losses in genes that may indicate sensitivity to immunotherapy (*LRP1B, CDK12, MLH1*) and one patient had germline and somatic *BRCA2* alterations. *Conclusions*: Most cases, whether primary or metastatic, harboured therapeutically relevant alterations, including those associated with PARP inhibitor sensitivity, immunotherapy sensitivity and resistance to androgen pathway targeting agents. The observed intra-patient heterogeneity and presence of genomic alterations in multiple growth pathways in individual cases suggests that a precision medicine model in prostate cancer needs to simultaneously incorporate multiple pathway-targeting agents. Our whole genome approach allowed for structural variant assessment in addition to the ability to rapidly reassess an individual's molecular landscape as knowledge of relevant biomarkers evolve. This retrospective oncological assessment highlights the genomic complexity of prostate cancer and the potential impact of assessing genomic data for an individual at any stage of the disease.

Keywords: prostate cancer; precision medicine; whole genome sequencing; optical mapping; therapy

1. Introduction

Worldwide, prostate cancer (PCa) is the most commonly diagnosed non-cutaneous cancer in men and a leading cause of cancer-related male deaths [1]. Treatment strategies range from observation alone to multi-modal treatment and vary based on clinical and pathological factors such as tumour stage (T Stage), prostate specific antigen (PSA) level, Gleason or International Society of Urological Pathology (ISUP) score and life expectancy. PCa is a heterogeneous disease, and these clinical factors alone cannot predict outcomes accurately. Early disease is potentially curable whereas eventual treatment resistance is an intractable problem in metastatic disease. In both early and advanced disease, escalation of treatment including combination therapies, such as androgen deprivation therapy (ADT) administered with docetaxel with or without radiotherapy to the primary has resulted in improved outcomes [2–5]. However, the escalated treatment comes at the cost of increased toxicity and only a subset of men garner benefit. As such, predictive biomarkers for optimal treatment selection are needed at all stages of the disease.

PCa progression is driven by genomic alterations and, as such, large sequencing efforts have focused on elucidating the succession of events driving its pathogenesis and progression. These sequencing efforts aim to establish new prognostic and therapeutic targets [6–11]. Thus far, these studies have focused on primary tumours from localized cancers and/or heavily pre-treated disease that has become resistant to ADT, termed castrate-resistant prostate cancer (CRPC). It has been established that intra- and inter-patient heterogeneity is high [12–16], though certain critical events may occur early in some patients and propagate. In general, genomic changes are thought to accumulate in response to treatment as the disease progresses and the importance of structural variants (SVs) in advanced prostate cancer is an evolving area of research [10,11].

A goal of previous studies is to advance "precision medicine" in PCa. Robinson et al. found that 89% of CRPC samples harboured a clinically actionable genomic alteration [6]. However, clinical trials utilizing the precision medicine paradigm of selecting a targeted drug based on molecular criteria have yielded mixed results. For example, though phosphoinositide 3-kinase (PI3K)/Protein Kinase B (Akt) pathway activating alterations are commonly reported in PCa, PI3K inhibitors have demonstrated limited efficacy to date [17,18]. However, a randomized phase II study of abiraterone +/−ipatasertib, an Akt inhibitor, in metastatic CRPC did find improved antitumoral activity in the combination arm, particularly in men with *PTEN* loss [19]. Similarly, poly ADP ribose polymerase (PARP) inhibitors have shown promise in selected men with CRPC and homologous recombination deficiency [20–23] but not all mutations in the homologous recombination pathway predict a response [21].

Although these large genomic studies have expanded the knowledge of molecular drivers of treatment-naïve primary and metastatic CRPC, they have generally viewed the data as a cohort without looking at cumulative alterations and their potential therapeutic impact within the individuals. Likewise, hormone sensitive (HSPC) metastatic disease has also been largely neglected. In this study, we performed whole genome sequencing (WGS) on men with confirmed PCa in order to assess the collective genomic events in individual cases and their impact on real-world therapeutic decisions. Recognizing the importance of SVs in prostate cancer and the limitations of WGS in detecting large genomic rearrangements, we also performed whole genome optical mapping (WGM) on a subset of the samples.

2. Results

2.1. Shared Genomic Landscape

In this study, we retrospectively analysed 13 PCa cases that had micro- or macro-metastatic disease at the time of sampling for genomic interrogation. Patient clinical and pathological characteristics are summarized in Table 1. Sixteen tumour samples comprised of nine primary and seven metastatic biopsies and the sites of concurrent or subsequent metastases included: bone (seven cases), lymph nodes (four cases), and brain (one case), while a single case had biochemically relapsed without evidence of macro-metastatic disease on conventional imaging. Figure 1 summarizes the commonalities and differences in the genomic landscape between our primary and metastatic samples, while placing our cases in context with the current knowledge based on large PCa WGS efforts. For the latter, we focused on the study published by Wedge et al. in 2018 for 112 patients (92 primary and 20 metastatic) with the metastases evenly distributed between HSPC and CRPC and biased towards lymph node metastasis (15/20) [8].

Common predisposing germline variants (Table S1) in our samples include the *EHBP1* rs721048 (c.1185 + 30064G > A) intronic variant in five (38%) and *FGFR4* rs35185519011 (c.1162G > A, p.Gly388Arg) in ten (77%) cases. Reported in 9% of the healthy population [24], the *EHBP1* rs721048 A-allele has been associated with a more aggressive PCa [25]. The functional variant in *FGFR4*, although present in 30% of the healthy population, may predispose PCa patients to an accelerated disease course [26]. Ten patients had one of two SNPs (rs1859962, rs8072254) in non-coding regions of the 17q24.3 locus previously associated with PCa susceptibility [27].

Common somatic alterations include *ETS* fusions (seven cases) and *TP53* alterations (six cases). Tumour mutational burden (TMB) was generally low, ranging from 0.73 to 5.79 mutations/Megabase (mut/Mb) (IQR 1.30–2.09), and did not correlate with disease stage at sampling (Figure 1, Table S2). Percent genome altered (PGA) ranged from 2.2% to 63.9% (IQR 2.79–19.4%) (Table S2).

We observed a prevalence (11/13 cases) of somatic copy number alterations (SCNA) affecting at least one DNA damage response (DDR) pathway gene (Table S4). Losses in *FANCA*, which helps recruit DNA repair proteins to areas of DNA damage [28], were present in five (38%) cases, while one case harboured germline and somatic *BRCA2* alterations. With variation depending on the gene sets tested for and stage of disease, DDR gene alterations occur in approximately 20% of PCas with *BRCA2* alterations reported for 3% of prostatic and 12% of metastatic samples [6,7,29]. Aside from DDR, the most commonly impacted pathways were Phosphoinositide 3-kinase (PI3K, 7/13 (54%) cases), Mitogen-activated protein kinase (MAPK, 10 (77%) cases) and Wnt (9 (69%) cases) (Table 2). PI3K and MAPK are intracellular and extracellular signalling pathways, respectively, that are key to the regulation of the cell cycle and, like certain DDR pathways, are therapeutically targetable (manipulable) with inhibitory drugs [30,31]. The Wnt signalling pathway is a cellular pathway involved in cell growth, embryogenesis and cell cycle progression, the activation of which has been implicated in progression to CRPC and treatment resistance [32]. Previous studies have found that approximately 25% of primary PCas harbour PI3K or MAPK pathway alterations while nearly 50% of metastatic CRPC samples have PI3K alterations [6,7] and 32% MAPK amplifications [30]. In our study, 6 of the 7 samples with somatic alterations impacting PI3K were in the primary tissue, and MAPK alterations were seen in 4/7 (57%) of the metastases and 6/8 (75%) of the primaries.

Overall, SCNAs and SVs, rather than single nucleotide variants (SNVs) and small insertions and deletions (sequences of no more than 50 nucleotides in length, indels), were more commonly acquired in PCa relevant genes (Tables S1–S6). The addition of WGM identified 120 SVs not identified by WGS alone, several of which overlapped with oncogenic and/or tumour suppresser genes (Table 3, Table S6).

In particular, large insertions and duplications were typically missed by our short-read WGS approach. However, no recurrent WGM-derived SVs were observed across the cases.

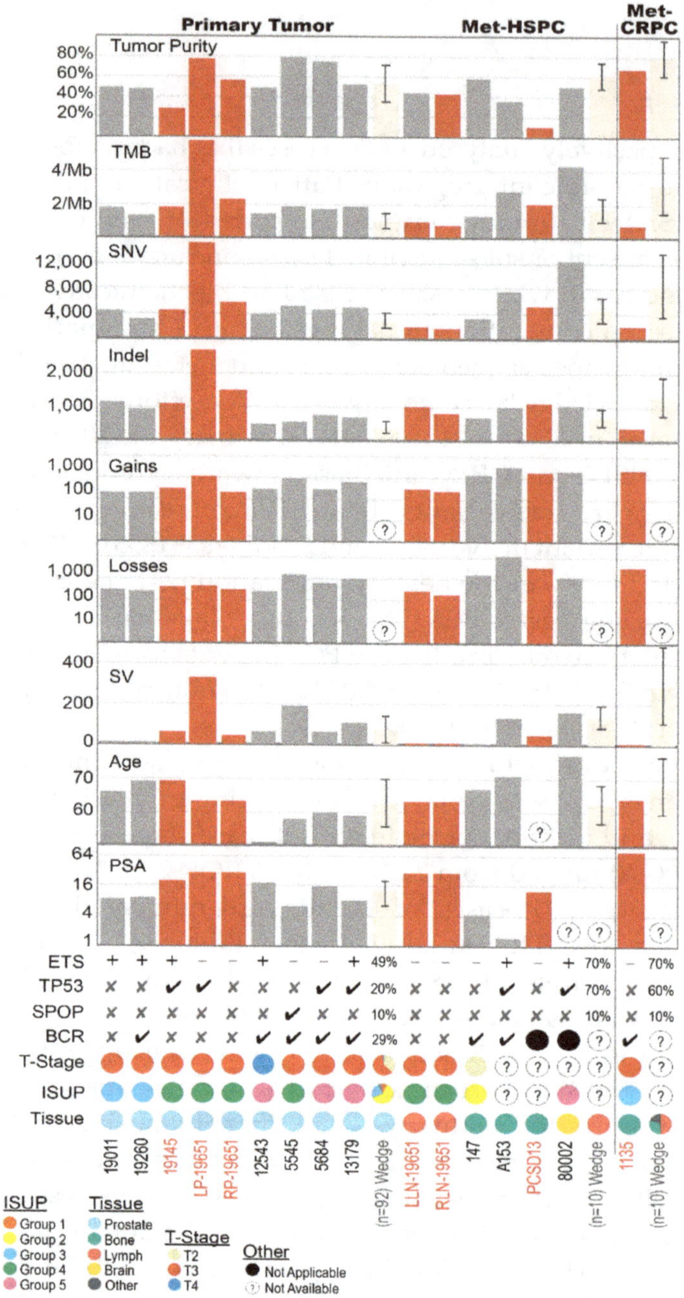

Figure 1. Summary of genomic landscape relevant to tumour purity and related to clinical and pathological features for 16 samples from 13 patients, and further compared to the Wedge et al. data. Met-HSPC: metastatic hormone sensitive PCa; met-CRPC: metastatic castration-resistant PCa; TMB: Tumour mutational burden; SNV: single nucleotide variants; Indel: small insertion or deletion; Gains and Losses: somatic copy number alterations (SCNA); SV: Structural variation including large insertions or deletions, inversions, translocations and duplications; PSA: prostate-specific antigen (ug/L); ETS: presence of ETS fusion event; TP53: presence of *TP53* alteration including SNV, SCNA or SV; SPOP: presence of *SPOP* SNV; BCR: biochemical recurrence; ISUP: International Society of Urological Pathologists cancer grade (correlates to Gleason scores). Error bars for Wedge et al. data reflect +/− one standard deviation of the sub-group totals. Sample identifiers in red, with matching red bar plots, are indicative of patients pre-treated with ADT.

Recurrent non-coding events in key PCa-associated genes have been reported [8,11,33–37], including transcription factor (TF) binding sites. Alterations at key non-coding sites within our cases are summarised in Table 4. Common to CRPC, SCNAs or SVs upstream of the androgen receptor (AR) gene were not seen in our cases, which is unsurprising given the hormone sensitive status of most of our patients. All but two of our samples contained non-coding AR binding site mutations (Table 4). Overall, 20% of the somatic SNVs or indels affected at least one TF binding cluster. However, no sample was significantly enriched for mutations within TF binding clusters and no TFs were enriched for mutations. Notably, 0.3% of the 10.5 million TF binding clusters analysed correspond to *JUN*, an average of 1.2% (0.5–1.5%) of somatic SNV in *JUN* binding clusters. JUN is a transcription factor that antagonizes AR signalling [38].

Excluding COSMIC Mutational Signature 1 common to all cancers, we observed a predominance of Mutational Signatures 3 and/or 8 (Figure 2A) that generally reduced in proportion from the clonal to subclonal stages of tumour evolution (Figure 2B). Known to be associated with DDR gene alterations [39–41], Signature 8 was particularly common in the primary 8/9 (89%) versus metastatic 3/7 (43%) samples, with notable loss in both of case 19651's lymph node metastases. In contrast, Signature 5, which is seen in most cancer types, particularly in smokers [39], and Signature 16, most often associated with liver cancer, both increased in the subclonal stage of tumour evolution.

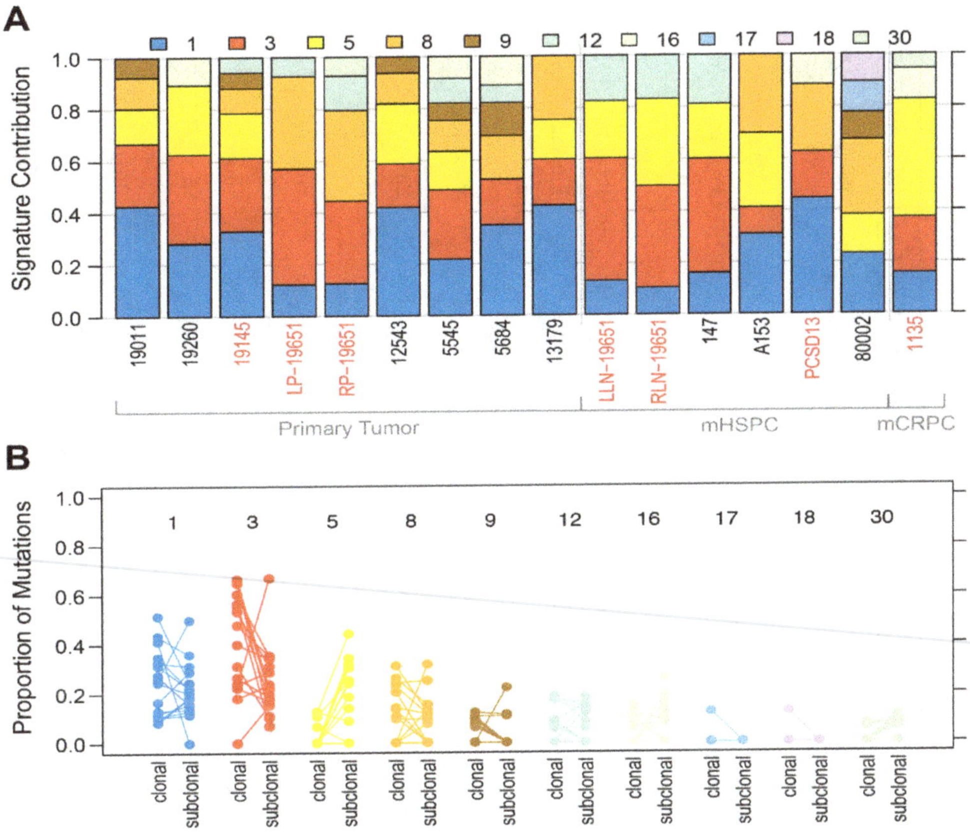

Figure 2. COSMIC Mutational Signatures (**A**) Proportion of signatures in each sample, for Signatures with >5% contribution; (**B**) Clonal vs. subclonal signature exposures. mHSPC: metastatic hormone-sensitive prostate cancer; mCRPC: metastatic castration-resistant prostate cancer.

When viewed in detail, each patient had unique features with potential therapeutic implications. This highlights the relevance of genomic information for guiding therapeutic decisions, including data derived from primary tumour tissue. Here, we discuss how the course of treatment for each patient may have been influenced by the availability of their genomic data.

Table 1. Clinical and pathological characteristics.

Diagnosis				Time of Sample Collection for Genomic Interrogation								Relapse and Outcomes			
Patient ID	Age	Stage	Initial Treatment	ISUP	Clinical State	PSA	ECOG	Symptoms	Sample Site	ADT Prior	CRPC?	Time to BCR (mos)	Rx for BCR	Time to Mets (mos)	Duration Follow-Up (mos)
1135	64	T3N0	RP	3	Rl	80.7	1	Yes	Bone	Yes	Yes	33	ADT	68	68
19651	63	T3N1	ADT, RP, aRT	4	Dx	28	0	No	Prostate, nodes	Yes (6wks)	No	NR	NA	NR	20
147	67	T2N0	RP	2	Rl	4.4	0	Yes	Bone	No	No	84	Nil	107	135
19260	69	T3N1	RP	3	Dx	9.2	0	No	Prostate	No	No	16	sRT	NR	27
5545	58	T3N0	RP	4	Dx	6.3	0	No	Prostate	No	No	6	sRT	24	72
5684	60	T3N0	RP	5	Dx	15.7	0	No	Prostate	No	No	36	ADT	120	132
19145	69	T3N1	RP, aRT	4	Dx	20	0	No	Prostate	Yes (4wks)	No	NR	NR	NA	33
19011	66	T3N1	RP, aRT	5	Dx	8.9	0	No	Prostate	No	No	NR	NA	NA	35
12543	51	T4N0	RP, aRT	5	Dx	18.6	0	No	Prostate	No	No	72	ADT	NA	120
13179	59	T3N0	RP, aRT, ADT	5	Dx	8.4	0	No	Prostate	No	No	51	ADT	51	51
PCSD13	69	TxNxM1	ADT	-	Dx	12.8	2	Yes	Bone	Yes (8wks)	No	NA	NA	NA	9
A153	71	T2N0	RP	3	Rl	1.5	0	Yes	Bone	No	No	93	Nil	105	120
80002	77	TxNxM1	Resection, ADT	5	Dx	-	1	Yes	Brain	No	No	NA	NA	NA	1

Dx = Diagnosis; Sample = time of tissue biopsy for genomic interrogation; ADT = Androgen deprivation therapy; RP = radical prostatectomy; aRT = adjuvant radiotherapy; sRT = salvage radiotherapy; Rl = Relapse; ECOG = Eastern Cooperative Oncology Group Performance Status; wks: weeks; BCR = Biochemical relapse; mos = months; NR = Not relapsed; NA = Not applicable.

Table 2. Genomic alterations affecting key genes in the PI3K, MAPK and WNT signaling pathways.

PI3K Pathway			MAPK Pathway			WNT Pathway		
Gene	Cases	Event	Gene	Cases	Event	Gene	Cases	Event
PTEN	554512543, 1914519145	SNVSCNASV	*BRAF*	1926019651LP, 13179, 1135, 147, A153, 8000219145,19651LP+RP, 80002	SNVSCNASV	*APC*	19651LP, 5545, A15319651LP+RP, 12543, 5545, A153	SCNASV
PIK3CA	19651LP, 13179	SCNA	*EGFR*	13179, 80002	SCNA	*CTNNB1*	19651LP, 13179	SCNA
PIK3CB	13179	SCNA	*KRAS*	19145, 5545, 5684	SCNA	*RNF43*	80002, 14780002, 147	SCNASV
PIK3R1	5684, 13179	SCNA	*MAP3K1*	5684, 13179,A153, 19651RP+LP	SCNASV	*WNT5A*	19651LP, 13179, 8000219260	SCNASV
AKT1	PCSD13	SNV, SCNA	*RAF1*	19651LP, 13179, 147, 80002	SCNA	*MED12*	19011	Germline SNV

Table 3. Structural variants identified by optical mapping as compared to whole genome sequencing. INS: Insertion; DEL: deletion; DUP: duplication; INV: inversion; Intra-Chr: intrachromosomal translocation; Inter-Chr: interchromosomal translocation.

Disease State of Sample	Sample ID	SVs from Whole Genome Optical Mapping							% Missed by Whole Genome Sequencing						
		Total	INS	DEL	DUP	INV	Intra-Chr	Inter-Chr	Total	INS	DEL	DUP	INV	Intra-Chr	Inter-Chr
Primary Tumor	5545	39	0	27	3	0	7	2	36	-	37	67	-	29	0
	13179	2	0	2	0	0	0	0	100	-	100	-	-	-	-
	5684	5	3	2	0	0	0	0	100	100	100	-	-	-	-
	12543	10	1	5	0	0	1	3	60	0	40	-	-	100	67
	19651LP	91	5	33	3	1	19	30	29	60	39	0	0	11	27
Met HSPC	A153	8	6	1	1	0	0	0	100	100	100	100	-	-	-
	147	5	4	0	1	0	0	0	100	100	-	100	-	-	-
	19651LLN	10	0	10	0	0	0	0	100	-	100	-	-	-	-
	80002	70	2	25	13	1	9	20	54	50	52	100	100	56	25
MetCRPC	1135	6	2	4	0	0	0	0	100	100	100	-	-	-	-

Table 4. Sites of recurrent non-coding alterations reported in the literature with potential clinical relevance.

Nearby Gene	Variant Positions	Data from Literature	Reference	Patient IDs
NEAT1	Chr11:65,190,268-65,213,009	13/112 cases, 6/20 mets all with previous ADT. *NEAT1* produces a long non-coding RNA that regulates several growth pathways and overexpression is associated with PCa progression	Wedge [8]	5545
FOXA1	Promoter, Chr14:37587200-37597201	14 coding and 6 non-coding mutations; regulates AR signalling	Wedge	5684
FOXA1	Chr14:37886261-37888565, 37903630-37906634, 38035667-38036817, 38053354-38056060, 38056084-38059097, 38127358-38128083	*FOXA1* is a co-factor for AR. These are *cis*-regulatory elements	Zhou [34]	5684
AR	Upstream promoter	Tandem duplications, 70–87% mCRPC vs. <2% primary PCa	Viswanathan [11]	Nil
AR	ChrX: 66117800-66128800 (66.10–66.20 bin)	I peak, long range enhancer of AR, only 1/54 primary samples (Viswanathan); Copy number gain results in proliferation in low androgen condition and enzalutamide resistance	Takeda [35], Viswanathan	Nil
AR	Transcription Factor Binding Sites	Recurrently altered in primary PCa	Morova [33]	1135, 5545, 5684, 12543, 13179, 19011, 19145, 19260, 80002, 19651 (LP, RP, RLN), A153, PCSD13
MYC	Chr8: 128.14–128.28, 128.47–128.54, 128.54–128.62	8q24 risk loci PCa, associated with MYC enhancer activity	Ahmadiyeh [37], Yeager [36]	19651LP, 12543, A153

2.2. Primary Prostate Samples with Synchronous Lymph Node Metastases: 19011, 19260, 19145 and 19651

These cases each presented with elevated PSA levels and prostate adenocarcinomas confirmed on biopsy. Only 19651 had evidence of nodal metastases on conventional imaging preoperatively. However, at radical prostatectomy with lymph node dissection, all had pathologically involved nodes. Genomic alterations of potential relevance are summarized in Figure 3 (19011, 19260, 19145) and Figure 4 (19651). Though nodal involvement at presentation is associated with a high PCa mortality rate [42], the optimal management strategy for these men has not been established. Retrospective data suggest that adjuvant ADT with radiotherapy compared to ADT or observation is beneficial for men with lymph node metastases identified at radical prostatectomy [43]. Based on their ISUP grade group or Gleason score and tumour (T) stage, 19011, 19145 and 19651 also meet eligibility criteria for the STAMPEDE trial arms C and G that have shown benefit for adding docetaxel or abiraterone respectively to ADT [3,44,45]. Though some studies of men with high-risk localized PCa treated with neoadjuvant and/or adjuvant docetaxel demonstrate improved outcomes, these improvements occur in a small proportion, with significant toxicity to many [4,46,47]. These studies have all been based on clinical risk factors, thus, there is an urgent need for biomarkers that better select men likely to benefit, thereby avoiding over- and undertreatment.

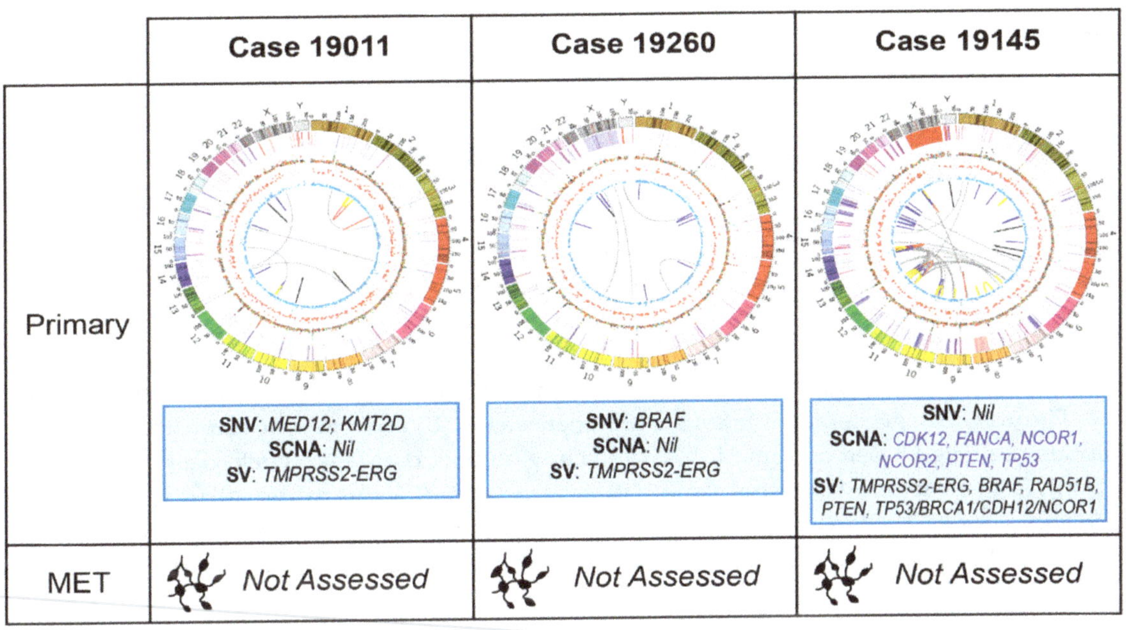

Figure 3. Summary of genomic alterations in primary prostate samples with synchronous lymph node metastases (Cases 19011, 19260 and 19145). Relevant somatic variants by type listed with SCNAs: blue indicates loss. Circos plots depict mutational load in each tumour sample. The outermost (first) track: autosome (chromosomes 1 to Y) ideograms with centromeres shown in red and the pter-qter orientation in a clockwise direction (length in Mbp); second track: somatic copy-number gains (red) and losses (blue); third track: somatic SNV allele frequencies (not corrected for tumour purity) coloured according to their mutation changes per Alexandrov et al. [39]; fourth and fifth tracks: allele frequencies (not corrected for tumour purity) of small deletions (red) and insertions (blue); innermost circle: acquired genomic rearrangements, including deletions (blue), tandem duplications (red), inversions (orange), insertions (black) and interchromosomal translocations (grey). MET: metastases.

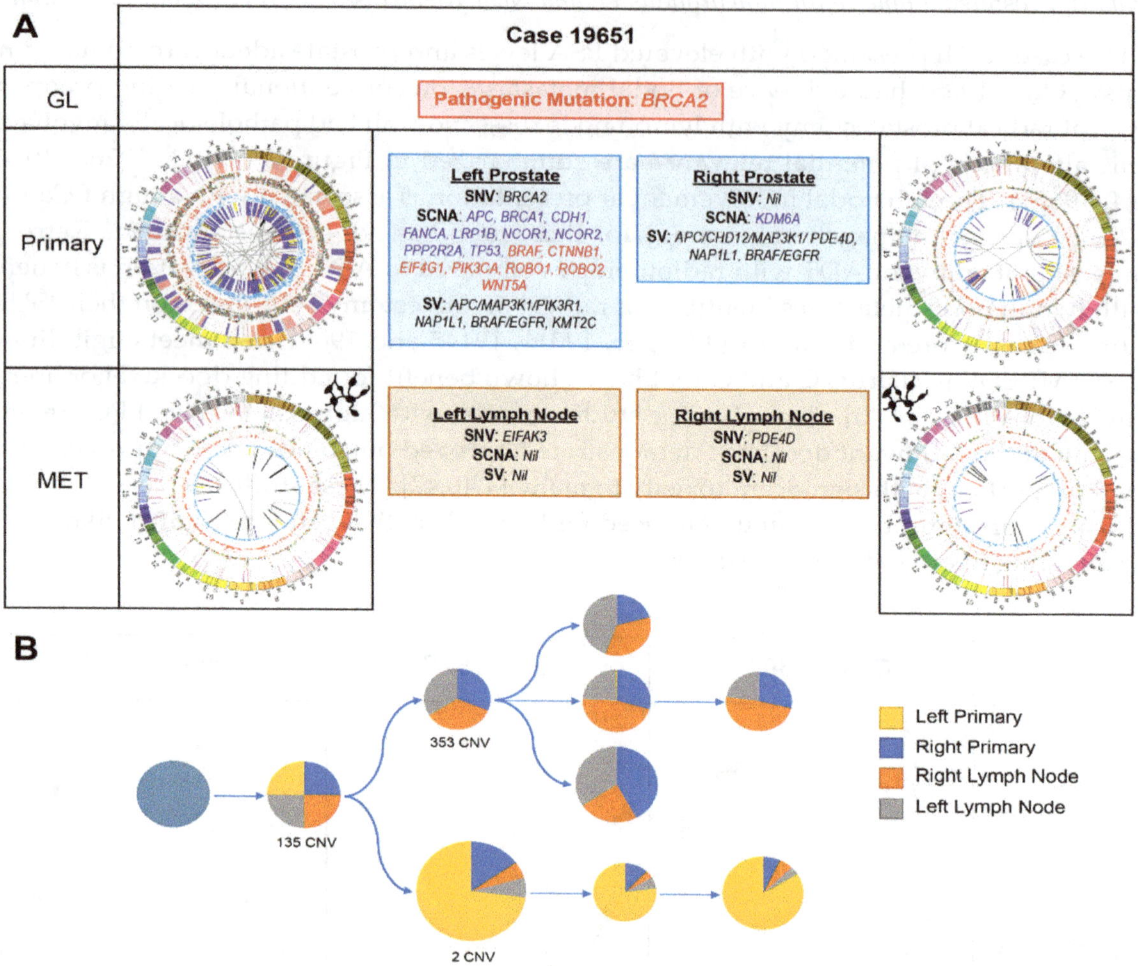

Figure 4. Case 19651. (**A**) Summary of relevant genomic alterations (germline and somatic); Circos plots as per Figure 3. GL: germline mutations; MET: metastases; (**B**) Phylogenetic reconstruction of cancer evolution predicted based on somatic SNV and copy number data. Each circle is a predicted tumour subclone, from the leftmost ancestral clone, with pie charts representing cancer cell fractions (proportion of the four samples harbouring the corresponding clone). Sizes of the circles are proportionate to the number of additional small somatic mutations acquired. Number of SCNAs acquired are indicated.

2.2.1. Case 19011: Left Prostate Tumour Core Biopsy

This *TMPRSS2-ERG* positive case had a somatic missense mutation in *MED12* (c.3670C > G; p.Leu1224Val), that is potentially pathogenic in many cancers, including prostate [48], via its upregulation of Wnt/β-catenin signalling [49]. A non-coding somatic SNV upstream of *CTNNB1* that is within the binding region of 188 TFs, may indicate misregulation of this gene involved in Wnt/β-catenin signalling [50]. No therapeutically relevant SCNA or SV was identified. PGA was low (2.7%).

Although no targetable alteration is seen in this case, the lack of mutations and low PGA may still be valuable in guiding decision-making. This patient is unlikely to respond to targeted therapies, like PARP inhibitors, but also to non-targeted agents that rely upon high mutational loads, such as immune checkpoint inhibition. The lack of poor prognostic markers, such as *TP53* loss, could mean this low volume, locally advanced PCa may respond well to aggressive local therapy without escalation to systemic therapy (e.g., addition of docetaxel). A low PGA is associated with a lower risk of BCR following definitive local therapy [51]. Despite meeting criteria for perioperative therapy trials, his genomic profile suggests aggressive local therapy will be sufficient. However, should he relapse however, the alterations in Wnt pathway-associated regions could confer resistance to AR targeting agents [32].

2.2.2. Case 19260: Right Prostate Tumour Core Biopsy

Patient 19260 was also treatment-naïve at the time of his prostatectomy and sampling for WGS. He biochemically relapsed 16 months postoperatively at which time he had salvage radiotherapy with a good PSA response.

TMPRSS2-ERG fusion positive with a low PGA (2.4%), this case presented with a pathogenic somatic missense mutation in *BRAF* (c1406G > T; p.Gly469Val). Known to confer increased kinase activity [48], this mutation may sensitise the patient to BRAF +/− MEK inhibitor therapy. Of interest in CRPC [30], with a report of response to targeted therapy in a *BRAF* mutant patient [52], clinical trials of MEK inhibitors are currently underway (NCT02881242). Though not relevant to this patient's upfront treatment, it could prove useful in the event of relapse.

2.2.3. Case 19145: Left Prostate Tumour Core Biopsy

This *TMPRSS2-ERG* positive tumour had a high PGA (10.2%), but lacked any known deleterious somatic mutation. SCNAs/SVs of note include heterozygous losses in *PTEN, FANCA, CDK12, TP53, NCOR1* and *NCOR2*, an inter-chromosomal translocation with breakpoints overlapping *RAD51B* and *PTEN* and a large heterozygous deletion overlapping with *TP53* and *NCOR1*.

Responses to PARP inhibition have been seen in patients with *FANCA* alterations [23,53] and preclinical data suggest that *PTEN* loss sensitises cancers to PARP inhibitors, with reported cases of exceptional responses to olaparib [54,55]. However, resistance to single agent PARP inhibition has been described in Pten/p53 deficient mouse models, though a synergistic response was seen upon PARP inhibition in combination with PI3K inhibition. [56]. *NCOR1* and *NCOR2* are transcriptional corepressors that negatively regulate androgen receptor (AR) signalling and androgen-induced cell proliferation [57–59]; losses in these genes increase with disease progression and are associated with anti-androgen and ADT resistance [60,61]. *TP53* loss may also predict inferior responses to novel androgen signalling inhibitors (ASIs), such as enzalutamide and abiraterone, in CRPC [62]. CDK12 loss may predict sensitivity to immune checkpoint inhibiting therapies [63].

Many of the observed alterations in this case have therapeutic potential but are still the subject of early phase clinical trials. The presence of the *NCOR1/2* losses, however, may indicate a vulnerability in this patient for early development of CRPC. His four week course of ADT preoperatively may have induced treatment resistant clones even at this early stage. These losses together with *TP53* loss and high PGA indicate this patient may develop early resistance to ADT and, given his high-risk disease at presentation, he would be an ideal candidate for escalation of his initial treatment with chemotherapy.

2.2.4. Case 19651: Bilateral Prostate and Internal Iliac Node Tumour Core Biopsies

Reporting a family history of PCa, via his father, and breast cancer in his mother and sister, it was not surprising that this patient carries a pathogenic germline *BRCA2* stop-gain mutation (rs80359031; c.7988A > T; p.Glu2663Val) confirmed to predispose carriers to BRCA-associated cancers.

The somatic heterogeneity across the four tumour samples is striking (Figures 1 and 4A). Of the 78 overlapping SNVs (out of 24,195) present across all four samples, none had notable therapeutic relevance. Phylogenetic reconstruction of this cancer's evolution reveals distinct differences between the left primary and the other three samples (Figure 4B). Notably, the left prostatic primary acquired a somatic pathogenic *BRCA2* stop-gain mutation ((c.6308C > G; p.Ser2103Ter), variant allele frequency (VAF; 26%). Additionally, genes associated with several different growth signalling pathways, including MAPK/ERK, TGF-β, PI3K and WNT, are impacted by SCNAs in the left primary but there are few events in the other samples. No relevant SVs within the left lymph node were noted on WGM. As expected with the combined germline and somatic *BRCA2* mutations, there was a high rate of large deletions in the left primary [10], including a 3Mb deletion overlapping multiple tumour suppressor genes (TSGs) including *BTG* and *DCN*.

Inter- and intra-patient heterogeneity have been well-described in PCa [13] and most recently in multi-focal primary tumours [64], with significant therapeutic implications. The germline mutation not only informs screening for secondary cancers and testing in relatives, *BRCA2* mutations may also be associated with a worse prognosis [65–69] and confer sensitivity to platinum-based chemotherapy [70] and PARP-inhibitors [23,53]. However, there is increasing evidence that responses are markedly improved with biallelic loss and many of the PARP inhibitor clinical trials have refined their inclusion criteria to include only patients with biallelic alterations. Acquiring a somatic *BRCA2* mutation in a single primary tumour could result in a differential response to targeted therapies that would not be predicted based on the typical single site sampling performed in clinical practice.

Aside from the germline *BRCA2* mutation, there is no unifying therapeutically relevant event across all four samples. Having had short-term ADT preoperatively, losses in *NCOR1* and *NCOR2* as well as other SCNAs associated with CRPC within the left primary raise the possibility that early ADT resistance is developing after minimal treatment.

In practice, knowledge of this patient's genomic landscape at baseline may have prompted his treating clinician to escalate his treatment with combination systemic therapy such as the rucaparib arm of the STAMPEDE trial. The loss of *NCOR1* and *NCOR2* and the poorer prognosis conferred by his *TP53* and *BRCA2* status represent potential indications for early chemohormonal therapy (ADT with docetaxel chemotherapy) despite him having low-volume, node only metastases [3,4,46,71]. *BRCA2* alterations may also sensitize this patient to radiotherapy due to impaired DDR. Therefore, had his genomic data been available early, an upfront strategy with radiotherapy to his primary in combination with ADT and docetaxel may have been used. At progression, he may be considered for a clinical trial with a PARP inhibitor, potentially in combination with another agent given his somatic *BRCA2* discordance. A metastatic biopsy at a site of progression could prove useful in determining whether new sites of disease harbour the somatic *BRCA2* alteration.

2.3. Primary Prostate Samples with Relapse Post Radical Prostatectomy: 12543, 5545, 5684, and 13179

At the time of surgery, none of these cases had evidence of metastatic disease on staging scans. All men subsequently relapsed with incurable disease, including bone metastases (5545, 5684 and 13179) and persistent BCR with eventual CRPC (12543). While TMBs were similar (range 1.4–1.9), there was more marked variability in their PGAs (range 3.1–26%). Genomic alterations with patient-specific relevance are summarized in Figure 5.

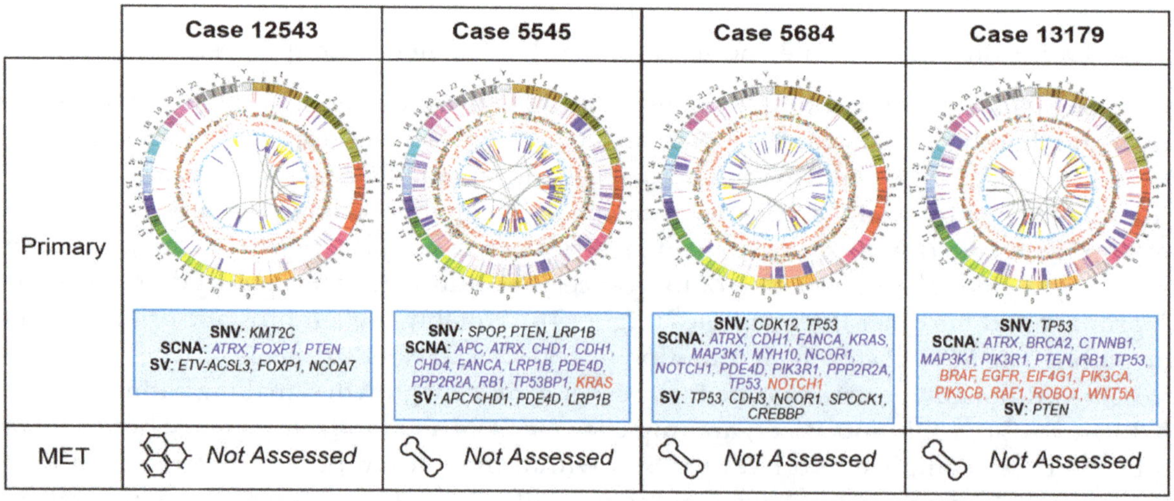

Figure 5. Summary of relevant genomic alterations for cases with subsequent metastatic relapse post radical prostatectomy (cases 12543, 5545, 5684, 13179); Circos plots as per Figure 3, with red text indicating SCNA loss.

2.3.1. Case 12543: Left Prostate Tumour Core Biopsy

This patient's tumour is characterized by *KMT2C* mutation, copy number losses (supported by large deletion) in *PTEN* and *FOXP1* and an *ETV1-ACSL3* fusion. *ETV1-ACSL3* fusion may account for this patient's prolonged ADT sensitivity (no evidence of metastatic disease following 10 years on ADT for BCR). *ACSL3* is an androgen responsive gene and thus, this fusion may lead to a strong reliance on androgen signalling [72]. Despite *PTEN* loss, loss of *FOXP1* may restore androgen receptor signalling, further enhancing this patient's response to ADT despite the *PTEN* loss [73]. At development of CRPC, this reliance on AR signalling may be exploited further with the addition of a novel ASI to his ADT, rather than docetaxel.

2.3.2. Case 5545: Left Prostate Tumour Core Biopsy

This case is characterized by a deleterious somatic *SPOP* missense variant (rs193921065, c.399C > G; p.Phe133Leu; VAF 44%) [7] and a large hemizygous deletion encompassing *CHD1*. We also predict the *LRB1B* mutation (c.3178A > G; p.Cys1060Arg) to be deleterious. Notable copy number losses include *TP53BP1* and the TSG *RB1* and the DDR genes *FANCA* and *PPP2R2A*, while a deletion overlapped *LRP1B*. Unique to WGM, we identified a large deletion involving *FILIP1L*, a gene commonly hypermethylated in PCa [74].

Point mutations in *SPOP* occur in approximately 11% of primary PCas [7] and are commonly associated with *CHD1* loss [75]. This combination of alterations is associated with increased abiraterone sensitivity in CRPC [76]. These tumours are also characterized by increased genomic instability due to error-prone double-strand DNA break repair, which results in more SVs, as seen in this case, and potential vulnerability to DNA damaging treatment such as irradiation, PARP inhibition and platinum chemotherapy [77]. Loss of *FANCA*, a gene involved in homologous recombination, may also sensitise this cancer to PARP inhibition. A recent retrospective study found that *LRP1B* alterations may predict for sensitivity to pembrolizumab [78].

SPOP/CHD1 co-altered clones persist across the disease spectrum in studies of serial patient samples [76]. Therefore, knowledge of this case's genomic data from radical prostatectomy would lead to a preference for abiraterone over docetaxel at development of CRPC. These alterations may also increase his responsiveness to PARP inhibition, though evidence is limited and preclinical models have shown that this vulnerability is reliant on elevated 53BP1 protein levels [77] and so the copy number loss in *TP53BP1* may counteract this vulnerability. This combination of alterations highlights the importance of understanding the entire genomic landscape in an individual.

2.3.3. Case 5684: Right Prostate Tumour Core Biopsy

This case harbours a small frameshift deletion in *TP53* between exons 11 and 12, in addition to heterozygous copy number loss and a deletion on SV analysis. He also presented with SCNA in *CDH1* and alterations in other DDR genes including: an SNV in *CDK12* and SCNAs in *PPP2R2A* and *FANCA*. Losses in genes affecting proliferative pathways include those in *PIK3R1*, the loss of which activates the PI3K pathway [79] and *MAP3K1*, which is associated with MEK signalling [80]. The inclusion of WGM for 5684 revealed a large insertion overlapping *SPOCK1*, which encodes a protein found to promote tumorigenesis and metastases in PCa [81]. WGM also identified an insertion in *CREBBP*, a coactivator of AR that is usually overexpressed in CRPC and the upregulation of which is associated with ADT resistance [82].

TP53 loss confers a worse prognosis and improved outcomes with chemotherapy compared to novel ASI agents [62]. Knowledge of his primary tumour *TP53* status may have guided ordering of therapies with a preference for chemotherapy, particularly upon progression to CRPC. A study of co-targeting PARP and Wee1 kinase with olaparib and AZD1775 is currently underway for *TP53* mutated solid tumours (NCT02576444). The losses in *PIK3R1* and *MAP3K1* may confer sensitivity to PI3K and MEK inhibitors respectively though these agents would only be used on a suitable clinical trial.

2.3.4. Case 13179: Right Prostate Tumour Core Biopsy

This *TMPRSS2-ERG* positive tumour is characterised by a high PGA at 26%, pathogenic somatic SNV in *TP53* (rs28934575, c.733G > A; p.Gly245Ser), as well as copy number loss of *PTEN*. Additional losses in *MAP3K1*, *PIK3R1* and *TP53* were observed, along with somatic alterations in the MAPK and PI3K pathways (Figure 5).

Co-loss of *TP53* and *PTEN* is associated with more aggressive disease, which is consistent with this patient's clinical course. Knowledge of these molecular features may have triggered more aggressive treatment upfront. Within current treatment paradigms, this may have included radiotherapy with ADT and docetaxel [5,71]. Additionally, the number of alterations in multiple targetable pathways, particularly PI3K (PI3K/AKT inhibitors) and MAPK/ERK (BRAF/MEK inhibitors), highlights the need to contextualise genomic events rather than viewing them in isolation. It is likely that this patient's treatment regimen would need to involve a tailored combination strategy if a targeted, precision-medicine approach was to be considered.

2.4. Bone Metastatic Samples: 147, A153, PCSD13 and 1135

Sampling for genomic analyses occurred at bone biopsy. Patients 147 and A153 had not yet had systemic therapy, while 1135 had CRPC, having commenced intermittent ADT for BCR 3 years postoperatively. PCSD13 presented with de novo metastatic disease manifesting as hip pain. Investigations revealed multiple bone metastases and an elevated PSA. Selected genomic events are summarized in Figure 6.

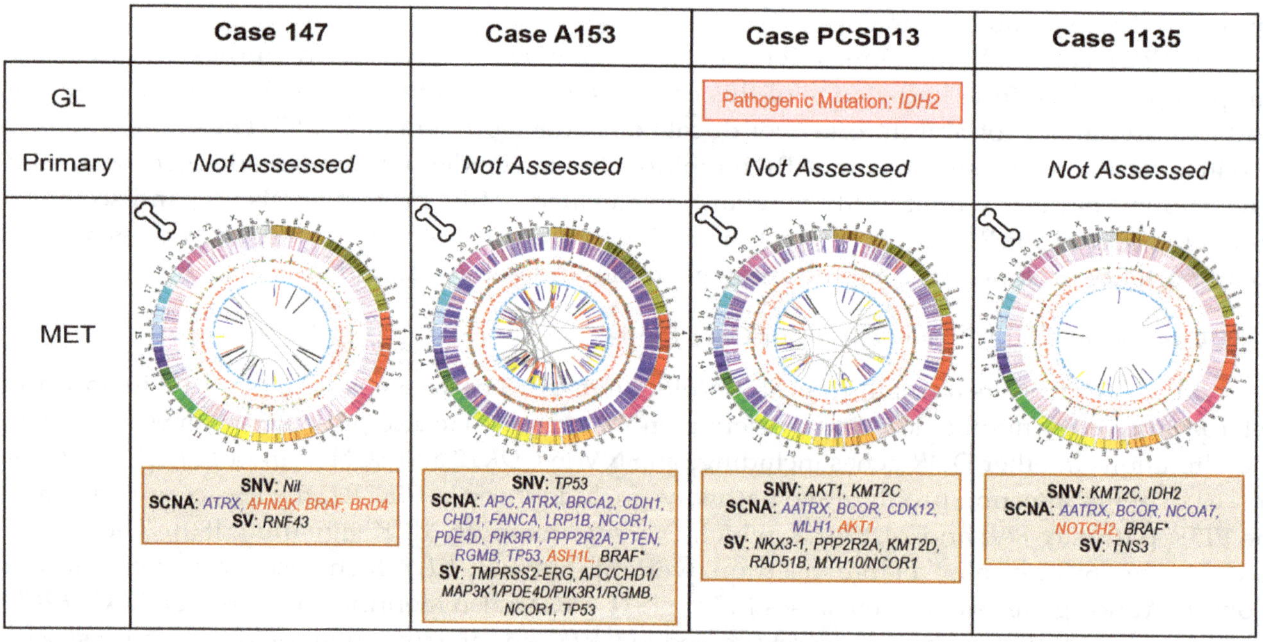

Figure 6. Summary of relevant genomic alterations for cases with metastatic disease at the time of sampling (cases 147, A153, PCSD13, 1135); Circos plots as per Figure 3.

2.4.1. Case 147: Biopsy Left Pubic Bone Corresponding to Sclerotic Region on Imaging

This case did not have any relevant somatic SNVs or WGS-identified SVs. SCNAs included gains in *BRAF*, *AHNAK* and *BRD4*.

It is unknown, yet unlikely, whether the copy number gain in *BRAF* would be sufficient to sensitize the patient to BRAF inhibition. The low level of relevant alterations in this case may explain his less aggressive disease course with a late clinical relapse (10 years post prostatectomy). The gains in *BRD4* and *AHNAK* may have contributed to metastasis formation: BRD4, part of the Bromodomain and Extraterminal (BET) protein family, regulates tumour cell migration and invasion through transcription of *AHNAK* [83]. Small molecule BRD4-selective degraders inhibit metastatic potential in PCa cell lines and a Phase I clinical trial of birabresib which included CRPC patients has been completed [84]. BRD4 is also involved in the non-homologous end joining (NHEJ) DDR pathway and higher protein levels from pre-treatment biopsies are associated with poor outcomes following radical radiotherapy in localized disease [85].

2.4.2. Case A153: Biopsy Right Iliac Crest Corresponding to Metastatic Deposit on Imaging

This *TMPRSS2-ERG* positive metastatic tumour harboured a pathogenic *TP53* mutation (rs121912656, c.734G > T; p.Gly245Val) and a high PGA (25.5%). SCNAs include losses in *APC, PTEN, CHD1, BRCA2, FANCA, PIK3R1* and *LRP1B*. A complex SV on chromosome 5 encompassing *PPAP2A, PDE4D, MAP3K1* and *IL6ST,* was previously associated with a worse prognosis [8].

TP53 loss is associated with a worse prognosis and decreased response to abiraterone in CRPC. *APC* loss, through its activation of Wnt signalling, may promote ASI resistance [32,62]. These two features would make docetaxel a better option than an ASI in the first instance for this patient at metastatic relapse. *BRCA2* and *FANCA* alterations were predictive for sensitivity to olaparib in the TOPARP studies [23,53] and, as previously discussed, *PTEN* and *CDH1* losses may sensitize this patient to PARP inhibition [54,77].

2.4.3. Case PCSD13: Biopsy Left Femur during Total Hip Replacement for Pathological Fracture

PCSD13 presented with a pathogenic germline *IDH2* mutation (rs121913502, c.419G > A; p.Arg140Gln). Reported to have an allele frequency of 0.00003 in The Genome Aggregation Database (gnomAD) [86], while associated with several other cancers, this mutation has not yet been reported in PCa [87]. In addition to an SNV in *AKT1*, there is a copy number gain in this gene. There are losses in the DDR genes *CDK12* and *MLH1*, and SVs also overlap multiple DDR genes. The COSMIC Mutational Signatures in this case show a subclonal increase in the proportion of Signature 3, whereas the majority of the other samples showed a decrease in this signature, which is associated with failure of double-strand DNA repair (Figure 2B).

The *AKT1* alterations may have contributed to his early ADT resistance (within 3 months of starting ADT) and confer sensitivity to AKT inhibitors [19]. These alterations could influence decisions on escalating ADT treatment with the addition of abiraterone, an androgen targeting drug, or docetaxel. However, the crosstalk between AR and PI3K/AKT signalling is well-established, [88,89] and additional pressure on the androgen axis in the context of an *AKT1* amplification may only drive further growth via the PI3K pathway. In the absence of a clinical trial with an AKT inhibitor, the addition of docetaxel rather than an AR targeting agent may have been more prudent. Immune checkpoint inhibition may have been another treatment option for this patient with his *CDK12* and *MLH1* SCNAs. This patient succumbed to his cancer shortly after developing CRPC.

2.4.4. Case 1135: Biopsy Right Posterior Iliac Crest Corresponding to Metastatic Deposit on Imaging

Despite having CRPC at the time of biopsy, case 1135 had very few alterations of interest with a TMB of 0.73 and PGA of 3.1%. This tumour contained SNVs in *KMT2C* and *IDH2* (rs121913502, c.419G > A; p.Arg140Gln) and SCNAs in *BCOR, NCOA7,* and *NOTCH2*. No significant SVs were identified with WGS but a homozygous deletion overlapping *TNS3* was identified using WGM.

The somatic SNV in *IDH2* is the same as the germline alteration seen in PCSD13 that has not been reported in PCa. It is unclear whether this mutation would drive the progression of this patient's cancer and if IDH inhibitor therapy, used to treat IDH-mutant AML, would be relevant. Based on preclinical studies, *KMT2C* alterations may confer sensitivity to PARP inhibition via its effects on the epigenetic status and expression of DDR genes. However, alterations in *KMT2C* are frequent in PCa [7] and responses to PARP inhibition only occur in a small proportion of patients [23]; therefore, it is unlikely this SNV alone will be enough to predict sensitivity to PARP monotherapy. ATRX is a DDR pathway gene while *BCOR, NCOA7* and *NOTCH2* are involved in androgen signalling. However, these alterations do not yet have any targeted therapeutic strategies for CRPC. While the impact of the deletion in *TNS3* is again unclear, it is noted that Tensins are a family of scaffolding proteins that regulate cell motility and growth and *TNS3* in involved in MET signalling [90], a target of the tyrosine kinase inhibiting drug, cabozantinib. Overall, though this case's alterations do not yet have any therapeutic relevance, the knowledge of molecular features in PCa is rapidly evolving and future findings may bring useful drugs to light.

2.5. Case 80002: Core Biopsy at Resection of Brain Metastasis

Patient 80002 presented with a solitary brain metastasis that was surgically resected. His PSA was elevated and morphology of the tumour specimen was consistent with an adenocarcinoma of prostatic origin; immunohistochemistry (IHC) markers for neuroendocrine differentiation were negative.

The relevant genomic features of this *TMPRSS2-ERG* fusion positive case are summarized in Figure 7 and include: *TP53* mutation (rs1057519999, c.716A > C; p.Asn239Thr) and SCNAs in *CDK12, RAD51C, RNF43, TP53,* and *BRAF*. This tumour presented with a high rate of SVs, including a large deletion overlapping *TP53,* a partial deletion of *LRP1B,* and an interchromosomal translocation involving *CTNNA1,* the downregulation of which is associated with a worse prognosis in PCa [91]. Using our WGM approach, we identified additional large heterozygous deletions. Two overlap TSGs including *TP53* and *KCTD11,* and another overlaps with *TBX3* [92] and *NRF2.* NRF2 has been shown to suppress PCa cell mitosis and migration [93,94]. Another large deletion on chromosome 2 overlapped *HOXD10* and *HOXD3.* Decreased HOXD10 expression promotes an aggressive phenotype in PCa in knockdown mice, as well on retrospective review of clinical outcomes [95] and *HOXD3* methylation predicts earlier BCR [96].

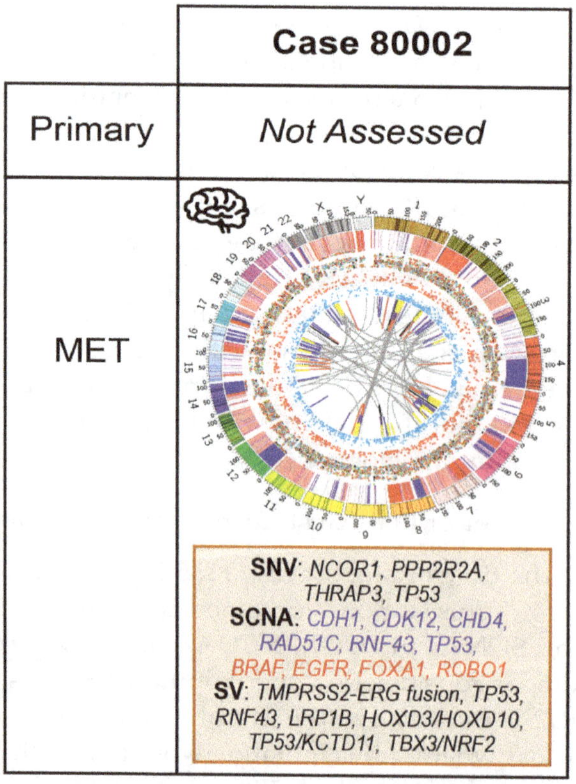

Figure 7. Summary of relevant genomic alterations for case 80002 with a brain metastasis at the time of sampling (80002) and Circos plots as per Figure 3.

Although COSMIC Mutational Signatures 1, 5, 8 and 9 are present, Signatures 17 and 18 contribute >5% each. Signature 18 may be associated with failure of base excision repair [97] and enriched in metastatic PCa [8]. Signature 17, predominantly found in gastric and oesophageal cancers, has been shown to co-occur with Signature 18 in mouse models of these cancers and this signature may be a by-product of oxidative damage [98,99].

Brain metastases are uncommon in prostate adenocarcinoma and tend to occur in cases with neuroendocrine differentiation [100]. However, gains in *FOXA1*, as seen in this case, are thought to protect against neuroendocrine trans-differentiation [101] and the *TMPRSS2-ERG* fusion supports the prostatic origin. This patient has a number of targets impacting androgen signalling, DDR and MAPK pathways. His clinical presentation would already support aggressive therapy with combination therapy and his genomic data include several poor prognostic features. The partial *LRP1B* deletion may produce sensitivity to pembrolizumab but the evidence for this is limited so this should only be considered as part of a clinical trial potentially upfront with docetaxel or later in his clinical course at development of CRPC. *KCTD11* is a negative regulator of hedgehog pathway signalling [102] and therefore its loss, identified using WGM, may increase signalling and imply this tumour would be sensitive to pathway inhibitors.

3. Materials and Methods

Included cases had adenocarcinoma of prostatic origin and were selected based on availability of tissue and matched blood specimens and micro- or overt metastatic disease either at the time of sampling or subsequent to radical prostatectomy. Patients sampled at the time of radical prostatectomy (primary tissue) had either pathologically confirmed lymph node metastases (19011, 19145, 19260, 19651) at diagnosis or subsequent metastatic relapse post-surgery (5545, 5684, 12543, 13179). Patients recruited at presentation of distant metastases had bone (1135, 147, A153, PCSD13) or brain (80002) tissue sampled.

All samples were obtained with written informed consent, as per the study approval granted from the St. Vincent's Human Research Ethics Committee (HREC), SVH/12/231 and HREC/12/SVH/323, Melbourne Health Human Research Ethics Committee HREC/12/MH/272 and Epworth Health 55512, or University of California Institute Review Board (IRB) approval 090401. Samples were shipped to the Garvan Institute of Medical Research in accordance with institutional Material Transfer Agreements (MTAs), and genomic screening and analysis were performed in accordance with approval granted by St. Vincent's Hospital HREC SVH/15/227 and governance review authorisation granted for human research at the Garvan Institute of Medical Research GHRP1522.

Primary tumour samples were collected at the time of radical prostatectomy and two core biopsies were taken from the prostate regions with cancer on preoperative biopsy. Lymph node tissue was collected at the time of radical prostatectomy from nodal masses with palpable tumour. Metastatic samples were obtained by image guided biopsy or at surgical resection (80002, PCSD13). All tissue samples were snap frozen. The presence of prostate cancer and its location within the samples was confirmed by a pathologist prior to dissection for DNA extraction. DNA was extracted from tissue and buffy coat or whole blood using one of two commercially available kits: the DNeasy blood and tissue kit protocol (Qiagen, Maryland), or for high molecular weight (HMW) DNA, the Bionano Prep Frozen Human Blood and Animal Tissue DNA isolation protocols (Bionano Genomics, San Diego document #30246 and #30077).

Demographic, clinical and pathological data were collected for each patient and are summarised in Figure 1 and Table 1. The median patient age at the time of PCa diagnosis was 65 years (range 51–77). The median time to biochemical recurrence (BCR) for those that underwent definitive first-line treatment and subsequently relapsed ($n = 8$) was 43.5 months (range 6–93); six of these patients relapsed with metastatic disease detectable on standard imaging at a median time of 86.5 months from initial diagnosis (range 24–120).

3.1. *Whole Genome Sequencing (WGS)*

DNA from tumour and matched blood underwent 2 × 150 bp sequencing on an Illumina HiSeq X Ten instrument (Kinghorn Centre for Clinical Genomics, Garvan Institute of Medical Research) averaging over 80× and 40× coverage, respectively. Read adapters were trimmed using Illumina's Bcl2fastq Conversion software (Illumina) and filtered to remove low quality bases (<Q15), short reads (<70 bp) and missing read pairs using cutadapt v1.9 [103]. Remaining reads were aligned to GRCh38 reference using bwa-mem v0.7.15 [104], with the ALT-aware mode. Alignment statistics were calculated using QualiMap v2.1.3 [105] and stromal contamination was calculated using Sequenza [106]. Sequencing statistics are summarized in Table S2. The sequencing data for the tumor and blood samples are available in the NCBI BioSample database under the following range of accessions: SAMN14209964–SAMN14209992.

3.2. *WGS Variant Calling*

The GATK pipeline version 3.5-0 was used for small variant calling [107]. We defined small variants as single nucleotide variants (SNVs) and insertions or deletions (indels) ≤ 50 bases and structural variants (SVs) as events ≥ 50 bases. Analysis-ready alignment per sample was called for SNVs and indels (GVCF mode) using GATK HaplotypeCaller (GVCF mode; [107]). Per-sample GVCFs were used for joint genotyping across genomes (GATK GenotypeGVCFs). Joint-called SNVs and indels were filtered via machine learning variant quality score recalibration and passed loci were kept. High-confidence somatic variants were called for each tumour-blood pair using MuTect2 [108]. A combination of GRIDSS and LUMPY was used for the detection of germline and somatic SVs [109,110]; potentially relevant SVs were manually inspected using Integrative Genomics Viewer (IGV) [111]. For somatic copy number alterations (SCNAs), binned copy number and segmentation profiles were determined using the copy number calling pipeline in the CNVkit package; gains (CN > 2) and losses (CN < 2) were assessed on calls adjusted for tumour purity [112].

3.3. *WGS Variant Annotation*

Germline and somatic SNVs and indels were annotated using Annovar [113] and pathogenic variants were manually inspected using IGV [111]. Missense mutations were further classified as potential oncogenic drivers using CanDrA [114] with PCa-specific databases.

The 30 SNV-derived Catalogue Of Somatic Mutations In Cancer (COSMIC) Mutational Signatures were annotated using the SomaticSignatures package in R [115]. Estimation of clonality and clonal segregation of somatic mutations were computed using PhyloWGS [116] and TITAN program [117].

3.4. *Tumour Mutational Burden and Percentage Genome Alteration*

TMB was calculated by counting the total number of small somatic mutations and dividing by genome size (3088 megabases (Mb)). PGA was calculated based on the cumulative number of base pairs altered for each gain or loss in the autosome (Chromosomes 1–22) per patient divided by the reference autosomal genome size (2875 Mb).

3.5. *Whole Genome Optical Mapping*

HMW DNA were fluorescently-labelled using either nicking enzyme Nt.BspQI (New England Biolabs) or non-nicking enzyme DLE-1 (BNG, Part #20351), according to the Bionano Prep Labeling NLRS Protocol (Document #30024) or Direct Label & Stain protocol (Document #30206), respectively. Samples prepared with BspQI (1135, 147, A153) were imaged using the Bionano Genomics (BNG) Irys system (San Diego, CA), while those prepared with DLE-1 (80002, 19651, 12543, 13179, 5545, 5684) were imaged using the BNG Saphyr system, to generate single molecule optical maps.

De novo assembly of single molecules into consensus genome maps was performed with the Bionano Solve (≥v3.2) software with aligner RefAligner (≥7437) [118–120]. Custom sets of parameters were used for this purpose and are included as File S1.

3.6. WGM Derived Genomic Rearrangements

SVs were identified relative to the human reference genome, GRCh38, whose genome maps were bioinformatically deduced based on predicted Nt.BspQI (GCTCTTCN) or DLE-1 (CTTAAG) motif sites. SV detection was performed as part of the Bionano Solve pipeline. Details of the underlying algorithm are described in the software's accompanying documentation (Document # 30110B).

3.7. WGM Derived Data Filtering

Filtering steps were performed on the resulting SVs. First, SVs that did not pass the Bionano recommended confidence level for the corresponding SV type were excluded; that is, all SVs other than inversion must have confidence > 0.1 and both breakpoints of an inversion event must have confidence > 0.01. Second, only rare SVs were included, defined as being observed in < 10% of a cohort of ~150 "normal" samples provided by Bionano [121]. Finally, "somatic" SVs were identified as those supported by a minimum of y_t molecules in the tumour sample but not observed in more than y_n molecules in the matching-normal sample, where $y = -0.3 + 0.13 * x$ and x being the effective coverage of the corresponding sample. This formula is recommended by Bionano as detailed in their Variant Annotation Pipeline v1.0 (BNG document # 30190). The minimum coverage cut-offs for somatic SV calling are summarized in Table S8. The WGM data are available at the following Doi: 10.25833/7wqs-gb12 [122].

3.8. Generation of a Prostate Cancer-Related Gene List

In addition to identifying annotated pathogenic and likely pathogenic alterations as well as the top genes affected by SCNAs, we reviewed alterations involving potential PCa driver genes and non-coding events associated with prostate cancer. A list of 159 PCa-associated genes was compiled from recent studies that identified recurrently mutated genes in primary and metastatic samples (Table S7) [6–9]. The list included commonly altered genes with potential functional relevance from The Cancer Genome Atlas (TCGA) primary PCa data [7,123], potential driver genes identified in primary and metastatic samples by Wedge et al. [8] and genes recurrently mutated in metastatic disease as identified by Robinson et al. [6] and Armenia et al. [9]. A list of non-coding events was compiled from recent published data (Table 4).

3.9. Other Analyses

The full list of binding clusters of 340 TFs compiled by the ENCODE project was obtained from the University of California Santa Cruz data repository (encRegTfbsClistered table; last updated 16 May 2019) and examined for somatic variants using a custom R script. Somatic variants within AR binding sites were evaluated against published putative binding sites observed in the LNCaP prostate cancer cell line (NCBI Gene Expression Omnibus accession GSE83860; [33]). The Circos plots in Figures 3–7 were generated using the CIRCOS software (v0.69-6) [124] based on SNV/indel data from MUTECT, copy number data from CNVkit, and SV data from GRIDSS. Phylogenetic reconstruction of tumour evolution for patient 19651 was performed using phyloWGS [116] based on SNV/indel data from MUTECT and copy number data from TITAN. Analyses of COSMIC Mutational Signature [125] clonal evolution was performed using the R package Palimpsest v1 [126] which utilized SNV data from MUTECT for estimates of mutation signature and SNV allele frequency data from MUTECT along with copy number segmentation data from Sequenza [106] for estimates of clonality.

4. Discussion

These real-world clinical cases demonstrate that clinically relevant mutations occur even in treatment-naïve patients across the spectrum of disease from high-risk primaries to metastatic cases. While the pathways impacted in these cases align with those identified in larger scale genomic studies, the coexistence of multiple alterations has not been explored. These findings raise several points.

Firstly, studies of neoadjuvant or adjuvant docetaxel in men with high-risk localized disease undertaking radical prostatectomy or definitive radiotherapy with ADT have had conflicting results [4, 46,71] but a subgroup of men appear to benefit. Poor prognostic genomic findings, such as *TP53* deletions or deleterious *BRCA2* alterations at baseline may be useful in selecting men for additional treatment. Similarly, not all men require escalated treatment beyond ADT for HSPC but biomarkers to guide treatment selection remain limited. The findings of *TP53* and/or Wnt pathway activating alterations in 5/8 (63%) of our primary samples highlight a potential biomarker for selecting men that should be considered for escalated therapy, preferably with docetaxel rather than a novel ASI [32,62,127]. Though speculative in the hormone sensitive setting, there is mounting evidence these alterations could be useful in guiding treatment selection in CRPC. Secondly, we observed events in minimally treated patients, such as *NCOR1* and *NCOR2* losses, that may be associated with ADT resistance. These alterations again may identify patients at risk for early development of CRPC who may need escalated therapy upfront. Thirdly, pathway mutations typically enriched in metastatic CRPC, particularly PI3K and MAPK pathway SCNAs, were frequently seen in our patients and represent potential targets for neoadjuvant intervention in high risk localized and/or de novo metastatic HSPC clinical trials.

The addition of WGM in our study did not identify a current therapeutic target but it did identify SVs impacting oncogenic and tumour suppressing genes that were not identified by using WGS alone. Though we did identify non-coding events affecting the promoters, enhancers and TF binding sites of relevant genes, their therapeutic relevance has yet to be elucidated. However, as WGS and WGM data accumulate and annotations improve, we may find new relevant mutations and begin to understand how they may be integrated into clinical practice. Additionally, the use of complementary genomic technologies such as RNA-sequencing and chromatin immunoprecipitation sequencing may improve our ability to translate genomic data into real-world clinical decision-making.

In this retrospective study, we assess the current status of genome profiling, specifically WGS and WGM, to inform decision-making for 13 patients presenting with metastatic PCa. Our findings suggest that, despite being a cancer associated with a low TMB, individual PCas can harbour complex series of mutations affecting multiple growth pathways. Therefore, the precision medicine model of identifying one target to treat is unlikely to succeed. Given its heterogeneity and despite comprising only a very small fraction of the I-PREDICT study cohort [128], PCa may be the ideal cancer to test the paradigm of using genomics to identify and treat multiple targets simultaneously.

5. Conclusions

Our analyses demonstrate that whole genomic interrogation of PCas may provide invaluable information at any stage of the disease. Most of our cases had alterations affecting multiple signalling pathways highlighting the utility of a comprehensive molecular assessment in tailoring treatment strategies to an individual. Moreover, WGM identified SVs disrupting prostate cancer relevant genes that were not apparent on our WGS analyses. Many non-coding and WGM events were identified but their therapeutic relevance is yet to be established. Though these data add to our current knowledge, further research is needed, potentially integrating additional genomic technologies, to identify new treatment targets and predictive biomarkers. While several potential biomarkers that may influence treatment decisions were found in these patients, most have yet to be validated in prospective clinical trials.

Author Contributions: Conceptualization, V.M.H., E.K.F.C., M.C., A.M.J., C.A.M.J., A.A.K, C.M.H. and P.I.C..; methodology, V.M.H., M.C., E.K.F.C., W.J., T.G., R.J.L., and D.C.P.; formal analysis, V.M.H., M.C, E.K.F.C., W.J., T.G.; resources, V.M.H., M.C., C.A.M.J., P.D.S., N.C., R.J.L., A.M.F.K., C.A.M.J., A.-M.H., C.M.H., A.A.K.; data curation, M.C., E.K.F.C.; writing—original draft preparation, M.C.; writing—review and editing, V.M.H., M.C., E.K.F.C., A.M.J., A.M.F.K., W.J., T.G., C.M.H., R.J.L.; visualization, E.K.F.C., M.C., V.M.H.; supervision, V.M.H.; project administration, V.M.H.; funding acquisition, V.M.H., A.M.J, C.A.M.J., P.D.S., P.I.C., N.C., C.M.H. All authors have read and agreed to the published version of the manuscript.

Acknowledgments: This work is supported by the HPC resources generously provided by the National Computational Infrastructure (Raijin/Gadi), the Garvan Institute of Medical Research (Wolfpack) and the University of Sydney (Artemis). We would like to acknowledge the Bionano team for generation of Case 19651's WGM data and additional support. We also thank the patients for their participation and the Garvan Institute Biobank and its staff for access to the tumor samples.

References

1. Global Burden of Disease Cancer Collaboration; Fitzmaurice, C.; Allen, C.; Barber, R.M.; Barregard, L.; Bhutta, Z.A.; Brenner, H.; Dicker, D.J.; Chimed-Orchir, O.; Dandona, R.; et al. Global, Regional, and National Cancer Incidence, Mortality, Years of Life Lost, Years Lived With Disability, and Disability-Adjusted Life-Years for 32 Cancer Groups, 1990 to 2015: A Systematic Analysis for the Global Burden of Disease Study. *JAMA Oncol.* **2017**, *3*, 524–548. [CrossRef]
2. Sweeney, C.J.; Chen, Y.-H.; Carducci, M.; Liu, G.; Jarrard, D.F.; Eisenberger, M.; Wong, Y.-N.; Hahn, N.; Kohli, M.; Cooney, M.M.; et al. Chemohormonal Therapy in Metastatic Hormone-Sensitive Prostate Cancer. *N. Engl. J. Med.* **2015**, *373*, 737–746. [CrossRef]
3. James, N.D.; Sydes, M.R.; Clarke, N.W.; Mason, M.D.; Dearnaley, D.P.; Spears, M.R.; Ritchie, A.W.S.; Parker, C.C.; Russell, J.M.; Attard, G.; et al. Addition of docetaxel, zoledronic acid, or both to first-line hormone therapy in prostate cancer (STAMPEDE): survival results from an adaptive, multiarm, multistage, platform randomised controlled trial. *Lancet* **2016**, *387*, 1163–1177. [CrossRef]
4. Rosenthal, S.A.; Hu, C.; Sartor, O.; Gomella, L.G.; Amin, M.B.; Purdy, J.; Michalski, J.M.; Garzotto, M.G.; Pervez, N.; Balogh, A.G.; et al. Effect of Chemotherapy With Docetaxel With Androgen Suppression and Radiotherapy for Localized High-Risk Prostate Cancer: The Randomized Phase III NRG Oncology RTOG 0521 Trial. *J. Clin. Oncol.* **2019**, *37*, 1159–1168. [CrossRef] [PubMed]
5. Parker, C.C.; James, N.D.; Brawley, C.D.; Clarke, N.W.; Hoyle, A.P.; Ali, A.; Ritchie, A.W.S.; Attard, G.; Chowdhury, S.; Cross, W.; et al. Systemic Therapy for Advanced or Metastatic Prostate cancer: Evaluation of Drug Efficacy (STAMPEDE) investigators Radiotherapy to the primary tumour for newly diagnosed, metastatic prostate cancer (STAMPEDE): A randomised controlled phase 3 trial. *Lancet* **2018**, *392*, 2353–2366. [CrossRef]
6. Robinson, D.; Van Allen, E.M.; Wu, Y.-M.; Schultz, N.; Lonigro, R.J.; Mosquera, J.-M.; Montgomery, B.; Taplin, M.-E.; Pritchard, C.C.; Attard, G.; et al. Integrative clinical genomics of advanced prostate cancer. *Cell* **2015**, *161*, 1215–1228. [CrossRef] [PubMed]
7. Cancer Genome Atlas Research Network. The molecular taxonomy of primary prostate cancer. *Cell* **2015**, *163*, 1011–1025. [CrossRef]
8. Wedge, D.C.; Gundem, G.; Mitchell, T.; Woodcock, D.J.; Martincorena, I.; Ghori, M.; Zamora, J.; Butler, A.; Whitaker, H.; Kote-Jarai, Z.; et al. Sequencing of prostate cancers identifies new cancer genes, routes of progression and drug targets. *Nat. Genet.* **2018**, *50*, 682–692. [CrossRef]
9. Armenia, J.; Wankowicz, S.A.M.; Liu, D.; Gao, J.; Kundra, R.; Reznik, E.; Chatila, W.K.; Chakravarty, D.; Han, G.C.; Coleman, I.; et al. The long tail of oncogenic drivers in prostate cancer. *Nat. Genet.* **2018**, *50*, 645–651. [CrossRef]
10. Quigley, D.A.; Dang, H.X.; Zhao, S.G.; Lloyd, P.; Aggarwal, R.; Alumkal, J.J.; Foye, A.; Kothari, V.; Perry, M.D.; Bailey, A.M.; et al. Genomic hallmarks and structural variation in metastatic prostate cancer. *Cell* **2018**, *174*, 758–769. [CrossRef]
11. Viswanathan, S.R.; Ha, G.; Hoff, A.M.; Wala, J.A.; Carrot-Zhang, J.; Whelan, C.W.; Haradhvala, N.J.; Freeman, S.S.; Reed, S.C.; Rhoades, J.; et al. Structural Alterations Driving Castration-Resistant Prostate Cancer Revealed by Linked-Read Genome Sequencing. *Cell* **2018** *174*, 433–447. [CrossRef] [PubMed]

12. Gerlinger, M.; Rowan, A.J.; Horswell, S.; Math, M.; Larkin, J.; Endesfelder, D.; Gronroos, E.; Martinez, P.; Matthews, N.; Stewart, A.; et al. Intratumor heterogeneity and branched evolution revealed by multiregion sequencing. *N. Engl. J. Med.* **2012**, *366*, 883–892. [CrossRef]
13. Boutros, P.C.; Fraser, M.; Harding, N.J.; de Borja, R.; Trudel, D.; Lalonde, E.; Meng, A.; Hennings-Yeomans, P.H.; McPherson, A.; Sabelnykova, V.Y.; et al. Spatial genomic heterogeneity within localized, multifocal prostate cancer. *Nat. Genet.* **2015**, *47*, 736–745. [CrossRef] [PubMed]
14. Ciccarese, C.; Massari, F.; Iacovelli, R.; Fiorentino, M.; Montironi, R.; Di Nunno, V.; Giunchi, F.; Brunelli, M.; Tortora, G. Prostate cancer heterogeneity: Discovering novel molecular targets for therapy. *Cancer Treat. Rev.* **2017**, *54*, 68–73. [CrossRef] [PubMed]
15. Attard, G.; Clark, J.; Ambroisine, L.; Mills, I.G.; Fisher, G.; Flohr, P.; Reid, A.; Edwards, S.; Kovacs, G.; Berney, D.; et al. Transatlantic Prostate Group Heterogeneity and clinical significance of ETV1 translocations in human prostate cancer. *Br. J. Cancer* **2008**, *99*, 314–320. [CrossRef] [PubMed]
16. Kristiansen, A.; Bergström, R.; Delahunt, B.; Samaratunga, H.; Guðjónsdóttir, J.; Grönberg, H.; Egevad, L.; Lindberg, J. Somatic alterations detected in diagnostic prostate biopsies provide an inadequate representation of multifocal prostate cancer. *Prostate* **2019**, *79*, 920–928. [CrossRef]
17. Hotte, S.J.; Joshua, A.M.; Torria, V.; Macfarlane, R.J.; Basappa, N.S.; Winquist, J.P.; Mukherjee, S.; Gregg, R.W.; Kollmannsberger, C.K.; Finch, D.L.; et al. NCIC CTG, IND-205: A phase II study of PX-866 in patients with recurrent or metastatic castration-resistant prostate cancer (CRPC). *J. Clin. Oncol.* **2013**, *31*, 5042. [CrossRef]
18. Hong, D.S.; Bowles, D.W.; Falchook, G.S.; Messersmith, W.A.; George, G.C.; O'Bryant, C.L.; Vo, A.C.H.; Klucher, K.; Herbst, R.S.; Eckhardt, S.G.; et al. A multicenter phase I trial of PX-866, an oral irreversible phosphatidylinositol 3-kinase inhibitor, in patients with advanced solid tumors. *Clin. Cancer Res.* **2012**, *18*, 4173–4182. [CrossRef]
19. de Bono, J.S.; De Giorgi, U.; Rodrigues, D.N.; Massard, C.; Bracarda, S.; Font, A.; Arranz Arija, J.A.; Shih, K.C.; Radavoi, G.D.; Xu, N.; et al. Randomized Phase II Study Evaluating Akt Blockade with Ipatasertib, in Combination with Abiraterone, in Patients with Metastatic Prostate Cancer with and without PTEN Loss. *Clin. Cancer Res.* **2019**, *25*, 928–936. [CrossRef]
20. Sandhu, S.K.; Schelman, W.R.; Wilding, G.; Moreno, V.; Baird, R.D.; Miranda, S.; Hylands, L.; Riisnaes, R.; Forster, M.; Omlin, A.; et al. The poly(ADP-ribose) polymerase inhibitor niraparib (MK4827) in BRCA mutation carriers and patients with sporadic cancer: A phase 1 dose-escalation trial. *Lancet Oncol.* **2013**, *14*, 882–892. [CrossRef]
21. Marshall, C.H.; Sokolova, A.O.; McNatty, A.L.; Cheng, H.H.; Eisenberger, M.A.; Bryce, A.H.; Schweizer, M.T.; Antonarakis, E.S. Differential Response to Olaparib Treatment Among Men with Metastatic Castration-resistant Prostate Cancer Harboring BRCA1 or BRCA2 Versus ATM Mutations. *Eur. Urol.* **2019**, *76*, 452–458. [CrossRef] [PubMed]
22. Sandhu, S.K.; Omlin, A.; Hylands, L.; Miranda, S.; Barber, L.J.; Riisnaes, R.; Reid, A.H.; Attard, G.; Chen, L.; Kozarewa, I.; et al. Poly(ADP-ribose) polymerase (PARP) inhibitors for the treatment of advanced germline BRCA2 mutant prostate cancer. *Ann. Oncol.* **2013**, *24*, 1416–1418. [CrossRef] [PubMed]
23. Mateo, J.; Carreira, S.; Sandhu, S.; Miranda, S.; Mossop, H.; Perez-Lopez, R.; Nava Rodrigues, D.; Robinson, D.; Omlin, A.; Tunariu, N.; et al. DNA-Repair Defects and Olaparib in Metastatic Prostate Cancer. *N. Engl. J. Med.* **2015**, *373*, 1697–1708. [CrossRef] [PubMed]
24. 1000 Genomes Project Consortium; Auton, A.; Brooks, L.D.; Durbin, R.M.; Garrison, E.P.; Kang, H.M.; Korbel, J.O.; Marchini, J.L.; McCarthy, S.; McVean, G.A.; et al. A global reference for human genetic variation. *Nature* **2015**, *526*, 68–74. [CrossRef] [PubMed]
25. Gudmundsson, J.; Sulem, P.; Rafnar, T.; Bergthorsson, J.T.; Manolescu, A.; Gudbjartsson, D.; Agnarsson, B.A.; Sigurdsson, A.; Benediktsdottir, K.R.; Blondal, T.; et al. Common sequence variants on 2p15 and Xp11.22 confer susceptibility to prostate cancer. *Nat. Genet.* **2008**, *40*, 281–283. [CrossRef]
26. Bange, J.; Prechtl, D.; Cheburkin, Y.; Specht, K.; Harbeck, N.; Schmitt, M.; Knyazeva, T.; Müller, S.; Gärtner, S.; Sures, I.; et al. Cancer progression and tumor cell motility are associated with the FGFR4 Arg(388) allele. *Cancer Res.* **2002**, *62*, 840–847.
27. Zhang, X.; Cowper-Sal lari, R.; Bailey, S.D.; Moore, J.H.; Lupien, M. Integrative functional genomics identifies an enhancer looping to the SOX9 gene disrupted by the 17q24.3 prostate cancer risk locus. *Genome Res.* **2012**, *22*, 1437–1446. [CrossRef]

28. Wang, W. Emergence of a DNA-damage response network consisting of Fanconi anaemia and BRCA proteins. *Nat. Rev. Genet.* **2007**, *8*, 735–748. [CrossRef]
29. Lang, S.H.; Swift, S.L.; White, H.; Misso, K.; Kleijnen, J.; Quek, R.G.W. A systematic review of the prevalence of DNA damage response gene mutations in prostate cancer. *Int. J. Oncol.* **2019**, *55*, 597–616. [CrossRef]
30. Nickols, N.G.; Nazarian, R.; Zhao, S.G.; Tan, V.; Uzunangelov, V.; Xia, Z.; Baertsch, R.; Neeman, E.; Gao, A.C.; Thomas, G.V.; et al. MEK-ERK signaling is a therapeutic target in metastatic castration resistant prostate cancer. *Prostate Cancer Prostatic Dis.* **2019**, *22*, 531–538. [CrossRef]
31. Crumbaker, M.; Khoja, L.; Joshua, A.M. AR signaling and the PI3K pathway in prostate cancer. *Cancers* **2017**, *9*, 34. [CrossRef] [PubMed]
32. Isaacsson Velho, P.; Fu, W.; Wang, H.; Mirkheshti, N.; Qazi, F.; Lima, F.A.S.; Shaukat, F.; Carducci, M.A.; Denmeade, S.R.; Paller, C.J.; et al. Wnt-pathway Activating Mutations Are Associated with Resistance to First-line Abiraterone and Enzalutamide in Castration-resistant Prostate Cancer. *Eur. Urol.* **2020**, *77*, 14–21. [CrossRef] [PubMed]
33. Morova, T.; McNeill, D.R.; Lallous, N.; Gönen, M.; Dalal, K.; Wilson, D.M.; Gürsoy, A.; Keskin, Ö.; Lack, N.A. Androgen receptor-binding sites are highly mutated in prostate cancer. *Nat. Commun.* **2020**, *11*, 1–10. [CrossRef] [PubMed]
34. Zhou, S.; Hawley, J.R.; Soares, F.; Grillo, G.; Teng, M.; Madani Tonekaboni, S.A.; Hua, J.T.; Kron, K.J.; Mazrooei, P.; Ahmed, M.; et al. Noncoding mutations target cis-regulatory elements of the FOXA1 plexus in prostate cancer. *Nat. Commun.* **2020**, *11*, 441. [CrossRef] [PubMed]
35. Takeda, D.Y.; Spisák, S.; Seo, J.-H.; Bell, C.; O'Connor, E.; Korthauer, K.; Ribli, D.; Csabai, I.; Solymosi, N.; Szállási, Z.; et al. A somatically acquired enhancer of the androgen receptor is a noncoding driver in advanced prostate cancer. *Cell* **2018**, *174*, 422–432. [CrossRef] [PubMed]
36. Yeager, M.; Orr, N.; Hayes, R.B.; Jacobs, K.B.; Kraft, P.; Wacholder, S.; Minichiello, M.J.; Fearnhead, P.; Yu, K.; Chatterjee, N.; et al. Genome-wide association study of prostate cancer identifies a second risk locus at 8q24. *Nat. Genet.* **2007**, *39*, 645–649. [CrossRef]
37. Ahmadiyeh, N.; Pomerantz, M.M.; Grisanzio, C.; Herman, P.; Jia, L.; Almendro, V.; He, H.H.; Brown, M.; Liu, X.S.; Davis, M.; et al. 8q24 prostate, breast, and colon cancer risk loci show tissue-specific long-range interaction with MYC. *Proc. Natl. Acad. Sci. USA* **2010**, *107*, 9742–9746. [CrossRef] [PubMed]
38. Hsu, C.-C.; Hu, C.-D. Transcriptional activity of c-Jun is critical for the suppression of AR function. *Mol. Cell. Endocrinol.* **2013**, *372*, 12–22. [CrossRef]
39. Alexandrov, L.B.; Nik-Zainal, S.; Wedge, D.C.; Aparicio, S.A.J.R.; Behjati, S.; Biankin, A.V.; Bignell, G.R.; Bolli, N.; Borg, A.; Børresen-Dale, A.-L.; et al. Signatures of mutational processes in human cancer. *Nature* **2013**, *500*, 415–421. [CrossRef]
40. Ma, J.; Setton, J.; Lee, N.Y.; Riaz, N.; Powell, S.N. The therapeutic significance of mutational signatures from DNA repair deficiency in cancer. *Nat. Commun.* **2018**, *9*, 1–12. [CrossRef]
41. Nik-Zainal, S.; Davies, H.; Staaf, J.; Ramakrishna, M.; Glodzik, D.; Zou, X.; Martincorena, I.; Alexandrov, L.B.; Martin, S.; Wedge, D.C.; et al. Landscape of somatic mutations in 560 breast cancer whole-genome sequences. *Nature* **2016**, *534*, 47–54. [CrossRef]
42. Eggener, S.E.; Scardino, P.T.; Walsh, P.C.; Han, M.; Partin, A.W.; Trock, B.J.; Feng, Z.; Wood, D.P.; Eastham, J.A.; Yossepowitch, O.; et al. Predicting 15-year prostate cancer specific mortality after radical prostatectomy. *J. Urol.* **2011**, *185*, 869–875. [CrossRef]
43. Touijer, K.A.; Karnes, R.J.; Passoni, N.; Sjoberg, D.D.; Assel, M.; Fossati, N.; Gandaglia, G.; Eastham, J.A.; Scardino, P.T.; Vickers, A.; et al. Survival Outcomes of Men with Lymph Node-positive Prostate Cancer After Radical Prostatectomy: A Comparative Analysis of Different Postoperative Management Strategies. *Eur. Urol.* **2018**, *73*, 890–896. [CrossRef]
44. James, N.D.; de Bono, J.S.; Spears, M.R.; Clarke, N.W.; Mason, M.D.; Dearnaley, D.P.; Ritchie, A.W.S.; Amos, C.L.; Gilson, C.; Jones, R.J.; et al. STAMPEDE Investigators Abiraterone for Prostate Cancer Not Previously Treated with Hormone Therapy. *N. Engl. J. Med.* **2017**, *377*, 338–351. [CrossRef]
45. James, N.; Woods, B.; Sideris, E.; Spears, M.R.; Dearnaley, D.P.; Mason, M.; Clarke, N.; Parmar, M.K.B.; Sydes, M.R.; Sculpher, M. STAMPEDE Investigators Addition of docetaxel to first-line long-term hormone therapy in prostate cancer (STAMPEDE): Long-term survival, quality-adjusted survival, and cost-effectiveness analysis. *J. Clin. Oncol.* **2018**, *36*, 162. [CrossRef]

46. Hurwitz, M.D.; Harris, J.; Sartor, O.; Xiao, Y.; Shayegan, B.; Sperduto, P.W.; Badiozamani, K.R.; Lawton, C.A.F.; Horwitz, E.M.; Michalski, J.M.; et al. Adjuvant radiation therapy, androgen deprivation, and docetaxel for high-risk prostate cancer postprostatectomy: Results of NRG Oncology/RTOG study 0621. *Cancer* **2017**, *123*, 2489–2496. [CrossRef]
47. Eastham, J.A.; Heller, G.; Halabi, S.; Monk, P.; Clinton, S.K.; Szmulewitz, R.Z.; Coleman, J.; Gleave, M.; Evans, C.P.; Hillman, D.W.; et al. CALGB 90203 (Alliance): Radical prostatectomy (RP) with or without neoadjuvant chemohormonal therapy (CHT) in men with clinically localized, high-risk prostate cancer (CLHRPC). *J. Clin. Oncol.* **2019**, *37*, 5079. [CrossRef]
48. Chang, M.T.; Asthana, S.; Gao, S.P.; Lee, B.H.; Chapman, J.S.; Kandoth, C.; Gao, J.; Socci, N.D.; Solit, D.B.; Olshen, A.B.; et al. Identifying recurrent mutations in cancer reveals widespread lineage diversity and mutational specificity. *Nat. Biotechnol.* **2016**, *34*, 155–163. [CrossRef] [PubMed]
49. Kim, S.; Xu, X.; Hecht, A.; Boyer, T.G. Mediator is a transducer of Wnt/beta-catenin signaling. *J. Biol. Chem.* **2006**, *281*, 14066–14075. [CrossRef] [PubMed]
50. Linch, M.; Goh, G.; Hiley, C.; Shanmugabavan, Y.; McGranahan, N.; Rowan, A.; Wong, Y.N.S.; King, H.; Furness, A.; Freeman, A.; et al. Intratumoural evolutionary landscape of high-risk prostate cancer: The PROGENY study of genomic and immune parameters. *Ann. Oncol.* **2017**, *28*, 2472–2480. [CrossRef]
51. Lalonde, E.; Ishkanian, A.S.; Sykes, J.; Fraser, M.; Ross-Adams, H.; Erho, N.; Dunning, M.J.; Halim, S.; Lamb, A.D.; Moon, N.C.; et al. Tumour genomic and microenvironmental heterogeneity for integrated prediction of 5-year biochemical recurrence of prostate cancer: A retrospective cohort study. *Lancet Oncol.* **2014**, *15*, 1521–1532. [CrossRef]
52. Prophet, M.; Xiao, K.; Gourdin, T.S.; Nagy, R.J.; Kiedrowski, L.A.; Ledet, E.; Sonpavde, G.; Sartor, A.O.; Lilly, M.B. Detection of actionable*BRAF* missense mutations by ctDNA-based genomic analysis in prostate cancer. *J. Clin. Oncol.* **2018**, *36*, 306. [CrossRef]
53. Mateo, J.; Porta, N.; Bianchini, D.; McGovern, U.; Elliott, T.; Jones, R.; Syndikus, I.; Ralph, C.; Jain, S.; Varughese, M.; et al. Olaparib in patients with metastatic castration-resistant prostate cancer with DNA repair gene aberrations (TOPARP-B): A multicentre, open-label, randomised, phase 2 trial. *Lancet Oncol.* **2020**, *21*, 162–174. [CrossRef]
54. Forster, M.D.; Dedes, K.J.; Sandhu, S.; Frentzas, S.; Kristeleit, R.; Ashworth, A.; Poole, C.J.; Weigelt, B.; Kaye, S.B.; Molife, L.R. Treatment with olaparib in a patient with PTEN-deficient endometrioid endometrial cancer. *Nat. Rev. Clin. Oncol.* **2011**, *8*, 302–306. [CrossRef]
55. Wang, J. Complete pathological remission after treatment with olaparib in a patient with PTEN-deficient sarcomatoid prostate cancer. *J. Mol. Cancer* **2018**, *1*, 17–19.
56. González-Billalabeitia, E.; Seitzer, N.; Song, S.J.; Song, M.S.; Patnaik, A.; Liu, X.-S.; Epping, M.T.; Papa, A.; Hobbs, R.M.; Chen, M.; et al. Vulnerabilities of PTEN-TP53-deficient prostate cancers to compound PARP-PI3K inhibition. *Cancer Discov.* **2014**, *4*, 896–904. [CrossRef] [PubMed]
57. Hodgson, M.C.; Astapova, I.; Cheng, S.; Lee, L.J.; Verhoeven, M.C.; Choi, E.; Balk, S.P.; Hollenberg, A.N. The androgen receptor recruits nuclear receptor CoRepressor (N-CoR) in the presence of mifepristone via its N and C termini revealing a novel molecular mechanism for androgen receptor antagonists. *J. Biol. Chem.* **2005**, *280*, 6511–6519. [CrossRef]
58. Cui, J.; Yang, Y.; Zhang, C.; Hu, P.; Kan, W.; Bai, X.; Liu, X.; Song, H. FBI-1 functions as a novel AR co-repressor in prostate cancer cells. *Cell Mol. Life Sci.* **2011**, *68*, 1091–1103. [CrossRef]
59. Wong, M.M.; Guo, C.; Zhang, J. Nuclear receptor corepressor complexes in cancer: Mechanism, function and regulation. *Am. J. Clin. Exp. Urol.* **2014**, *2*, 169–187.
60. Lopez, S.M.; Agoulnik, A.I.; Zhang, M.; Peterson, L.E.; Suarez, E.; Gandarillas, G.A.; Frolov, A.; Li, R.; Rajapakshe, K.; Coarfa, C.; et al. Nuclear Receptor Corepressor 1 Expression and Output Declines with Prostate Cancer Progression. *Clin. Cancer Res.* **2016**, *22*, 3937–3949. [CrossRef]
61. Lorenzin, F.; Demichelis, F. Evolution of the prostate cancer genome towards resistance. *JTGG J. Transl. Genet. Genom.* **2019**, *3*, 1–12. [CrossRef]
62. Maughan, B.L.; Guedes, L.B.; Boucher, K.; Rajoria, G.; Liu, Z.; Klimek, S.; Zoino, R.; Antonarakis, E.S.; Lotan, T.L. p53 status in the primary tumor predicts efficacy of subsequent abiraterone and enzalutamide in castration-resistant prostate cancer. *Prostate Cancer Prostatic Dis.* **2018**, *21*, 260–268. [CrossRef] [PubMed]

63. Wu, Y.-M.; Cieślik, M.; Lonigro, R.J.; Vats, P.; Reimers, M.A.; Cao, X.; Ning, Y.; Wang, L.; Kunju, L.P.; de Sarkar, N.; et al. Inactivation of CDK12 delineates a distinct immunogenic class of advanced prostate cancer. *Cell* **2018**, *173*, 1770–1782. [CrossRef] [PubMed]
64. Løvf, M.; Zhao, S.; Axcrona, U.; Johannessen, B.; Bakken, A.C.; Carm, K.T.; Hoff, A.M.; Myklebost, O.; Meza-Zepeda, L.A.; Lie, A.K.; et al. Multifocal primary prostate cancer exhibits high degree of genomic heterogeneity. *Eur. Urol.* **2019**, *75*, 498–505. [CrossRef] [PubMed]
65. Edwards, S.M.; Evans, D.G.R.; Hope, Q.; Norman, A.R.; Barbachano, Y.; Bullock, S.; Kote-Jarai, Z.; Meitz, J.; Falconer, A.; Osin, P.; et al. UK Genetic Prostate Cancer Study Collaborators and BAUS Section of Oncology Prostate cancer in BRCA2 germline mutation carriers is associated with poorer prognosis. *Br. J. Cancer* **2010**, *103*, 918–924. [CrossRef] [PubMed]
66. Castro, E.; Goh, C.; Leongamornlert, D.; Saunders, E.; Tymrakiewicz, M.; Dadaev, T.; Govindasami, K.; Guy, M.; Ellis, S.; Frost, D.; et al. Effect of BRCA Mutations on Metastatic Relapse and Cause-specific Survival After Radical Treatment for Localised Prostate Cancer. *Eur. Urol.* **2015**, *68*, 186–193. [CrossRef]
67. Na, R.; Zheng, S.L.; Han, M.; Yu, H.; Jiang, D.; Shah, S.; Ewing, C.M.; Zhang, L.; Novakovic, K.; Petkewicz, J.; et al. Germline Mutations in ATM and BRCA1/2 Distinguish Risk for Lethal and Indolent Prostate Cancer and are Associated with Early Age at Death. *Eur. Urol.* **2017**, *71*, 740–747. [CrossRef]
68. Castro, E.; Goh, C.; Olmos, D.; Saunders, E.; Leongamornlert, D.; Tymrakiewicz, M.; Mahmud, N.; Dadaev, T.; Govindasami, K.; Guy, M.; et al. Germline BRCA mutations are associated with higher risk of nodal involvement, distant metastasis, and poor survival outcomes in prostate cancer. *J. Clin. Oncol.* **2013**, *31*, 1748–1757. [CrossRef]
69. Annala, M.; Struss, W.J.; Warner, E.W.; Beja, K.; Vandekerkhove, G.; Wong, A.; Khalaf, D.; Seppälä, I.-L.; So, A.; Lo, G.; et al. Treatment Outcomes and Tumor Loss of Heterozygosity in Germline DNA Repair-deficient Prostate Cancer. *Eur. Urol.* **2017**, *72*, 34–42. [CrossRef]
70. Pomerantz, M.M.; Spisák, S.; Jia, L.; Cronin, A.M.; Csabai, I.; Ledet, E.; Sartor, A.O.; Rainville, I.; O'Connor, E.P.; Herbert, Z.T.; et al. The association between germline BRCA2 variants and sensitivity to platinum-based chemotherapy among men with metastatic prostate cancer. *Cancer* **2017**, *123*, 3532–3539. [CrossRef]
71. Oudard, S.; Latorzeff, I.; Caty, A.; Miglianico, L.; Sevin, E.; Hardy-Bessard, A.C.; Delva, R.; Rolland, F.; Mouret, L.; Priou, F.; et al. Effect of Adding Docetaxel to Androgen-Deprivation Therapy in Patients With High-Risk Prostate Cancer With Rising Prostate-Specific Antigen Levels After Primary Local Therapy: A Randomized Clinical Trial. *JAMA Oncol.* **2019**, *5*, 623–632. [CrossRef]
72. Migita, T.; Takayama, K.-I.; Urano, T.; Obinata, D.; Ikeda, K.; Soga, T.; Takahashi, S.; Inoue, S. ACSL3 promotes intratumoral steroidogenesis in prostate cancer cells. *Cancer Sci.* **2017**, *108*, 2011–2021. [CrossRef] [PubMed]
73. Hieronymus, H.; Iaquinta, P.J.; Wongvipat, J.; Gopalan, A.; Murali, R.; Mao, N.; Carver, B.S.; Sawyers, C.L. Deletion of 3p13-14 locus spanning FOXP1 to SHQ1 cooperates with PTEN loss in prostate oncogenesis. *Nat. Commun.* **2017**, *8*, 1–10. [CrossRef] [PubMed]
74. Desotelle, J.; Truong, M.; Ewald, J.; Weeratunga, P.; Yang, B.; Huang, W.; Jarrard, D. CpG island hypermethylation frequently silences FILIP1L isoform 2 expression in prostate cancer. *J. Urol.* **2013**, *189*, 329–335. [CrossRef] [PubMed]
75. Barbieri, C.E.; Baca, S.C.; Lawrence, M.S.; Demichelis, F.; Blattner, M.; Theurillat, J.-P.; White, T.A.; Stojanov, P.; Van Allen, E.; Stransky, N.; et al. Exome sequencing identifies recurrent SPOP, FOXA1 and MED12 mutations in prostate cancer. *Nat. Genet.* **2012**, *44*, 685–689. [CrossRef]
76. Boysen, G.; Rodrigues, D.N.; Rescigno, P.; Seed, G.; Dolling, D.; Riisnaes, R.; Crespo, M.; Zafeiriou, Z.; Sumanasuriya, S.; Bianchini, D.; et al. SPOP-Mutated/CHD1-Deleted Lethal Prostate Cancer and Abiraterone Sensitivity. *Clin. Cancer Res.* **2018**, *24*, 5585–5593. [CrossRef]
77. Shenoy, T.R.; Boysen, G.; Wang, M.Y.; Xu, Q.Z.; Guo, W.; Koh, F.M.; Wang, C.; Zhang, L.Z.; Wang, Y.; Gil, V.; et al. CHD1 loss sensitizes prostate cancer to DNA damaging therapy by promoting error-prone double-strand break repair. *Ann. Oncol.* **2017**, *28*, 1495–1507. [CrossRef]
78. Tucker, M.D.; Zhu, J.; Marin, D.; Gupta, R.T.; Gupta, S.; Berry, W.R.; Ramalingam, S.; Zhang, T.; Harrison, M.; Wu, Y.; et al. Pembrolizumab in men with heavily treated metastatic castrate-resistant prostate cancer. *Cancer Med.* **2019**, *8*, 4644–4655. [CrossRef]
79. Yu, J.; Zhang, Y.; McIlroy, J.; Rordorf-Nikolic, T.; Orr, G.A.; Backer, J.M. Regulation of the p85/p110 phosphatidylinositol 3′-kinase: Stabilization and inhibition of the p110alpha catalytic subunit by the p85 regulatory subunit. *Mol. Cell. Biol.* **1998**, *18*, 1379–1387. [CrossRef]

80. Xue, Z.; Vis, D.J.; Bruna, A.; Sustic, T.; van Wageningen, S.; Batra, A.S.; Rueda, O.M.; Bosdriesz, E.; Caldas, C.; Wessels, L.F.A.; et al. MAP3K1 and MAP2K4 mutations are associated with sensitivity to MEK inhibitors in multiple cancer models. *Cell Res.* **2018**, *28*, 719–729. [CrossRef]
81. Chen, Q.; Yao, Y.-T.; Xu, H.; Chen, Y.-B.; Gu, M.; Cai, Z.-K.; Wang, Z. SPOCK1 promotes tumor growth and metastasis in human prostate cancer. *Drug Des. Dev. Ther.* **2016**, *10*, 2311–2321. [PubMed]
82. Comuzzi, B.; Nemes, C.; Schmidt, S.; Jasarevic, Z.; Lodde, M.; Pycha, A.; Bartsch, G.; Offner, F.; Culig, Z.; Hobisch, A. The androgen receptor co-activator CBP is up-regulated following androgen withdrawal and is highly expressed in advanced prostate cancer. *J. Pathol.* **2004**, *204*, 159–166. [CrossRef] [PubMed]
83. Shafran, J.S.; Andrieu, G.P.; Györffy, B.; Denis, G.V. BRD4 Regulates Metastatic Potential of Castration-Resistant Prostate Cancer through AHNAK. *Mol. Cancer Res.* **2019**, *17*, 1627–1638. [CrossRef]
84. Lewin, J.; Soria, J.-C.; Stathis, A.; Delord, J.-P.; Peters, S.; Awada, A.; Aftimos, P.G.; Bekradda, M.; Rezai, K.; Zeng, Z.; et al. Phase Ib Trial With Birabresib, a Small-Molecule Inhibitor of Bromodomain and Extraterminal Proteins, in Patients With Selected Advanced Solid Tumors. *J. Clin. Oncol.* **2018**, *36*, 3007–3014. [CrossRef]
85. Li, X.; Baek, G.; Ramanand, S.G.; Sharp, A.; Gao, Y.; Yuan, W.; Welti, J.; Rodrigues, D.N.; Dolling, D.; Figueiredo, I.; et al. BRD4 Promotes DNA Repair and Mediates the Formation of TMPRSS2-ERG Gene Rearrangements in Prostate Cancer. *Cell Rep.* **2018**, *22*, 796–808. [CrossRef]
86. Karczewski, K.J.; Francioli, L.C.; Tiao, G.; Cummings, B.B.; Alföldi, J.; Wang, Q.; Collins, R.L.; Laricchia, K.M.; Ganna, A.; Birnbaum, D.P.; et al. Variation across 141,456 human exomes and genomes reveals the spectrum of loss-of-function intolerance across human protein-coding genes. *BioRxiv* **2019**.
87. Kotredes, K.P.; Razmpour, R.; Lutton, E.; Alfonso-Prieto, M.; Ramirez, S.H.; Gamero, A.M. Characterization of cancer-associated IDH2 mutations that differ in tumorigenicity, chemosensitivity and 2-hydroxyglutarate production. *Oncotarget* **2019**, *10*, 2675–2692. [CrossRef]
88. Mulholland, D.J.; Tran, L.M.; Li, Y.; Cai, H.; Morim, A.; Wang, S.; Plaisier, S.; Garraway, I.P.; Huang, J.; Graeber, T.G.; et al. Cell autonomous role of PTEN in regulating castration-resistant prostate cancer growth. *Cancer Cell* **2011**, *19*, 792–804. [CrossRef]
89. Carver, B.S.; Chapinski, C.; Wongvipat, J.; Hieronymus, H.; Chen, Y.; Chandarlapaty, S.; Arora, V.K.; Le, C.; Koutcher, J.; Scher, H.; et al. Reciprocal feedback regulation of PI3K and androgen receptor signaling in PTEN-deficient prostate cancer. *Cancer Cell* **2011**, *19*, 575–586. [CrossRef]
90. Qian, X.; Li, G.; Vass, W.C.; Papageorge, A.; Walker, R.C.; Asnaghi, L.; Steinbach, P.J.; Tosato, G.; Hunter, K.; Lowy, D.R. The Tensin-3 protein, including its SH2 domain, is phosphorylated by Src and contributes to tumorigenesis and metastasis. *Cancer Cell* **2009**, *16*, 246–258. [CrossRef]
91. Jiang, T.; Jiang, H.; Su, X.-M.; Zheng, L.; Li, Q.-L.; Zhang, Z.-W.; Li, X.-C. Expressions of E-cadherin and alpha-catenin in benign, malignant and metastatic prostate tumors. *Zhonghua Nan Ke Xue* **2012**, *18*, 499–503. [PubMed]
92. Chang, F.; Xing, P.; Song, F.; Du, X.; Wang, G.; Chen, K.; Yang, J. The role of T-box genes in the tumorigenesis and progression of cancer. *Oncol. Lett.* **2016**, *12*, 4305–4311. [CrossRef] [PubMed]
93. Xue, D.; Zhou, C.; Shi, Y.; Lu, H.; Xu, R.; He, X. Nuclear transcription factor Nrf2 suppresses prostate cancer cells growth and migration through upregulating ferroportin. *Oncotarget* **2016**, *7*, 78804–78812. [CrossRef] [PubMed]
94. Frohlich, D.A.; McCabe, M.T.; Arnold, R.S.; Day, M.L. The role of Nrf2 in increased reactive oxygen species and DNA damage in prostate tumorigenesis. *Oncogene* **2008**, *27*, 4353–4362. [CrossRef]
95. Mo, R.J.; Lu, J.M.; Wan, Y.P.; Hua, W.; Liang, Y.X.; Zhuo, Y.J.; Kuang, Q.W.; Liu, Y.L.; He, H.C.; Zhong, W.D. Decreased hoxd10 expression promotes a proliferative and aggressive phenotype in prostate cancer. *Curr. Mol. Med.* **2017**, *17*, 70–78. [CrossRef]
96. Kron, K.J.; Liu, L.; Pethe, V.V.; Demetrashvili, N.; Nesbitt, M.E.; Trachtenberg, J.; Ozcelik, H.; Fleshner, N.E.; Briollais, L.; van der Kwast, T.H.; et al. DNA methylation of HOXD3 as a marker of prostate cancer progression. *Lab. Investig.* **2010**, *90*, 1060–1067. [CrossRef]
97. Pilati, C.; Shinde, J.; Alexandrov, L.B.; Assié, G.; André, T.; Hélias-Rodzewicz, Z.; Ducoudray, R.; Le Corre, D.; Zucman-Rossi, J.; Emile, J.-F.; et al. Mutational signature analysis identifies MUTYH deficiency in colorectal cancers and adrenocortical carcinomas. *J. Pathol.* **2017**, *242*, 10–15. [CrossRef]
98. Tomkova, M.; Tomek, J.; Kriaucionis, S.; Schuster-Böckler, B. Mutational signature distribution varies with DNA replication timing and strand asymmetry. *Genome Biol.* **2018**, *19*, 1–12. [CrossRef]

99. Tomkova, M.; Renard, C.; Urban, L.; Kolli, S.; Ardin, M.; Pandey, M.; Zhivagui, M.; Huskova, H.; Olivier, M.; Marusawa, H.; et al. Abstract 4661: Deciphering the causes of the COSMIC mutational signature 17 by combining pan-cancer data with experimental mouse models. In *Tumor Biology*; American Association for Cancer Research: Amherst, MA, USA, 2019; p. 4661.
100. Hatzoglou, V.; Patel, G.V.; Morris, M.J.; Curtis, K.; Zhang, Z.; Shi, W.; Huse, J.; Rosenblum, M.; Holodny, A.I.; Young, R.J. Brain metastases from prostate cancer: An 11-year analysis in the MRI era with emphasis on imaging characteristics, incidence, and prognosis. *J. Neuroimag.* **2014**, *24*, 161–166. [CrossRef]
101. Kim, J.; Jin, H.; Zhao, J.C.; Yang, Y.A.; Li, Y.; Yang, X.; Dong, X.; Yu, J. FOXA1 inhibits prostate cancer neuroendocrine differentiation. *Oncogene* **2017**, *36*, 4072–4080. [CrossRef]
102. Zazzeroni, F.; Nicosia, D.; Tessitore, A.; Gallo, R.; Verzella, D.; Fischietti, M.; Vecchiotti, D.; Ventura, L.; Capece, D.; Gulino, A.; et al. KCTD11 tumor suppressor gene expression is reduced in prostate adenocarcinoma. *Biomed Res. Int.* **2014**, *2014*, 380398. [CrossRef] [PubMed]
103. Martin, M. Cutadapt removes adapter sequences from high-throughput sequencing reads. *EMBnet J.* **2011**, *17*, 10–12. [CrossRef]
104. Li, H.; Durbin, R. Fast and accurate short read alignment with Burrows-Wheeler transform. *Bioinformatics* **2009**, *25*, 1754–1760. [CrossRef] [PubMed]
105. Okonechnikov, K.; Conesa, A.; García-Alcalde, F. Qualimap 2: Advanced multi-sample quality control for high-throughput sequencing data. *Bioinformatics* **2016**, *32*, 292–294. [CrossRef] [PubMed]
106. Favero, F.; Joshi, T.; Marquard, A.M.; Birkbak, N.J.; Krzystanek, M.; Li, Q.; Szallasi, Z.; Eklund, A.C. Sequenza: Allele-specific copy number and mutation profiles from tumor sequencing data. *Ann. Oncol.* **2015**, *26*, 64–70. [CrossRef] [PubMed]
107. Van der Auwera, G.A.; Carneiro, M.O.; Hartl, C.; Poplin, R.; Del Angel, G.; Levy-Moonshine, A.; Jordan, T.; Shakir, K.; Roazen, D.; Thibault, J.; et al. From FastQ data to high confidence variant calls: The Genome Analysis Toolkit best practices pipeline. *Curr. Protoc. Bioinform.* **2013**, *43*, 1–11.
108. Cibulskis, K.; Lawrence, M.S.; Carter, S.L.; Sivachenko, A.; Jaffe, D.; Sougnez, C.; Gabriel, S.; Meyerson, M.; Lander, E.S.; Getz, G. Sensitive detection of somatic point mutations in impure and heterogeneous cancer samples. *Nat. Biotechnol.* **2013**, *31*, 213–219. [CrossRef]
109. Cameron, D.L.; Schröder, J.; Penington, J.S.; Do, H.; Molania, R.; Dobrovic, A.; Speed, T.P.; Papenfuss, A.T. GRIDSS: Sensitive and specific genomic rearrangement detection using positional de Bruijn graph assembly. *Genome Res.* **2017**, *27*, 2050–2060. [CrossRef]
110. Layer, R.M.; Chiang, C.; Quinlan, A.R.; Hall, I.M. LUMPY: A probabilistic framework for structural variant discovery. *Genome Biol.* **2014**, *15*, R84. [CrossRef]
111. Thorvaldsdóttir, H.; Robinson, J.T.; Mesirov, J.P. Integrative Genomics Viewer (IGV): High-performance genomics data visualization and exploration. *Brief. Bioinform.* **2013**, *14*, 178–192. [CrossRef]
112. Talevich, E.; Shain, A.H.; Botton, T.; Bastian, B.C. CNVkit: Genome-Wide Copy Number Detection and Visualization from Targeted DNA Sequencing. *PLoS Comput. Biol.* **2016**, *12*, e1004873. [CrossRef] [PubMed]
113. Wang, K.; Li, M.; Hakonarson, H. ANNOVAR: Functional annotation of genetic variants from high-throughput sequencing data. *Nucleic Acids Res.* **2010**, *38*, e164. [CrossRef] [PubMed]
114. Mao, Y.; Chen, H.; Liang, H.; Meric-Bernstam, F.; Mills, G.B.; Chen, K. CanDrA: Cancer-specific driver missense mutation annotation with optimized features. *PLoS ONE* **2013**, *8*, e77945. [CrossRef] [PubMed]
115. Gehring, J.S.; Fischer, B.; Lawrence, M.; Huber, W. SomaticSignatures: Inferring mutational signatures from single-nucleotide variants. *Bioinformatics* **2015**, *31*, 3673–3675. [CrossRef] [PubMed]
116. Deshwar, A.G.; Vembu, S.; Yung, C.K.; Jang, G.H.; Stein, L.; Morris, Q. PhyloWGS: Reconstructing subclonal composition and evolution from whole-genome sequencing of tumors. *Genome Biol.* **2015**, *16*, 1–29. [CrossRef]
117. Ha, G.; Roth, A.; Khattra, J.; Ho, J.; Yap, D.; Prentice, L.M.; Melnyk, N.; McPherson, A.; Bashashati, A.; Laks, E.; et al. TITAN: Inference of copy number architectures in clonal cell populations from tumor whole-genome sequence data. *Genome Res.* **2014**, *24*, 1881–1893. [CrossRef]
118. Lam, E.T.; Hastie, A.; Lin, C.; Ehrlich, D.; Das, S.K.; Austin, M.D.; Deshpande, P.; Cao, H.; Nagarajan, N.; Xiao, M.; et al. Genome mapping on nanochannel arrays for structural variation analysis and sequence assembly. *Nat. Biotechnol.* **2012**, *30*, 771–776. [CrossRef]
119. Hastie, A.R.; Dong, L.; Smith, A.; Finklestein, J.; Lam, E.T.; Huo, N.; Cao, H.; Kwok, P.-Y.; Deal, K.R.; Dvorak, J.; et al. Rapid genome mapping in nanochannel arrays for highly complete and accurate de novo sequence assembly of the complex Aegilops tauschii genome. *PLoS ONE* **2013**, *8*, e55864. [CrossRef]

120. Hastie, A.R.; Lam, E.T.; Pang, A.W.C.; Zhang, X.; Andrews, W.; Lee, J.; Liang, T.Y.; Wang, J.; Zhou, X.; Zhu, Z.; et al. Rapid Automated Large Structural Variation Detection in a Diploid Genome by NanoChannel Based Next-Generation Mapping. *BioRxiv* **2017**.
121. Levy-Sakin, M.; Pastor, S.; Mostovoy, Y.; Li, L.; Leung, A.K.Y.; McCaffrey, J.; Young, E.; Lam, E.T.; Hastie, A.R.; Wong, K.H.Y.; et al. Genome maps across 26 human populations reveal population-specific patterns of structural variation. *Nat. Commun.* **2019**, *10*, 1–14. [CrossRef]
122. Bionano Data. Available online: https://protect-au.mimecast.com/s/QtA0COMK24uZZWrtEuAv2?domain=dx.doi.org (accessed on 2 March 2020).
123. Gonzalez-Perez, A.; Perez-Llamas, C.; Deu-Pons, J.; Tamborero, D.; Schroeder, M.P.; Jene-Sanz, A.; Santos, A.; Lopez-Bigas, N. IntOGen-mutations identifies cancer drivers across tumor types. *Nat. Methods* **2013**, *10*, 1081–1082. [CrossRef]
124. Krzywinski, M.; Schein, J.; Birol, I.; Connors, J.; Gascoyne, R.; Horsman, D.; Jones, S.J.; Marra, M.A. Circos: An information aesthetic for comparative genomics. *Genome Res.* **2009**, *19*, 1639–1645. [CrossRef] [PubMed]
125. Alexandrov, L.; Kim, J.; Haradhvala, N.J.; Huang, M.N.; Ng, A.W.T.; Boot, A.; Covington, K.R.; Gordenin, D.A.; Bergstrom, E.; Lopez-Bigas, N.; et al. The repertoire of mutational signatures in human cancer. *Nature.* **2020**, *578*, 94–101. [CrossRef] [PubMed]
126. Shinde, J.; Bayard, Q.; Imbeaud, S.; Hirsch, T.Z.; Liu, F.; Renault, V.; Zucman-Rossi, J.; Letouzé, E. Palimpsest: An R package for studying mutational and structural variant signatures along clonal evolution in cancer. *Bioinformatics* **2018**, *34*, 3380–3381. [CrossRef] [PubMed]
127. De Laere, B.; Oeyen, S.; Mayrhofer, M.; Whitington, T.; van Dam, P.-J.; Van Oyen, P.; Ghysel, C.; Ampe, J.; Ost, P.; Demey, W.; et al. TP53 Outperforms Other Androgen Receptor Biomarkers to Predict Abiraterone or Enzalutamide Outcome in Metastatic Castration-Resistant Prostate Cancer. *Clin. Cancer Res.* **2019**, *25*, 1766–1773. [CrossRef] [PubMed]
128. Sicklick, J.K.; Kato, S.; Okamura, R.; Schwaederle, M.; Hahn, M.E.; Williams, C.B.; De, P.; Krie, A.; Piccioni, D.E.; Miller, V.A.; et al. Molecular profiling of cancer patients enables personalized combination therapy: The I-PREDICT study. *Nat. Med.* **2019**, *25*, 744–750. [CrossRef]

12

The Disturbed Iron Phenotype of Tumor Cells and Macrophages in Renal Cell Carcinoma Influences Tumor Growth

Matthias Schnetz [1], Julia K. Meier [1], Claudia Rehwald [1], Christina Mertens [1], Anja Urbschat [2], Elisa Tomat [3], Eman A. Akam [3], Patrick Baer [4], Frederik C. Roos [5], Bernhard Brüne [1,6,7,8] and Michaela Jung [1,*]

1 Institute of Biochemistry I, Goethe-University Frankfurt, Theodor-Stern-Kai 7, 60590 Frankfurt am Main, Germany; matthias.schnetz@t-online.de (M.S.); meier@biochem.uni-frankfurt.de (J.K.M.); rehwald@biochem.uni-frankfurt.de (C.R.); c.mertens86@gmail.com (C.M.); B.Bruene@biochem.uni-frankfurt.de (B.B.)

2 Institute for Biomedicine, Aarhus University, C. F. Møllers Allé 6, 8000 Aarhus, Denmark; anja.urbschat@staff.uni-marburg.de

3 Department of Chemistry and Biochemistry, University of Arizona, 1306 E. University Blvd., Tucson, AZ 85721-0041, USA; tomat@email.arizona.edu (E.T.); EAKAM@mgh.harvard.edu (E.A.A.)

4 Division of Nephrology, Department of Internal Medicine III, Goethe-University Frankfurt, Theodor-Stern-Kai 7, 60590 Frankfurt am Main, Germany; p.baer@em.uni-frankfurt.de

5 Clinic of Urology, Goethe-University Frankfurt, Theodor-Stern-Kai 7, 60590 Frankfurt am Main, Germany; Frederik.Roos@kgu.de

6 German Cancer Consortium (DKTK), partner site Frankfurt/Mainz, 60590 Frankfurt am Main, Germany

7 Frankfurt Cancer Institute, Goethe-University Frankfurt, 60596 Frankfurt am Main, Germany

8 Project Group Translational Medicine and Pharmacology TMP, Fraunhofer Institute for Molecular Biology and Applied Ecology, 60596 Frankfurt am Main, Germany

* Correspondence: m.jung@biochem.uni-frankfurt.de

Abstract: Accumulating evidence suggests that iron homeostasis is disturbed in tumors. We aimed at clarifying the distribution of iron in renal cell carcinoma (RCC). Considering the pivotal role of macrophages for iron homeostasis and their association with poor clinical outcome, we investigated the role of macrophage-secreted iron for tumor progression by applying a novel chelation approach. We applied flow cytometry and multiplex-immunohistochemistry to detect iron-dependent markers and analyzed iron distribution with atomic absorption spectrometry in patients diagnosed with RCC. We further analyzed the functional significance of iron by applying a novel extracellular chelator using RCC cell lines as well as patient-derived primary cells. The expression of iron-regulated genes was significantly elevated in tumors compared to adjacent healthy tissue. Iron retention was detected in tumor cells, whereas tumor-associated macrophages showed an iron-release phenotype accompanied by enhanced expression of ferroportin. We found increased iron amounts in extracellular fluids, which in turn stimulated tumor cell proliferation and migration. In vitro, macrophage-derived iron showed pro-tumor functions, whereas application of an extracellular chelator blocked these effects. Our study provides new insights in iron distribution and iron-handling in RCC. Chelators that specifically scavenge iron in the extracellular space confirmed the importance of macrophage-secreted iron in promoting tumor growth.

Keywords: renal cell carcinoma; iron; macrophages; chelation therapy

---

1. Introduction

Iron is the most abundant transition metal in the human body and drives a variety of mechanisms considered as hallmarks of cancer. Due to its role as critical cofactor for the rate-limiting step of DNA synthesis, iron controls cell division, DNA repair, and chromatin remodeling [1]. Iron is essential for basic cellular processes such as mitochondrial respiration and the enhanced metabolic turnover under cancerous conditions is controlled by iron-sulfur cluster proteins [2]. Considering the poor bioavailability of iron and its potent role in tumorigenesis, the interplay of different proteins important for iron import, storage, and export has to be tightly regulated through the interplay of various proteins, including the major iron storage protein ferritin with its subunits ferritin light chain (FTL) and ferritin heavy chain (FTH), the iron exporter ferroportin (FPN), transferrin receptor 1 (TfR1) for iron uptake, and iron-regulatory proteins 1 and 2 (IRP1/2) [3].

The kidney plays a unique role in systemic iron homeostasis by filtering and reabsorbing iron as well as providing the main body source of erythropoietin, which promotes hemoglobin synthesis [4]. It was previously shown that renal iron overload in anemic patients requiring chronic transfusions enhanced the incidence of renal cell carcinoma (RCC) development [5]. Repeated injections of iron led to RCC development with increased metastasis to the lungs and lymph nodes in experimental models [6]. Recently, the expression of TfR1 was associated with progression and mortality in clear cell RCC (ccRCC), identifying TfR1 as a novel RCC biomarker and potential therapeutic target [7]. Despite these compelling observations and the fact that RCC is one of the 15 most common cancers in humans as well as the third most common cause of death among urological cancers in 2018 [8], the role of iron for renal cancer was not investigated in detail so far. As RCC is considered to be resistant against conventional chemo- and radiation therapy, medical therapeutic options are currently still limited, thus making nephrectomy the first treatment approach in localized disease [9]. For metastatic disease state, treatment options include systemic therapy with multitarget tyrosine kinase inhibitors (TKIs), including sunitinib, cabozantinib, and pazopanib as well as mammalian target of rapamycin (mTOR) inhibitors such as everolimus or temsirolimus, offering only modest benefits [10]. Novel promising approaches for the treatment of metastatic RCC include immunotherapy and immune checkpoint inhibitors (ICI) targeting the cytotoxic-T-lymphocyte-associated antigen 4 (CTLA-4) and programmed death-1 (PD-1) with monoclonal antibodies [11]. Herein, besides to monotherapy a combinatory immunotherapy with checkpoint inhibitors has recently been approved on the base of a clinical phase-3 trial [12]. However, it is clear that there is still an urgent need for a deeper understanding of the molecular processes underlying RCC, which could provide new strategies to interfere during cancer therapy or might help to better determine patient prognosis.

Based on its concentration-dependent toxicity under physiological conditions, cellular iron homeostasis has to be strictly regulated [13]. This balance is shown to be compromised in the tumor microenvironment [14]. The malignant state of cancer cells is associated with a deregulation in cellular iron homeostasis, particularly in the expression of iron-regulated genes to fuel their higher metabolic iron demand needed for division, growth, and survival [14]. Cancer cells of various tumor entities develop an iron retaining phenotype by upregulating FTL, FTH [15,16], TfR1 [7,17], and IRP1/2 [18], while downregulating the iron exporter FPN [17]. These alterations result in increased tumor growth, aggressiveness and a poor patient outcome [14,19]. However, it still remains partly unclear how cancer cells acquire iron from the tumor microenvironment. One of the key players of iron homeostasis are macrophages (MΦ), which play a dual, activation-dependent role in iron homeostasis [20]. While classical, pro-inflammatory MΦ sequester iron to restrict iron availability for bacterial growth [21], alternatively activated anti-inflammatory MΦ recycle iron from dying cells by enhanced phagocytic activity [22]. Due to their physiological function, alternatively activated MΦ promote tissue repair, cell proliferation, and angiogenesis [23]. In the context of carcinogenesis, tumor associated MΦ (TAM) are major players when looking at abundance [24] and pro-tumoral function [25]. TAMs show characteristics of both pro-inflammatory MΦ that create an inflammatory environment during early stages of tumor development as well as anti-inflammatory MΦ [25,26] during later stages that suppress anti-tumor immunity and stimulate tumor neovascularization as well as metastasis [27,28]. Accordingly, TAMs were shown to positively associate with tumor progression and worse patient prognosis [29–31].

Although the control of iron availability in the tumor microenvironment seems to be crucial for tumor development, the distribution of iron within cellular compartments of the tumor, in particular tumor cells and TAMs, as well their association with tumor outcome have not been investigated so far in renal cancer. In the present study, we provide evidence that iron-dependent genes are highly expressed in renal cancer and are associated with tumor pT-stage (tumor size and invasion as defined by UICC) and tumor grade. We further show that TAMs adopt an iron-release phenotype with increased expression of the iron exporter FPN, whereas tumor cells retain intracellular iron. *In vitro* assays with patient-derived extracellular fluids as well as novel extracellular iron chelators showed the iron-dependence of renal tumor growth and metastasis.

2. Results

2.1. Iron Homeostasis Is Altered in RCC

In order to determine whether renal iron homeostasis is altered in RCC, we first analyzed mRNA expression of several iron-dependent genes, including *FPN, FTL, FTH, IRP2,* and *TfR1* in whole tissue homogenates of our patient cohort (Table 1).

Table 1. Patient cohort. The patient cohort is composed of 64 patients, grouped into three major renal tumor types ccRCC, pRCC, and chRCC. Patient parameters age, sex, pT-stage and grade are depicted in the table.

Number of Patients	ccRCC	pRCC	chRCC
	56	7	7
Age (years)			
mean	64 ± 10	68 ± 11	63 ± 10
median	64 ± 10	71 ± 11	62 ± 10
range	44–85	48–79	48–75
sex			
female	24%	29%	80%
male	76%	71%	20%
pT-stage			
pT1-pT2	55%		
pT3-pT4	45%		
Grade			
G1-G2	84%		
G3-G4	16%		

We found a significantly increased mRNA expression in tumor tissue compared to adjacent healthy tissue for all genes (Figure 1A–E). We performed hematoxylin staining in both healthy adjacent tissue and RCC subtypes of clear cell RCC (ccRCC), papillary RCC (pRCC) as well as chromophobe RCC (chRCC) that were included in our patient cohort (Figure S1A), and analyzed the *CAIX* mRNA expression, which was shown to be upregulated in more than 90% of RCC cases [32] (Figure S1B). Accordingly, *CAIX* mRNA expression was significantly upregulated in ccRCC and pRCC tumor subtypes, whilst varying in chRCC compared to adjacent healthy tissue. We next analyzed the mRNA expression of iron-dependent genes in relation to tumor grade (G1-G2 vs. G3-G4) and tumor pT-stage (pT1 pT2 vs. pT3-pT4). *FPN* mRNA expression was significantly increased in all tumor pT-stages and tumor grades compared to adjacent healthy tissue with the notion of enhanced expression in higher tumor pT-stage (Figure 1F). This expression pattern was also observed for mRNA expression of *TfR1* (Figure 1G).

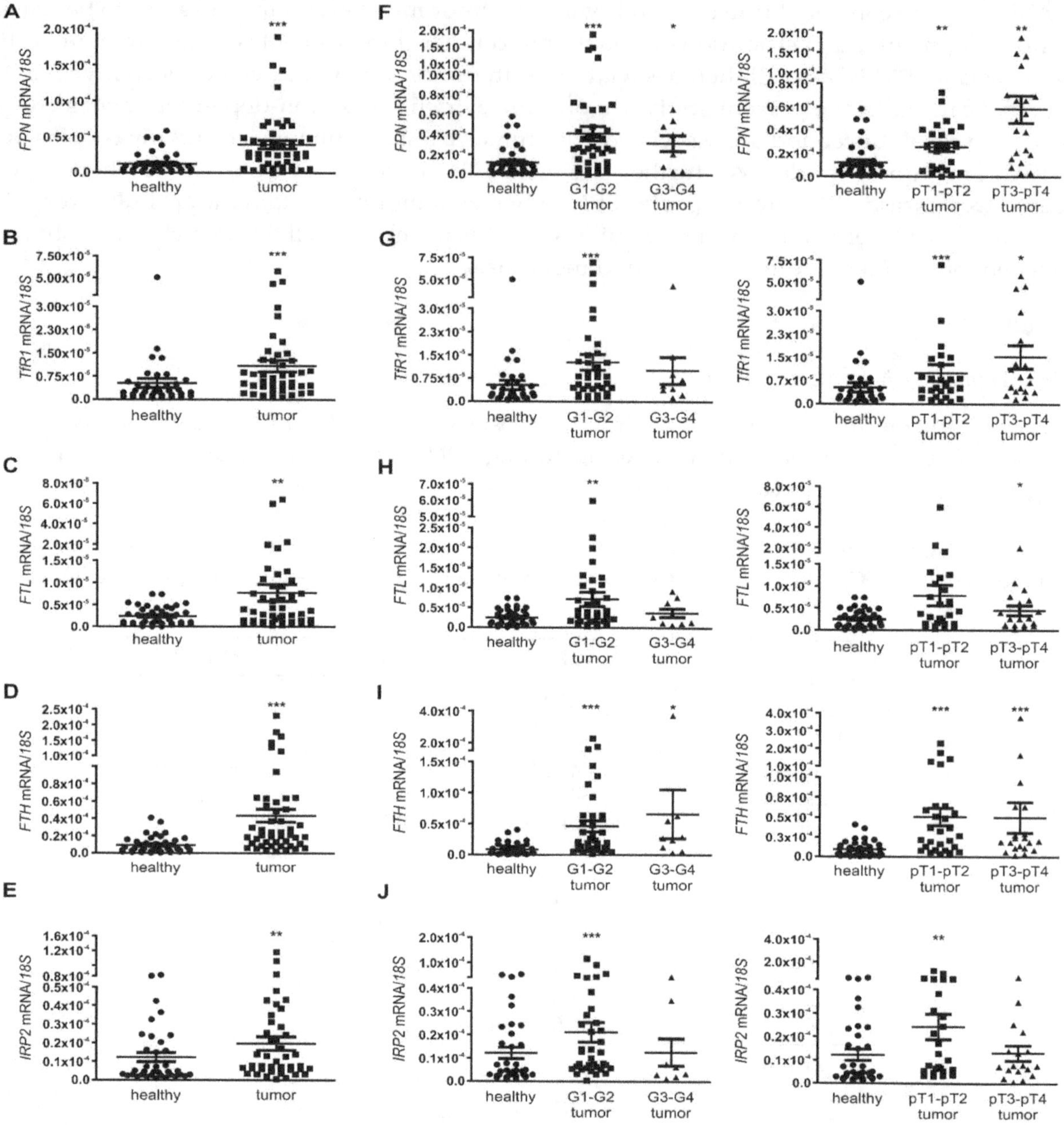

Figure 1. Expression of iron-regulated genes in human renal cancer samples. mRNA expression normalized to the housekeeping gene *18S* in whole tissue homogenates of renal tumor tissue and adjacent healthy tissue of (**A**) *FPN* ($n = 48$), (**B**) *TfR1* ($n = 47$), (**C**) *FTL* ($n = 48$), (**D**) *FTH* ($n = 48$), and (**E**) *IRP2* ($n = 46$). (**F–J**) Left: mRNA expression of (**F**) *FPN*, (**G**) *TfR1*, (**H**) *FTL*, (**I**) *FTH*, and (**J**) *IRP2* correlated to low (G1-G2) and high (G3-G4) tumor grade. Right: mRNA expression of (**F**) *FPN*, (**G**) *TfR1*, (**H**) *FTL*, (**I**) *FTH*, and (**J**) *IRP2* correlated to low (pT1–pT2) and high (pT3–pT4) tumor pT-stage. Number of tested patients differ between genes due to patients with failed measurements of initially low sample RNA amount. No samples have been excluded as outliers. Graphs are displayed as means ± SEM with * $p < 0.05$, ** $p < 0.01$, *** $p < 0.001$.

For *FTL, FTH,* and *IRP2,* we found an increased mRNA expression in lower tumor grades (G1-G2) and lower tumor pT-stage (pT1–pT2), but either similar or lower expression within the group of higher tumor grades (G3-G4) and higher tumor pT-stage (pT3–pT4; Figure 1H–J).

Since RCC subtypes significantly differ regarding in the prognosis and treatment [33], we analyzed the mRNA expression of iron-dependent gene expression in patients with ccRCC, pRCC, or chRCC of our cohort (Figure 2A–E, left panel). While the defined iron-dependent genes were significantly upregulated within the ccRCC subgroup in comparison to adjacent healthy tissue, mRNA expression in the pRCC and the chRCC subtype varied, depending on the analyzed gene. Expression of *FPN, FTH,* and *IRP2* was higher in all RCC subtypes compared to adjacent healthy tissue, whereas *FTL* remained unaltered in the chRCC subtype and *TfR1* was lower in pRCC subtypes. In order to verify our data, especially regarding patients diagnosed with pRCC and chRCC, where less patients were included in our cohort, we analyzed publically available TCGA KIRC (ccRCC), KIRP (pRCC), and KICH (chRCC) data sets (Figure 2A–E, right panel). RNA expression in the TCGA data sets confirmed a significant upregulation of *FPN, FTL,* and *FTH* in ccRCC. In pRCC, *FPN, FTL,* and *FTH* are significantly higher expressed, while *IRP2* remained unaltered. Our data regarding reduced *TfR1* expression in pRCC and unaltered *FTL* expression in chRCC was corroborated using the TCGA data analysis.

As we showed an altered iron homeostasis in all histopathological subtypes, we next aimed at looking into the iron distribution in RCC tissue. We first analyzed the iron amount of tumor and adjacent healthy tissues by AAS measurements. Tumor tissue showed an overall significantly higher iron amount than adjacent healthy renal tissue (Figure 3A). When analyzing the histopathological subtypes, both ccRCC and chRCC showed a higher iron amount compared to adjacent healthy tissue, whereas in pRCC the total iron amount remained nearly unaltered (Figure 3B). To address the question of iron localization within the tissues, Perl's staining of tumor versus adjacent healthy tissue slides was used. In line with our AAS analysis, healthy renal tissue showed a low amount of iron deposits appearing in blue. Compared to the healthy adjacent tissue, a more intense staining in ccRCC was observed, whereas iron deposits in pRCC remained low (Figure 3C and Figure S2A–D). Intriguingly, the iron load in chRCC varies considerably between different patients (Figure S2D) with the notion of overall enhanced iron deposits in tumor tissue compared to adjacent healthy tissue. In ccRCC tissue, we hypothesize that the highly intense blue-colored cells might be tumor cells, whereas the diffuse positive staining around long-shaped cells in the stroma might be iron secreted by MΦ. There are also other positive-stained cells in the stroma that appear much smaller, which we believe might be lymphocytes that are also able to handle iron in the tumor stroma as previously described by Marques et al. in mammary carcinoma [34]. For pRCC we only detect low amounts of overall Perl's staining, with localized positive staining mostly in tumor cells, whereas we observed high amounts of iron deposits in chRCC, mostly within the tumor stroma. We and others previously showed that tumor cells are prone to adopt an iron retaining phenotype, whereas cells from the tumor stroma such as MΦ rather adopt an iron mobilization and iron releasing phenotype [34,35]. In order to verify the location of iron within different tumor compartments in RCC tissues, we sorted both tumor cells and tumor-associated MΦ from tumor tissue of all histopathological RCC subtypes and compared them to sorted epithelial cells and MΦ isolated from adjacent healthy tissue (Figure 3D,E). A significantly reduced intracellular iron amount in MΦ isolated from ccRCC and pRCC tissues was observed, whereas MΦ from chRCC tissues showed similar intracellular iron levels as cells from adjacent healthy tissue (Figure 3D). In contrast, tumor cells showed a significant increased iron amount in ccRCC and pRCC compared to adjacent renal epithelial cells. In chRCC, iron amount in tumor cells showed a larger variation resulting in a non-significant increase compared to renal epithelial cells isolated from adjacent healthy tissue (Figure 3E).

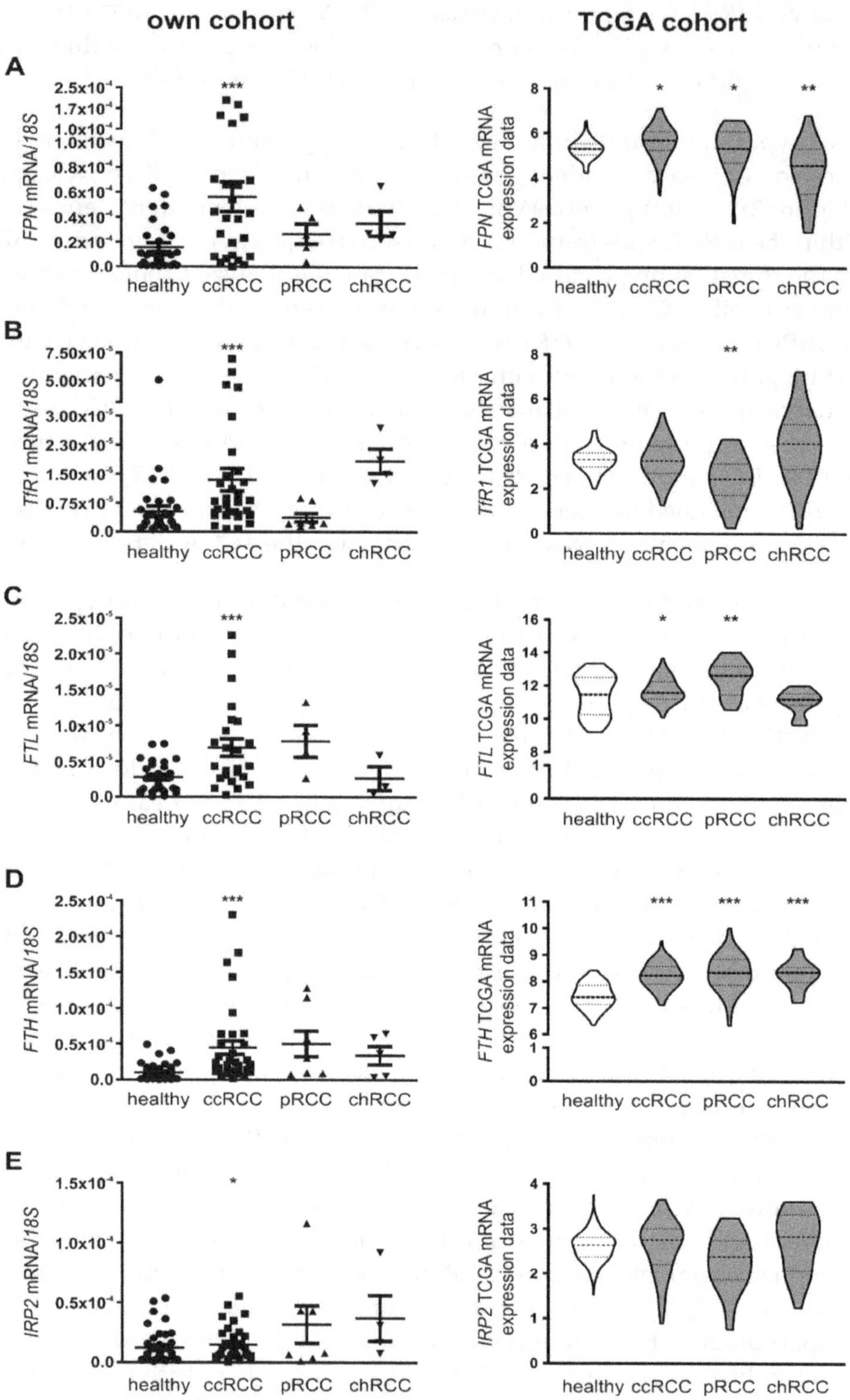

Figure 2. Profile of iron-regulated genes in histopathologically distinct RCC subtypes. mRNA expression of renal tumor and adjacent healthy samples in clear cell (ccRCC), papillary (pRCC), and chromophobe (chRCC) RCC of own patient cohort (left) compared to mRNA expression acquired from the TCGA database applying the ccRCC-KIRC ($n = 70$), pRCC-KIRP ($n = 31$), and chRCC-KICH ($n = 23$) datasets (right). Analyzed genes include (**A**) *FPN*, (**B**) *TfR1*, (**C**) *FTL*, (**D**) *FTH*, and (**E**) *IRP2*. Own cohort is normalized to housekeeping gene *18S* expression. Graphs are displayed as means ± SEM with * $p < 0.05$, ** $p < 0.01$, *** $p < 0.001$.

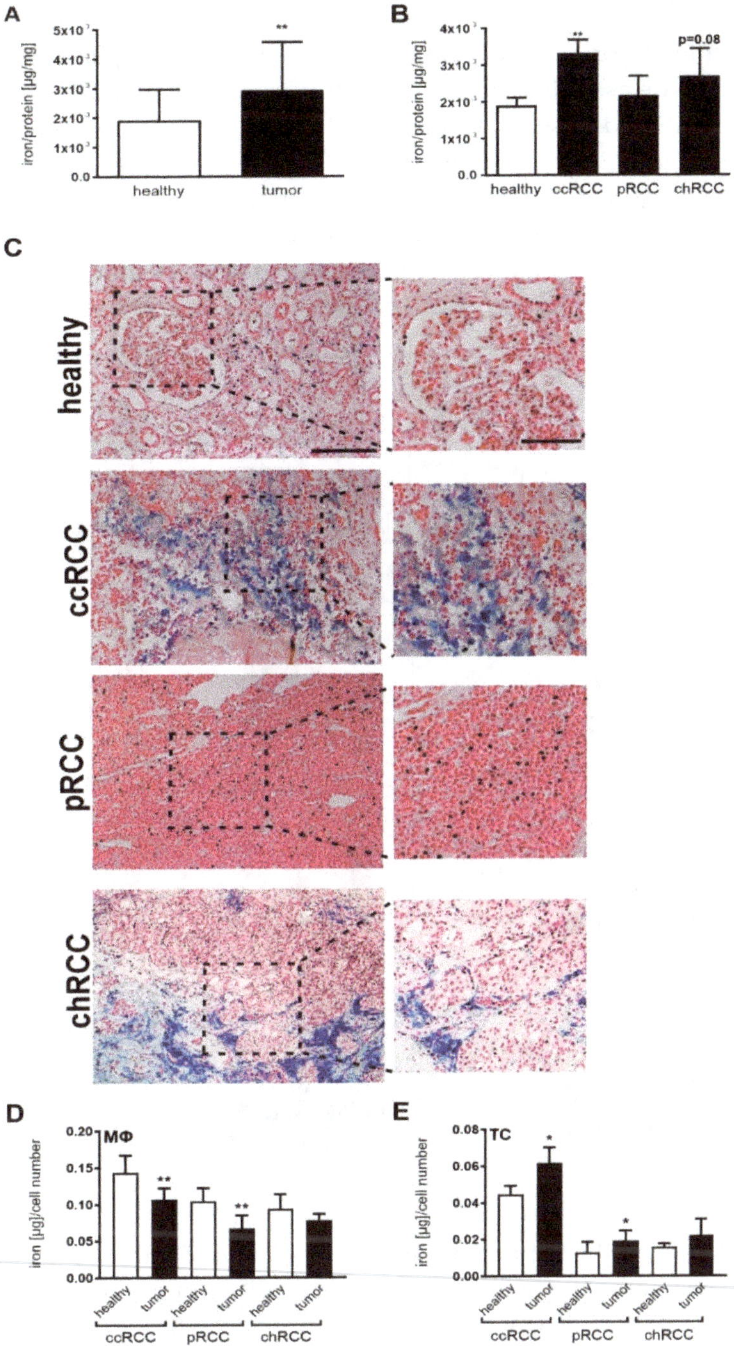

Figure 3. Iron homeostasis and distribution is altered in RCC. (**A**) Iron load normalized to protein amount in whole tissue homogenates of renal cancer tissue in comparison to adjacent healthy renal tissue measured by AAS ($n = 31$). (**B**) Iron load in whole tissue homogenates of clear cell (ccRCC; $n = 17$), papillary (pRCC; $n = 7$), and chromophobe (chRCC; $n = 7$) RCC in comparison to corresponding healthy renal tissue measured by AAS. (**C**) Representative pictures of Perl's staining of RCC tissue and adjacent healthy renal tissue of ccRCC, pRCC, and chRCC. Representative pictures (scale bar: 200 µm) with corresponding detailed pictures (scale bar: 100 µm) are given. (**D**,**E**) Macrophages (MΦ) and CD326+ cells were isolated by FACS-sorting from RCC tissue and adjacent healthy tissue. Intracellular iron load of (**D**) MΦ and (**E**) either tumor cells (TC) or epithelial cells from adjacent healthy tissue of ccRCC ($n = 7$), pRCC ($n = 13$), and chRCC ($n = 4$) measured by AAS. Statistical analysis was performed comparing tumor to adjacent healthy tissue within the histopathological subtypes. Graphs are displayed as means ± SEM. * $p < 0.05$, ** $p < 0.01$.

2.2. *Iron Promotes Renal Tumor Cell Growth*

In order to test the role of iron released into the tumor stroma, we generated extracellular fluids (EC fluids) from both tumor tissue as well as adjacent healthy tissue (Figure 4A). First, we analyzed the iron amount in EC fluids by AAS and observed significantly higher iron amounts in EC fluids isolated from tumor tissue as compared to EC fluids from adjacent healthy tissue (Figure 4B). We then stimulated renal tumor cells CAKI-1 (Figure 4C) and 786-O (Figure 4D) as well as primary patient-derived tumor tubular epithelial cells (TTEC; Figure 4E) with tumor EC fluids. Cellular proliferation was analyzed applying xCELLigence real-time measurements. Results showed that all tested cell lines as well as primary tumor cells positively responded to treatments with tumor EC fluids and augmented cellular proliferation upon stimulation.

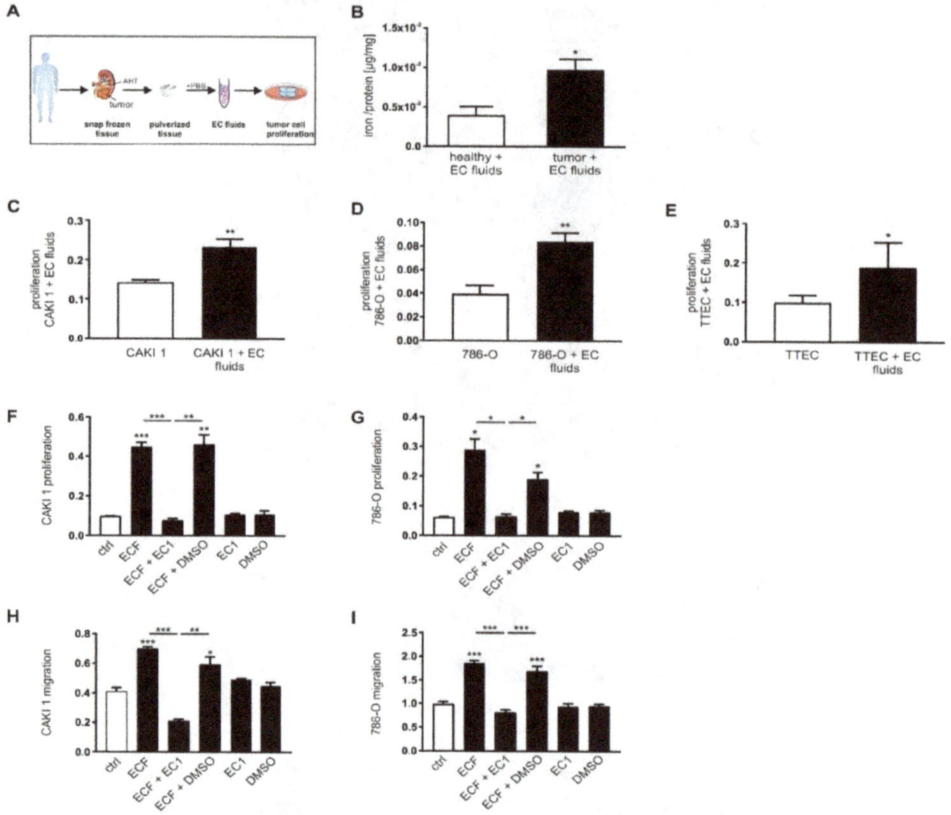

Figure 4. Extracellular iron induces proliferation and migration of tumor cells in vitro. (**A**) Schematic overview of how to generate extracellular (EC) fluids (ECF) from primary human renal tumor and adjacent healthy tissue. (**B**) Iron load measured by AAS relative to the total protein amount of EC fluids of ccRCC tissue compared to adjacent healthy renal tissue ($n = 8$). Proliferation of (**C**) CAKI-1 ($n = 7$), (**D**) 786-O ($n = 8$), and (**E**) primary human tumor tubular epithelial cells (TTEC) upon stimulation with EC fluids in vitro measured with the xCELLigence system ($n = 8$). Proliferation of **(F)** CAKI 1 ($n = 4$) and (**G**) 786-O ($n = 4$) cells as well as migration of (**H**) CAKI 1 ($n = 4$) and (**I**) 786-O cells ($n = 4$) upon stimulation with EC fluids in the presence or absence of an extracellular chelator (EC1, 100μM) or dimethyl sulfoxide (DMSO) as negative control measured with the xCELLigence system. Graphs are displayed as means ± SEM with * $p < 0.05$, ** $p < 0.01$, *** $p < 0.001$.

To further verify the role of extracellular iron on tumor proliferation and migration, we stimulated tumor cells with EC fluids in the presence of a specific extracellular chelator (EC1). This novel compound was designed for extracellular chelation as it features an established iron-binding unit as well as a negatively charged group to hinder cell membrane permeation (Figure S3A). In particular, the tridentate chelating unit of EC1 includes a thiosemicarbazone moiety that is common to many anti-proliferative iron chelators [36,37]; however, the incorporation of a negatively charged sulfonate group significantly limits the ability of EC1 to cross cellular membranes. As a result, EC1 is expected to chelate iron only in the extracellular space without affecting intracellular iron levels. The iron binding abilities were validated using optical absorption spectroscopy (Figure S3B). The effects of EC1 on cellular viability and proliferation were tested in vitro in CAKI-1 and 786-O cells in comparison to the unspecific chelator 2,2′-dipyridine (2′2-DPD) and the intracellularly activated prochelator $(TC3\text{-}S)_2$ [38–40]. Whereas EC1 showed no effect at concentrations up to 100 µM with regard to both, viability (Figure S3C,D) and cellular proliferation (Figure S3E,F) under basal growth conditions, both 2′2-DPD and $(TC3\text{-}S)_2$ showed increasingly adverse effects at higher concentrations regarding cellular viability and anti-proliferative capacity due to the fact that both are able to chelate intracellular iron. In contrast, EC1 showed toxicity effects only at very high concentrations (500 µM), which might be due to non-specific side effects. Supplementation of EC fluids with EC1 (100 µM) in order to specifically block iron secreted to the supernatant resulted in a significant inhibition of cellular proliferation and migration of both CAKI-1 (Figure 4F,H) and 786-O cells (Figure 4G,I).

2.3. *Tumor Proliferation by Macrophage-Secreted Iron Is Suppressed by EC1*

According to our previous observation that tumor-associated MΦ adopt an iron releasing phenotype (Figure 3D), we further established an in vitro setting to analyze the role of macrophage-secreted iron in conferring renal tumor cell growth (Figure 5A).

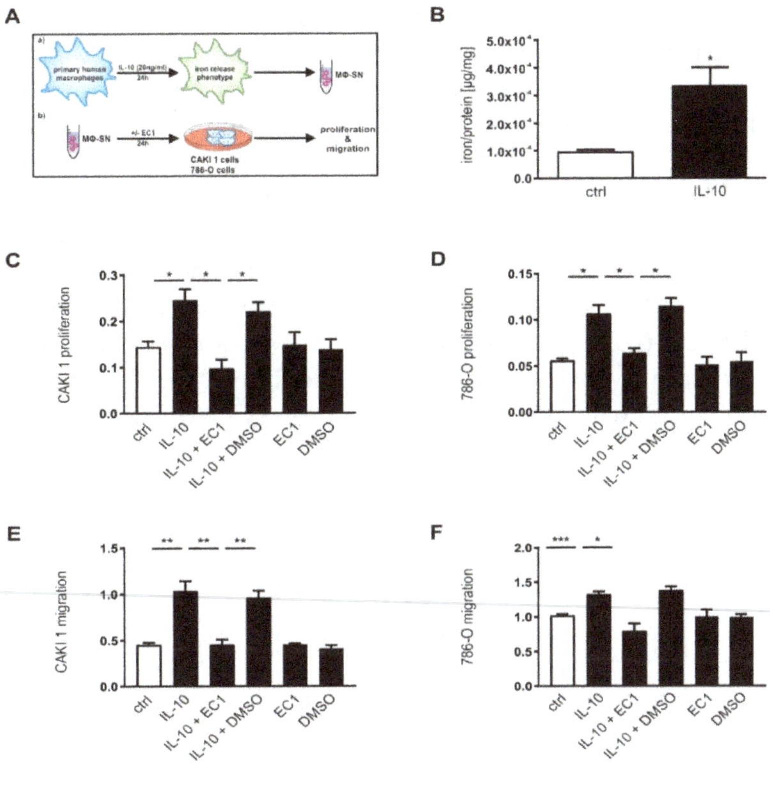

Figure 5. Macrophage-secreted iron induces proliferation and migration of tumor cells in vitro. (**A**) Schematic overview of how to generate conditioned medium from iron-releasing human MΦ. (**B**) Iron amount measured by AAS relative to the total protein amount in the supernatant of primary human MΦ, either left untreated (ctrl) or stimulated with IL-10 (20 ng/mL; 24 h) ($n = 5$). Proliferation of (**C**) CAKI 1 ($n = 4$) and (**D**) 786-O ($n = 4$) cells as well as migration of (**E**) CAKI 1 ($n = 4$) and (**F**) 786-O cells ($n = 4$) upon stimulation with the supernatant of IL-10-stimulated MΦ in the presence or absence of an extracellular chelator (EC1, 100 µM) or dimethyl sulfoxide (DMSO) as negative control measured with the xCELLigence system. Graphs are displayed as means ± SEM with * $p < 0.05$, ** $p < 0.01$, *** $p < 0.001$.

As previously published [41,42], IL-10 stimulation of primary human MΦ induced the release of iron into the supernatant measured by AAS (Figure 5B). We next applied macrophage-conditioned supernatants to renal tumor cells CAKI-1 (Figure 5C,E) and 786-O (Figure 5D,F) and observed enhanced proliferation (Figure 5C,D) as well as tumor cell migration (Figure 5E,F) measured by xCELLigence in real-time upon stimulation with IL-10-conditioned media.

To further verify the effect of EC1 on tumor proliferation and migration in the presence of macrophage-secreted iron, we stimulated tumor cells with MΦ-conditioned media supplemented by EC1 (100 μM). In line with our previous observations using EC fluids (Figure 4F–I), EC1 was able to significantly inhibit cellular proliferation and migrations of both CAKI-1 (Figure 5C,E) and 786-O cells (Figure 5D,F).

2.4. Macrophage-Derived Iron Is Exported Via the Iron Exporter FPN, Which Is Positively Associated with Poor Patient Outcome

We next asked whether the iron exporter FPN was expressed in tumor-associated MΦ. Therefore, FPN protein expression in MΦ by flow cytometry (Figure 6A) was measured, showing higher FPN expression in both tumor stroma (Figure 6B) as well as tumor-associated MΦ (Figure 6C) compared to stroma and MΦ from adjacent healthy tissue. In order to localize FPN protein within the tissue, multiplex-immunohistochemistry was applied, combining CD163 as macrophage marker, FPN, and DAPI as nuclear stain (Figure 6D), showing enhanced co-localization of CD163 and FPN in tumor tissue compared to adjacent healthy tissue. Taking our previous *FPN* mRNA data into consideration that showed enhanced *FPN* expression in tumor tissue compared to adjacent healthy tissue (Figures 1A and 2A), we next questioned the association of *FPN* expression with tumor grade (Figure 6E) and tumor (Figure 6F) of our own cohort (upper part) compared to the TCGA data set (lower part). In line with the TCGA data set, we observed association of FPN mRNA expression only with lower tumor grade (Figure 6E). For tumor pT-stage (Figure 6F), a positive association with lower tumor pT-stages (pT1–pT2) was noticed, which was more pronounced in higher tumor pT-stages (pT3–pT4). However, TCGA data suggests higher FPN expression in patients with low tumor grade (G1–G2) and tumor pT-stage (pT1–pT2). Accordingly, low tissue FPN expression correlated with a lower overall survival probability analyzed by the R2: Genomics Analysis and Visualization Platform applying the 'Tumor Kidney Renal Clear Cell Carcinoma—TCGA-533' data set (Figure 6G).

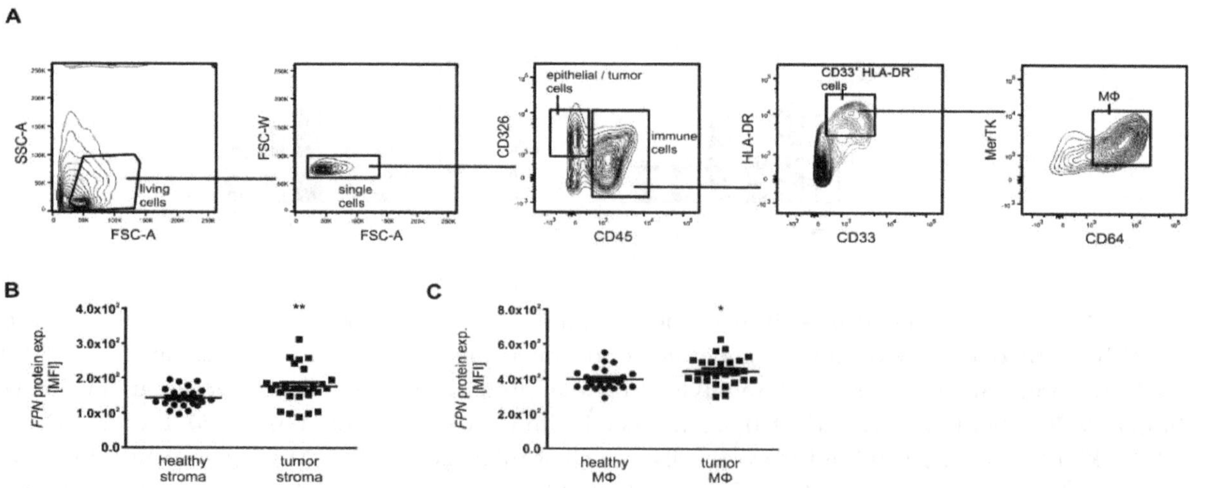

Figure 6. *Cont.*

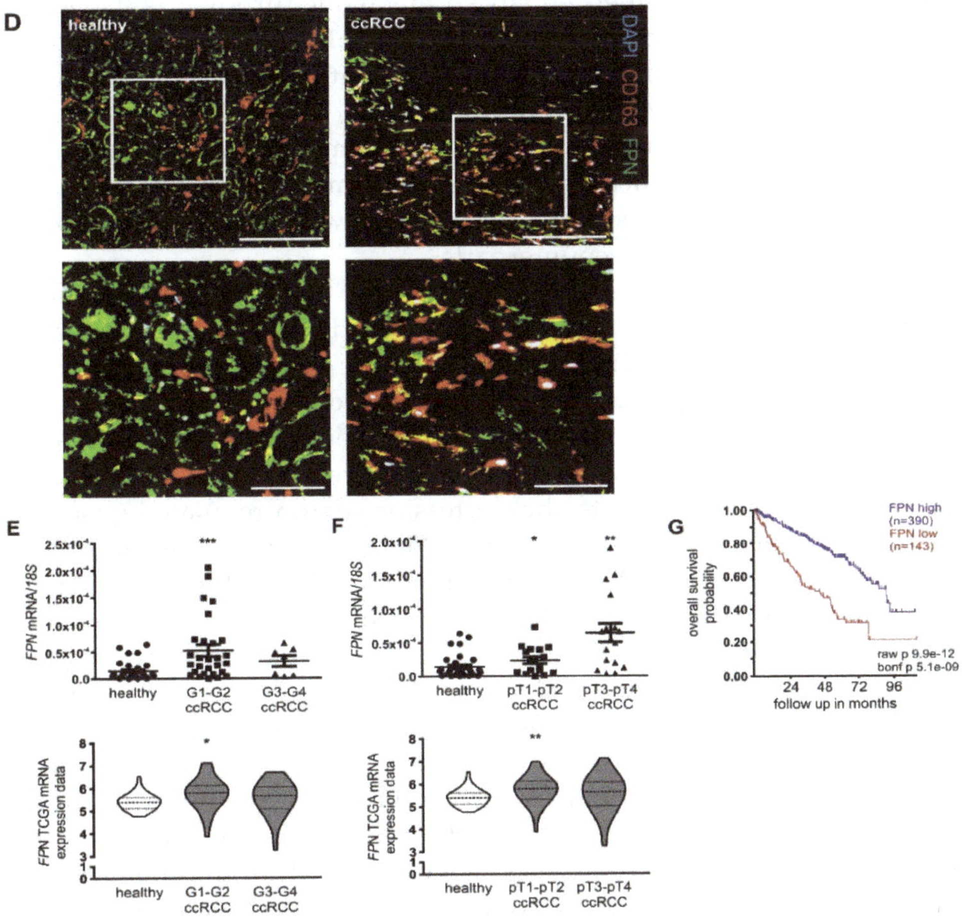

Figure 6. Tumor-associated MΦ express enhanced FPN protein. (**A**) FACS panel how to gate $CD45^+$ immune cells and $CD326^+$ epithelial/tumor cells. Immune cells were further gated for $CD33^+$/HLA-DR^+ cells of which $CD64^+$ and $MerTK^+$ MΦ were sub-selected. Cells were subsequently analyzed for their FPN protein expression, displayed as MFI (mean fluorescence intensity). (**B**) FPN protein expression as MFI of $CD45^-$/$CD326^-$ stroma cells ($n = 26$). (**C**) FPN protein expression as MFI of MΦ in tumor tissue compared to adjacent healthy tissue ($n = 26$). (**D**) Representative pictures for the MΦ marker CD163 and FPN protein expression in tumor tissue compared to healthy adjacent tissue applying confocal laser scanning miscroscopy. DAPI was used as nuclear stain. Scale bar: 200 µm. *FPN* mRNA expression normalized to *18S* expression correlated to (**E**) low (G1–G2) and high (G3–G4) tumor grade and (**F**) low (pT1–pT2) and high (pT3–pT4) tumor pT-stage in our patient cohort (upper panels; $n = 48$) compared to the TCGA data base, applying the ccRCC-KIRC data set (lower panels; $n = 70$). (**G**) Kaplan-Meier curve of high or low *FPN* expression from the R2 bioinformatics platform using the ccRCC-KIRC data set. Graphs are displayed as means ± SEM with * $p < 0.05$, ** $p < 0.01$, *** $p < 0.001$.

3. Discussion

We present evidence that iron metabolism is significantly altered in renal cancer. We observed elevated iron deposits in renal tumor tissue compared to adjacent healthy tissue as well as enhanced expression of iron-regulated genes in tumor tissue isolated from patients with renal cancer compared to adjacent healthy tissue. As iron is of importance for essentially all tumor hallmarks, we further investigated the role of iron in determining tumor cell proliferation and migration. In this setting, we also described and characterized the use of a novel extracellular iron chelator that scavenges iron in the extracellular space, thereby providing a valuable tool to investigate its role in the tumor microenvironment.

Numerous studies support a positive association between increased iron levels and cancer development, whereby cancer cells evolved specialized mechanisms for iron acquisition, storage, and mobilization in order to ensure their enhanced metabolic turnover [43]. Despite the fact that both availability as well as distribution of iron is strictly regulated under healthy conditions, cancers exert a profoundly dysregulated iron-handling capacity with altered expression of iron-regulated genes [15–17,44,45]. These observations are corroborated by the present study, detecting enhanced expression of iron-regulated genes in renal tumor tissue as compared to adjacent healthy tissue, which was most prominent in ccRCC. This effect was further confirmed by TCGA data base analysis. In this regard, we also found that cancer cells isolated from patients with renal cancer showed enhanced iron sequestration compared to their healthy counterparts.

Taking the unique role of the kidney in iron physiology into consideration [4], several markers, including erythropoietin [46] have been tested in RCC. Regardless of the initial promising effects, they only showed low predictive value. There are still no specific and reliable tumor markers neither for RCC diagnosis nor for monitoring post-operative disease outcome. Despite the apparent association of RCC with the development of systemic anemia in RCC patients [47], the role of iron in human RCC carcinogenesis is largely unknown and was only scarcely investigated so far. Because of the growing evidence on their tumor-promoting effects, the expression of iron-regulated genes could become an important factor among the markers of tumorigenesis. Along these lines, Greene at al. recently showed an association of TfR1 expression and RCC progression [7], with TfR1 levels being highest in benign primary tumors, subsequently dropping during the course of disease progression. TfR1 levels were therefore inversely associated with worse survival, but independent of tumor pathology. In line, we observed overall enhanced iron amounts in tumor tissue as compared to adjacent healthy tissue for all investigated renal cancer subtypes. Interestingly, iron amounts in chRCC varied considerably between different patients and needs to be further addressed in follow-up studies including higher patient number. Intriguingly, we also found initial differences in iron levels in adjacent healthy tissue for each histopathological subtype. These observations might arise both from the original localization of the tissue for individual samples as well as result from different basal iron levels of each individual patient. Therefore, healthy control tissue has to be controlled carefully to avoid misleading interpretation.

Nonetheless, modulating the iron-retaining tumor phenotype reduced growth and progression of both human and mouse carcinomas [48]. The use of iron chelators in the treatment of cancer inhibited DNA synthesis and caused a G1-S-phase cell cycle arrest, attenuated epithelial-mesenchymal-transition, and promoted cancer cell apoptosis [39]. Furthermore, chemically-induced and oncogene-driven cancer models corroborated these findings and stressed the relevance of iron for tumor development [49,50]. Numerous studies investigated methods to interfere with iron-handling in cancer cells, either by directly modulating iron-regulated genes [43] or by the use of iron chelators [37]. Nevertheless, a detailed knowledge of the effects of chelators within the tumor microenvironment (and on potential iron sources thereof) is still lacking [43]. In this study, we identified enhanced iron levels in extracellular fluids of tumor tissue in comparison to healthy adjacent tissue, suggesting that cells of the tumor microenvironment secreted iron in extracellular fluids. Due to their important role in tumor development and iron handling, we proposed that MΦ might adopt a pro-tumorigenic iron-releasing phenotype, whereby tumor growth is favored. Since MΦ are central players in systemic iron homeostasis, they have evolved unique mechanisms to recycle, store, and release iron to their local microenvironment. However, our data suggest differences in total tissue iron levels versus iron amounts of both MΦ and tumor cells for histopathological renal cancer subtypes. We hypothesize that even if the overall amount of iron is not changed in tumor tissue compared to adjacent healthy tissue in pRCC patients, the different distribution of iron within the tissue and in cells of the tumor mass, i.e. MΦ or tumor cells might add to the characteristics of iron as a pro-tumoral factor.

Macrophage iron homeostasis is functionally coupled to their heterogeneity and plasticity, with their polarization status being reflected also by their expression profiles of iron-regulated genes.

We previously showed that treatment of MΦ with LPS/IFNγ enhanced the retention of iron within the cell, whereas stimulation with anti-inflammatory cytokines such as IL-10 or IL-4 induced the release of iron [41]. This observation falls in line with a typical cytokine/chemokine profile of differentially polarized MΦ. We used this setting also in the present study to generate supernatant from IL-10-polarized iron-releasing MΦ. We tested the effect of iron, which was released by MΦ, in combination with an iron chelator that specifically binds iron in the extracellular space. EC1, which was designed and synthesized specifically for this study, is a thiosemicarbazone chelator featuring a sulfonate group that is negatively charged near neutral pH. While the tridentate (*O,N,S*) binding unit (see Figure S3A) ensures high-affinity iron coordination, the negative charge on the scaffold was incorporated to limit or hamper cellular membrane permeability. This strategy is particularly advantageous for the study of iron with respect to the crosstalk between TAMs and cancer cells. We found that the addition of EC1 reversed the positive effect of macrophage-conditioned media on the proliferation and migration of cancer cells. Although the exact molecular speciation of iron released in the macrophage supernatant remains to be determined, these experiments indicated that this iron pool is accessible by small-molecule chelators and could represent a hitherto unrecognized effect of these antiproliferative compounds in the tumor microenvironment.

Our previous studies using intracellularly active pro-chelators underscore the importance of macrophage-released iron for tumor cell proliferation [41]. Intriguingly, current research focuses primarily on the role of iron and iron-chelation therapy in tumor cells, whereas detailed knowledge on the crosstalk between tumor cells and tumor-associated MΦ as a possible source of iron is lacking. Taking into account that the presence of MΦ in tumor tissue is closely linked to tumor progression, we further analyzed the expression of the iron exporter FPN as a determinant of the iron releasing capacity of MΦ. We found enhanced expression of FPN in tumor MΦ compared to MΦ of adjacent healthy tissues, which was significantly associated with tumor pT-stage. However, these data could not be corroborated by TCGA data base analysis regarding overall patient survival. This discrepancy might arise from low cohort size of analyzed patients. Furthermore, it might also be necessary to distinguish FPN expression in stromal cells versus tumor cells as compared to whole tissue analysis. Recently, it was shown that tumor-associated MΦ also secrete iron in form of FT, which, in turn, stimulated tumor cell proliferation [44]. FTL expression in MΦ was further described as an independent prognostic marker in node-negative breast cancer. However, in the present study, we did not observe significant changes in FT protein expression in tumor-associated MΦ compared to MΦ isolated from adjacent healthy tissue. Recently, Marques et al. observed that FT expression was elevated in tumor-infiltrating lymphocytes, whereas no changes were detected for FT expression in tumor-associated MΦ [34]. The crucial implication of MΦ in tumor development and their role in iron distribution within the tumor microenvironment represents an important area of investigation in contemporary cancer biology.

Collectively, the results of the present study indicate that iron homeostasis is significantly disturbed in renal cancer with most of the investigated iron-regulated genes being associated with tumor grade and tumor pT-stage. Moreover, we observed that iron availability in the tumor microenvironment might be controlled by tumor-associated MΦ, which adopt an iron-release phenotype through increased expression of FPN. Application of chelators that are able to specifically scavenge iron in the extracellular space confirmed the importance of macrophage-secreted iron in promoting tumor cell proliferation and migration.

Future experimental in vivo studies should address the possibility to either interfere with iron availability in the tumor microenvironment or use macrophage-targeted chelation strategies. Moreover, more research is needed with regard to the questions of: i) the molecular networks that allow tumor cells to actually take up, store, and utilize iron and ii) the release of tumor cell-derived mediators that re-program stromal cells, i.e., MΦ, to serve as an iron source in order to maintain their enhanced metabolism and growth.

4. Materials and Methods

4.1. Ethics

Investigations were conducted in accordance with the ethical standards according to the Declaration of Helsinki and to national and international guidelines. Primary human tumor and adjacent healthy tissues were obtained from 64 patients with the approval of the ethics committees of the Goethe-University Hospital Frankfurt am Main (04/09 UGO 03/10) and the Philipps-University Hospital Marburg (122/14). Patients gave their written informed consent prior to surgery (UCT 122/14 and 04/09 UGO 03/10).

4.2. Participants

Patients included in this study underwent nephrectomy or partial nephrectomy for renal lesions histopathologically diagnosed with renal cancer between 2016 and 2019 at University Hospitals Frankfurt am Main and Marburg (see Table 1). Patients underwent preoperative staging either by computed tomography or Magnetic resonance imaging and surgery was performed before receiving other therapy. Tissue was collected immediately after surgery and processed for single cell suspensions, fixed in 4% paraformaldehyde (PFA) or stored at −80 °C. Pathological examination was performed by independent pathologists applying the UICC TNM classification of malignant tumors [51].

4.3. RNA Extraction and Quantitative Real-Time PCR (qRT-PCR)

Total RNA was extracted from homogenized tissue samples using peqGold RNAPure (VWR, Darmstadt, Germany, 732-3312) and transcribed using Maxima First Strand cDNA synthesis kit (Thermo Fisher, Dreieich, Germany, K1642). Gene expression profiles were determined by qPCR using the SYBR Green Supermix (Bio-Rad, Munich, Germany, 1725006CUST) on a CFX-Connect real-time-PCR detection system (Bio-Rad). Results were quantified using the Bio-Rad CFX-Manager (Bio-Rad, version 3) with 18S mRNA expression as housekeeping control. All primers except TfR1 Primer (Qiagen, Hilden, Germany, QT00094850) are listed in the supplemental information file and were purchased from Biomers (Ulm, Germany).

4.4. Data baSe Analysis

To show mRNA expression of *FPN, FTL, FTH, TfR1* and *IRP2* in different renal cancer subtypes, gene expression data of the Cancer Genome Atlas were analyzed (https://portal.gdc.cancer.gov/). Expression data of TCGA files were used of the following data sets: "Tumor Kidney Renal Clear Cell Carcinoma" (KIRC, $n = 533$), "Tumor Kidney Renal Papillary Cell Carcinoma" (KIRP, $n = 290$), and "Tumor Kidney Chromophobe" (KICH, $n = 66$). Cases with tumor and adjacent renal healthy tissue data available were included in the analysis (KIRC: $n = 70$; KIRP: $n = 31$; KICH: $n = 23$).

Kaplan-Meier plots were generated using the R2 Genomics Analysis and Visualization Platform (http://r2.amc.nl). The dataset "Tumor Kidney Renal Clear Cell Carcinoma" ($n = 533$) was chosen. Default settings of the KaplanScan including a log rank comparison between the groups were used to determine an optimum survival cut-off as described in the portal. The resulting p-value as well as the Bonferroni correction of the log rank comparison are included in the plots.

4.5. Atomic Absorption Spectroscopy (AAS)

Iron measurements were performed as previously described [35]. Whole tissue homogenates where either measured as whole homogenates and normalized to total protein amount or underwent FACS sorting with the final cell suspension being analyzed for its iron content and normalized to the total number of sorted cells.

4.6. Perl's Stain

Tissue slides were dewaxed in xylene and rehydrated in a series of alcohol solutions using decreasing concentrations. Perl's stain was performed using the Iron Stain Kit (Sigma Aldrich, Taufkirchen, Germany, HT20) according to the manufacturer's protocol. Slides were then washed in distilled water, counterstained with Nuclear Fast Red solution (Sigma Aldrich, N3020), rapidly dehydrated, and mounted in Entellan (Merck, Darmstadt, Germany, 107961). Pictures were acquired using an Axioskop 40 (Zeiss, Oberkochen, Germany).

4.7. Flow Cytometric Analyses

Tumors and adjacent healthy renal tissues were dissociated using the human Tumor Dissociation Kit (Miltenyi Biotec, Bergisch-Gladbach, Germany, 130-095-929) and GentleMACS System (Miltenyi Biotec). Samples were acquired with a LSRII/Fortessa flow cytometer (BD, Heidelberg, Germany) expressed as mean fluorescence intensity (MFI). CompBeads (BD) were used for single color compensation to create multi-color compensation matrices. For gating, fluorescence minus one (FMO) controls were used. Prior to experiments, all antibodies and secondary reagents were titrated to determine optimal concentrations.

For staining of FPN, extracellular staining of patient-derived single cell suspensions was performed, containing CD33 BV510 (BD, 563257), MerTK BV421 (Biolegend, San Diego, CA, USA, 367603), CD45 AF700 (Biolegend, 368513), CD 64 BV605 (Biolegend, 305033), CD206 PE-Cy7 (Biolegend, 321124), CD326 PE-CF594 (BD, 565399), HLA-DR APC-Cy7 (Biolegend, 307658), and FPN PE (Novus, Wiesbaden, Germany, NBP1-21502).

4.8. FACS Sorting and Processing of Sorted Cells

Single cell suspensions of tumor and adjacent healthy renal tissue were stained with an antibody cocktail containing CD33 BV510 (BD, 563257), MerTK BV421 (Biolegend, 367603), CD45 AF700 (Biolegend, 368513), CD64 BV605 (Biolegend, 305033), CD326 PE-CF594 (BD, 565399), HLA-DR APC-Cy7 (Biolegend, 307658). Cell suspensions were sorted using a FACS Aria (BD) FACS sorter, resulting in $CD45^-/CD326^+$ epithelial cells and $CD45^+/CD33^+/HLA\text{-}DR^+/CD64^+/MerTK^+$ MΦ from tumor and healthy tissue.

Cells were harvested for AAS (5000 cells) or used for RNA isolation (1000 cells). RNA isolation and transcription were performed using the RNeasy Micro Kit (Qiagen, 74004) and Sensiscript RT Kit (Qiagen, 205211) according to the manufacturer's kit protocols.

4.9. Cell Culture

Human renal cancer cell lines CAKI-1 and 786-O cells (kindly provided by PD Dr. Anja Urbschat) were cultured in Dulbecco's modified Eagle's medium (Gibco, Dreieich, Germany, 41965) supplemented with penicillin 100 U/mL (Sigma-Aldrich, P4333), streptomycin 100 mg/mL (Sigma-Aldrich, S8636), and 10% FCS (Capricorn Scientific, Ebersdorfergrund, Germany FBS-11A). Cells were regularly tested for mycoplasma contamination using Venor GeM Classic (Minerva Biolabs, Berlin, Germany, 11-1100).

4.10. Tumor Tubular Epithelial Cell Isolation

Human tubular epithelial cells (TTEC) were isolated as previously described [52]. Briefly, tumor tissue was minced, digested with collagenase/dispase (1 mg/mL), and passed through a 106 μm mesh. The tumor tissue solution was then incubated with collagenase (1 mg/mL), DNase (0.1 mg/mL) and MgCl2 (5 mmol/L). Cells were seeded on FCS-precoated plates and grown in M199 medium (Sigma Aldrich, M4530), supplemented with penicillin (100 U/mL), streptomycin (100 mg/mL), and 10% FBS. Meropenem (100 μg/mL, Sigma Aldrich, M2574) was added to the culture medium for the first 2–3 days after isolation. Passages from two to four were used for experiments.

4.11. EC Fluids Generation

Frozen tumor and adjacent healthy renal tissues were crushed into fragments <2 mm in diameter and suspended in 1:2 weight/volume of 2× phosphate-buffered saline (PBS). The solution was rotated at 4 °C for 3 h. The samples were then vortexed, and the centrifugation-cleared supernatants were used for experiments.

4.12. Generation of Conditioned Medium (CM) from Human MΦ

Human monocytes were isolated from commercially available, anonymized buffy coats (DRK-Blutspendedienst Baden-Württemberg-Hessen, Frankfurt, Germany) using Ficoll-Hypaque gradients (PAA Laboratories, Cölbe, Germany) as previously described [41]. Briefly, monocytes were differentiated into primary human MΦ with RPMI-1640 containing 5% AB-positive human serum (DRK-Blutspendedienst Baden-Württemberg-Hessen, Frankfurt, Germany). Prior to stimulation, cells were serum-starved for 24 h and stimulated with 20 ng/mL IL-10 (Peprotech, Hamburg, Germany) for 24 h to generate conditioned-media of polarized MΦ [41]. Conditioned-media from iron-releasing MΦ were collected and used for following proliferation and migration assays. Supernatant of unstimulated MΦ served as control.

4.13. Proliferation and Migration Assays

Proliferation and migration assays were performed using the xCELLigence RTCA DP instrument (OLS, Bremen, Germany) as previously described [53]. Proliferation was recorded continuously for 3 days and migration for 24 h. Data were acquired as a measure for time-dependent impedance changes. RTCA Software 1.2 (OLS) was used for acquisition and analysis.

4.14. Immunohistochemistry

Immunohistochemical staining was adapted from previously described protocols [35]. Formalin-fixed and paraffin-embedded patient tissues were stained with antibodies against FPN (Novus, NBP1-21502) and CD163 (Abcam, Cambridge, UK, ab182422) according to the manufacturer's protocol using the Opal 4-color-automation IHC-kit (PerkinElmer, Rodgau, Germany, NEL820001KT). Images were acquired using the LSM 800 microscope (Zeiss) and edited using ImageJ software.

4.15. Hematoxylin and Eosin Stain

For hematoxylin and eosin staining, formalin-fixed and paraffin-embedded tissues were rehydrated, stained using Mayer's hemalum solution (Merck, 109249), washed, counter-stained using Eosin (Merck, 102439), and mounted in Entellan (Merck, 107961). An Axioskop 40 (Zeiss) was used to acquire images.

4.16. XTT

Cytotoxicity of iron chelators was tested by a photometric XTT assay (Panreac, Darmstadt, Germany, A8088). Briefly, sub-confluent cells were exposed to iron chelators for 12 h. Subsequently, XTT reagent was added and absorbance was measured at 450 nm vs. 630 nm according to manufacturer's protocol. Experiments were conducted in quintuplicates. Cell viability was normalized to the untreated control.

4.17. Synthesis and Chemical Characterization of the Extracellular Chelator EC1

2-Hydroxybenzaldehyde (125 mg, 1.0 mmol) was added to a solution of sodium 4-(hydrazinecarbothioamido) benzenesulfonate (426 mg, 1.5 mmol) in water (1 mL). Ethanol (2 mL) was added and the solution was brought to reflux and stirred for 30 min. The reaction mixture was then allowed to cool to room temperature and the formed precipitate was filtered, washed with ethanol, and dried under vacuum. The identity and purity of the desired product (311 mg, 81% yield) were confirmed by high-resolution mass spectrometry via electrospray ionization (HRMS-ESI) and nuclear magnetic resonance (NMR) spectroscopy. HRMS-ESI (*m/z*): $[M - Na]^-$ calcd for $[C_{14}H_{12}N_3O_4S_2]^-$, 350.02747; found, 350.02741; $[M + H]^+$ calcd for $[C_{14}H_{13}N_3NaO_4S_2]^+$, 374.02397; found, 374.02401. ^1H NMR (500 MHz, DMSO-d_6) δ 11.79 (s, 1H), 10.07 (s, 1H), 9.98 (bs, 1H), 8.50 (s, 1H), 8.09 (bd, 1H), 7.64–7.44 (m, 4H), 7.24 (m, 1H), 6.95–6.78 (m, 2H). ^{13}C NMR (125 MHz, DMSO-d_6) δ 176.21, 157.17, 145.37, 140.65, 139.76, 131.86, 127.55, 125.85, 125.12, 120.69, 119.70, 116.53.

4.18. Chelator Solutions

2,2′-Dipyridine (2′2-DPD) was obtained commercially (Sigma Aldrich, D216305) and the intracellular prochelator $(TC3\text{-}S)_2$ was prepared as previously reported [54]. Extracellular chelator EC1 was synthesized as described above. For experiments in cell cultures, stock solutions were prepared at a standard concentration of 100 μM in dimethyl sulfoxide (DMSO) and were always prepared freshly in degassed DMSO.

4.19. Statistical Analysis

Statistical analysis was performed applying GraphPad Prism software (GraphPad Inc., San Diego, CA, USA, version 8.2.1). Variable distribution was tested for normality using the Kolmogorov-Smirnov test. Respectively, Gaussian distributed, and non-Gaussian distributed patient samples were statistical analyzed using two-tailed paired student's *t*-test or Wilcoxon matched-pairs signed-ranks test. In vitro experiments were analyzed using one-way ANOVA. Cell culture experiments were performed at least three times (independent experiments using technical replicates). Patient samples were used in experiments upon availability. P values were considered significant at * $p < 0.05$, ** $p < 0.01$, *** $p < 0.001$.

5. Conclusions

This study provides new insights of a significantly altered iron metabolism in renal cell carcinoma. Most of the studied iron-regulated genes are associated with tumor grade and tumor pT-stage. Moreover, our results suggest that tumor-associated macrophages adopt a pro-tumorigenic iron-releasing phenotype through increased expression of FPN. These tumor-associated macrophages are then able to fuel the increased iron demands of tumor cells by secreting iron in the tumor microenvironment.

EC1, a novel iron chelator, specifically scavenges iron in the extracellular space and was able to reverse pro-tumorigenic effects of macrophage-conditioned media on proliferation and migration of cancer cells, including primary patient-derived renal cancer cells. These results might pave the way towards further in vivo studies addressing the possibility to interfere with iron availability in the tumor microenvironment by targeted chelation strategies.

6. Patents

Issued patent: Tomat E.; Chang, T. M. "Redox-Directed Chelators Targeting Intracellular Metal Ions" U.S. Patent No. 9,486,423, November 8th, 2016.

Pending patent application: Tomat, E.; Chang, T.; Akam, E. A. "Redox-activated Pro-chelators" U.S. Patent Appl. No.: 16/200,286, November 26th, 2018.

Author Contributions: Conceptualization: M.J.; Methodology: M.S., C.R., C.M., E.T., E.A.A., M.J.; Software: M.S.; Validation: M.S., C.R., C.M., J.K.M., M.J.; Formal analysis: M.S., C.R., A.U., C.M., E.T., E.A.A., M.J.; Investigation: M.S., C.R., A.U., C.M., J.K.M., E.T., E.A.A., P.B., F.C.R., M.J.; Resources: A.U., P.B., F.R., B.B., M.J.; Data curation: M.J.; Writing—original draft preparation: M.S., E.T., B.B., M.J.; Writing—review and editing, M.S., E.T., B.B., M.J.; Visualization: M.S., M.J.; Supervision: M.J.; Project administration: M.J.; Funding acquisition: E.T., B.B., M.J. All authors have read and agreed to the published version of the manuscript.

Acknowledgments: The authors thank Aline Kraus and Yu-Shien Sung for assistance on the chemical characterization of EC1.

References

1. White, M.F.; Dillingham, M.S. Iron-sulphur clusters in nucleic acid processing enzymes. *Curr. Opin. Struct. Biol.* **2012**, *22*, 94–100. [CrossRef] [PubMed]
2. Wang, Y.; Yu, L.; Ding, J.; Chen, Y. Iron Metabolism in Cancer. *Int. J. Mol. Sci.* **2018**, *20*, 95. [CrossRef] [PubMed]
3. Pantopoulos, K.; Porwal, S.K.; Tartakoff, A.; Devireddy, L. Mechanisms of mammalian iron homeostasis. *Biochemistry* **2012**, *51*, 5705–5724. [CrossRef] [PubMed]
4. Haase, V.H. Hypoxic regulation of erythropoiesis and iron metabolism. *Am. J. Physiol. Ren. Physiol.* **2010**, *299*, F1–F13. [CrossRef] [PubMed]
5. Seminog, O.O.; Ogunlaja, O.I.; Yeates, D.; Goldacre, M.J. Risk of individual malignant neoplasms in patients with sickle cell disease: English national record linkage study. *J. R. Soc. Med.* **2016**, *109*, 303–309. [CrossRef] [PubMed]
6. Vargas-Olvera, C.Y.; Sánchez-González, D.J.; Solano, J.D.; Aguilar-Alonso, F.A.; Montalvo-Muñoz, F.; Martínez-Martínez, C.M.; Medina-Campos, O.N.; Ibarra-Rubio, M.E. Characterization of N-diethylnitrosamine -initiated and ferric nitrilotriacetate-promoted renal cell carcinoma experimental model and effect of a tamarind seed extract against acute nephrotoxicity and carcinogenesis. *Mol. Cell. Biochem.* **2012**, *369*, 105–117. [CrossRef] [PubMed]
7. Greene, C.J.; Attwood, K.; Sharma, N.J.; Gross, K.W.; Smith, G.J.; Xu, B.; Kauffman, E.C. Transferrin receptor 1 upregulation in primary tumor and downregulation in benign kidney is associated with progression and mortality in renal cell carcinoma patients. *Oncotarget* **2017**, *8*, 107052–107075. [CrossRef]
8. Bray, F.; Ferlay, J.; Soerjomataram, I.; Siegel, R.L.; Torre, L.A.; Jemal, A. Global cancer statistics 2018: GLOBOCAN estimates of incidence and mortality worldwide for 36 cancers in 185 countries. *CA Cancer J. Clin.* **2018**. [CrossRef]
9. Makhov, P.; Joshi, S.; Ghatalia, P.; Kutikov, A.; Uzzo, R.G.; Kolenko, V.M. Resistance to Systemic Therapies in Clear Cell Renal Cell Carcinoma: Mechanisms and Management Strategies. *Mol. Cancer Ther.* **2018**, *17*, 1355–1364. [CrossRef]
10. Gill, D.M.; Agarwal, N.; Vaishampayan, U. Evolving Treatment Paradigm in Metastatic Renal Cell Carcinoma. *Am. Soc. Clin. Oncol. Educ. Book* **2017**, *37*, 319–329. [CrossRef]
11. Amin, A.; Hammers, H. The Evolving Landscape of Immunotherapy-Based Combinations for Frontline Treatment of Advanced Renal Cell Carcinoma. *Front. Immunol.* **2018**, *9*, 3120. [CrossRef] [PubMed]
12. Cella, D.; Grünwald, V.; Escudier, B.; Hammers, H.J.; George, S.; Nathan, P.; Grimm, M.-O.; Rini, B.I.; Doan, J.; Ivanescu, C.; et al. Patient-reported outcomes of patients with advanced renal cell carcinoma treated with nivolumab plus ipilimumab versus sunitinib (CheckMate 214): A randomised, phase 3 trial. *Lancet Oncol.* **2019**, *20*, 297–310. [CrossRef]
13. Kohgo, Y.; Ikuta, K.; Ohtake, T.; Torimoto, Y.; Kato, J. Body iron metabolism and pathophysiology of iron overload. *Int. J. Hematol.* **2008**, *88*, 7–15. [CrossRef] [PubMed]
14. Torti, S.V.; Torti, F.M. Iron and cancer: More ore to be mined. *Nat. Rev. Cancer* **2013**, *13*, 342–355. [CrossRef]
15. Kirkali, Z.; Esen, A.A.; Kirkali, G.; Güner, G. Ferritin: A tumor marker expressed by renal cell carcinoma. *Eur. Urol.* **1995**, *28*, 131–134. [CrossRef]
16. Jézéquel, P.; Campion, L.; Spyratos, F.; Loussouarn, D.; Campone, M.; Guérin-Charbonnel, C.; Joalland, M.-P.; André, J.; Descotes, F.; Grenot, C.; et al. Validation of tumor-associated macrophage ferritin light chain as a prognostic biomarker in node-negative breast cancer tumors: A multicentric 2004 national PHRC study. *Int. J. Cancer* **2012**, *131*, 426–437. [CrossRef]
17. Brookes, M.J.; Hughes, S.; Turner, F.E.; Reynolds, G.; Sharma, N.; Ismail, T.; Berx, G.; McKie, A.T.; Hotchin, N.; Anderson, G.J.; et al. Modulation of iron transport proteins in human colorectal carcinogenesis. *Gut* **2006**, *55*, 1449–1460. [CrossRef]
18. Wang, W.; Deng, Z.; Hatcher, H.; Miller, L.D.; Di, X.; Tesfay, L.; Sui, G.; D'Agostino, R.B.; Torti, F.M.; Torti, S.V. IRP2 regulates breast tumor growth. *Cancer Res.* **2014**, *74*, 497–507. [CrossRef]
19. Ludwig, H.; Müldür, E.; Endler, G.; Hübl, W. Prevalence of iron deficiency across different tumors and its association with poor performance status, disease status and anemia. *Ann. Oncol.* **2013**, *24*, 1886–1892. [CrossRef]

20. Corna, G.; Campana, L.; Pignatti, E.; Castiglioni, A.; Tagliafico, E.; Bosurgi, L.; Campanella, A.; Brunelli, S.; Manfredi, A.A.; Apostoli, P.; et al. Polarization dictates iron handling by inflammatory and alternatively activated macrophages. *Haematologica* **2010**, *95*, 1814–1822. [CrossRef]
21. Cairo, G.; Recalcati, S.; Mantovani, A.; Locati, M. Iron trafficking and metabolism in macrophages: Contribution to the polarized phenotype. *Trends Immunol.* **2011**, *32*, 241–247. [CrossRef] [PubMed]
22. Recalcati, S.; Locati, M.; Marini, A.; Santambrogio, P.; Zaninotto, F.; De Pizzol, M.; Zammataro, L.; Girelli, D.; Cairo, G. Differential regulation of iron homeostasis during human macrophage polarized activation. *Eur. J. Immunol.* **2010**, *40*, 824–835. [CrossRef] [PubMed]
23. Murray, P.J.; Wynn, T.A. Protective and pathogenic functions of macrophage subsets. *Nat. Rev. Immunol.* **2011**, *11*, 723–737. [CrossRef] [PubMed]
24. Chevrier, S.; Levine, J.H.; Zanotelli, V.R.T.; Silina, K.; Schulz, D.; Bacac, M.; Ries, C.H.; Ailles, L.; Jewett, M.A.S.; Moch, H.; et al. An Immune Atlas of Clear Cell Renal Cell Carcinoma. *Cell* **2017**, *169*, 736–749. [CrossRef] [PubMed]
25. Chanmee, T.; Ontong, P.; Konno, K.; Itano, N. Tumor-associated macrophages as major players in the tumor microenvironment. *Cancers* **2014**, *6*, 1670–1690. [CrossRef] [PubMed]
26. Ikemoto, S.; Yoshida, N.; Narita, K.; Wada, S.; Kishimoto, T.; Sugimura, K.; Nakatani, T. Role of tumor-associated macrophages in renal cell carcinoma. *Oncol. Rep.* **2003**. [CrossRef]
27. Toge, H.; Inagaki, T.; Kojimoto, Y.; Shinka, T.; Hara, I. Angiogenesis in renal cell carcinoma: The role of tumor-associated macrophages. *Int. J. Urol.* **2009**, *16*, 801–807. [CrossRef]
28. Lewis, C.E.; Pollard, J.W. Distinct role of macrophages in different tumor microenvironments. *Cancer Res.* **2006**, *66*, 605–612. [CrossRef]
29. Komohara, Y.; Hasita, H.; Ohnishi, K.; Fujiwara, Y.; Suzu, S.; Eto, M.; Takeya, M. Macrophage infiltration and its prognostic relevance in clear cell renal cell carcinoma. *Cancer Sci.* **2011**, *102*, 1424–1431. [CrossRef]
30. Xu, L.; Zhu, Y.; Chen, L.; An, H.; Zhang, W.; Wang, G.; Lin, Z.; Xu, J. Prognostic value of diametrically polarized tumor-associated macrophages in renal cell carcinoma. *Ann. Surg. Oncol.* **2014**, *21*, 3142–3150. [CrossRef]
31. Sangaletti, S.; Di Carlo, E.; Gariboldi, S.; Miotti, S.; Cappetti, B.; Parenza, M.; Rumio, C.; Brekken, R.A.; Chiodoni, C.; Colombo, M.P. Macrophage-derived SPARC bridges tumor cell-extracellular matrix interactions toward metastasis. *Cancer Res.* **2008**, *68*, 9050–9059. [CrossRef] [PubMed]
32. Sandlund, J.; Oosterwijk, E.; Grankvist, K.; Oosterwijk-Wakka, J.; Ljungberg, B.; Rasmuson, T. Prognostic impact of carbonic anhydrase IX expression in human renal cell carcinoma. *BJU Int.* **2007**, *100*, 556–560. [CrossRef] [PubMed]
33. Nguyen, D.P.; Vertosick, E.A.; Corradi, R.B.; Vilaseca, A.; Benfante, N.E.; Touijer, K.A.; Sjoberg, D.D.; Russo, P. Histological subtype of renal cell carcinoma significantly affects survival in the era of partial nephrectomy. *Urol. Oncol.* **2016**, *34*, 259.e1–259.e8. [CrossRef] [PubMed]
34. Marques, O.; Porto, G.; Rêma, A.; Faria, F.; Cruz Paula, A.; Gomez-Lazaro, M.; Silva, P.; Martins da Silva, B.; Lopes, C. Local iron homeostasis in the breast ductal carcinoma microenvironment. *BMC Cancer* **2016**, *16*, 187. [CrossRef]
35. Mertens, C.; Mora, J.; Ören, B.; Grein, S.; Winslow, S.; Scholich, K.; Weigert, A.; Malmström, P.; Forsare, C.; Fernö, M.; et al. Macrophage-derived lipocalin-2 transports iron in the tumor microenvironment. *Oncoimmunology* **2018**, *7*, e1408751. [CrossRef]
36. Jung, M.; Weigert, A.; Tausendschön, M.; Mora, J.; Ören, B.; Sola, A.; Hotter, G.; Muta, T.; Brüne, B. Interleukin-10-induced neutrophil gelatinase-associated lipocalin production in macrophages with consequences for tumor growth. *Mol. Cell. Biol.* **2012**, *32*, 3938–3948. [CrossRef]
37. Mertens, C.; Akam, E.A.; Rehwald, C.; Brüne, B.; Tomat, E.; Jung, M. Intracellular Iron Chelation Modulates the Macrophage Iron Phenotype with Consequences on Tumor Progression. *PLoS ONE* **2016**, *11*, e0166164. [CrossRef]
38. Yu, Y.; Kalinowski, D.S.; Kovacevic, Z.; Siafakas, A.R.; Jansson, P.J.; Stefani, C.; Lovejoy, D.B.; Sharpe, P.C.; Bernhardt, P.V.; Des Richardson, R. Thiosemicarbazones from the old to new: Iron chelators that are more than just ribonucleotide reductase inhibitors. *J. Med. Chem.* **2009**, *52*, 5271–5294. [CrossRef]
39. Utterback, R.D.; Tomat, E. Developing Ligands to Target Transition Metals in Cancer. *Encycl. Inorg. Bioinorg. Chem.* **2019**. [CrossRef]

40. Akam, E.A.; Chang, T.M.; Astashkin, A.V.; Tomat, E. Intracellular reduction/activation of a disulfide switch in thiosemicarbazone iron chelators. *Metallomics* **2014**, *6*, 1905–1912. [CrossRef]
41. Akam, E.A.; Utterback, R.D.; Marcero, J.R.; Dailey, H.A.; Tomat, E. Disulfide-masked iron prochelators: Effects on cell death, proliferation, and hemoglobin production. *J. Inorg. Biochem.* **2018**, *180*, 186–193. [CrossRef] [PubMed]
42. Greene, B.T.; Thorburn, J.; Willingham, M.C.; Thorburn, A.; Planalp, R.P.; Brechbiel, M.W.; Jennings-Gee, J.; Wilkinson, J.; Torti, F.M.; Torti, S.V. Activation of caspase pathways during iron chelator-mediated apoptosis. *J. Biol. Chem.* **2002**, *277*, 25568–25575. [CrossRef] [PubMed]
43. Jung, M.; Mertens, C.; Tomat, E.; Brüne, B. Iron as a Central Player and Promising Target in Cancer Progression. *Int. J. Mol. Sci.* **2019**, *20*, 273. [CrossRef] [PubMed]
44. Alkhateeb, A.A.; Han, B.; Connor, J.R. Ferritin stimulates breast cancer cells through an iron-independent mechanism and is localized within tumor-associated macrophages. *Breast Cancer Res. Treat.* **2013**, *137*, 733–744. [CrossRef]
45. Kukulj, S.; Jaganjac, M.; Boranic, M.; Krizanac, S.; Santic, Z.; Poljak-Blazi, M. Altered iron metabolism, inflammation, transferrin receptors, and ferritin expression in non-small-cell lung cancer. *Med. Oncol.* **2010**, *27*, 268–277. [CrossRef]
46. Nseyo, U.O.; Williams, P.D.; Murphy, G.E. Clinical significance of erythropoietin levels in renal carcinoma. *Urology* **1986**, *28*, 301–306. [CrossRef]
47. Dowd, A.A.; Ibrahim, F.I.; Mohammed, M.M. Renal cell carcinoma as a cause of iron deficiency anemia. *Afr. J. Urol.* **2014**, *20*, 25–27. [CrossRef]
48. Jiang, X.P.; Elliott, R.L.; Head, J.F. Manipulation of iron transporter genes results in the suppression of human and mouse mammary adenocarcinomas. *Anticancer Res.* **2010**, *30*, 759–765.
49. Coombs, G.S.; Schmitt, A.A.; Canning, C.A.; Alok, A.; Low, I.C.C.; Banerjee, N.; Kaur, S.; Utomo, V.; Jones, C.M.; Pervaiz, S.; et al. Modulation of Wnt/β-catenin signaling and proliferation by a ferrous iron chelator with therapeutic efficacy in genetically engineered mouse models of cancer. *Oncogene* **2012**, *31*, 213–225. [CrossRef]
50. Hrabinski, D.; Hertz, J.L.; Tantillo, C.; Berger, V.; Sherman, A.R. Iron repletion attenuates the protective effects of iron deficiency in DMBA-induced mammary tumors in rats. *Nutr. Cancer* **1995**, *24*, 133–142. [CrossRef]
51. Brierley, J.; Gospodarowicz, M.K.; Wittekind, C. *TNM Classification of Malignant Tumours*, 8th ed.; Brierley, J., Gospodarowicz, M.K., Wittekind, C., O'Sullivan, B., Eds.; John Wiley & Sons, Inc: Oxford, UK, 2017; ISBN 9781119263562.
52. Baer, P.C.; Nockher, W.A.; Haase, W.; Scherberich, J.E. Isolation of proximal and distal tubule cells from human kidney by immunomagnetic separation. Technical note. *Kidney Int.* **1997**, *52*, 1321–1331. [CrossRef] [PubMed]
53. Jung, M.; Ören, B.; Mora, J.; Mertens, C.; Dziumbla, S.; Popp, R.; Weigert, A.; Grossmann, N.; Fleming, I.; Brüne, B. Lipocalin 2 from macrophages stimulated by tumor cell-derived sphingosine 1-phosphate promotes lymphangiogenesis and tumor metastasis. *Sci. Signal.* **2016**, *9*, ra64. [CrossRef] [PubMed]
54. Chang, T.M.; Tomat, E. Disulfide/thiol switches in thiosemicarbazone ligands for redox-directed iron chelation. *Dalton Trans.* **2013**, *42*, 7846–7849. [CrossRef] [PubMed]

13

Repurposing of α1-Adrenoceptor Antagonists: Impact in Renal Cancer

Meredith Mihalopoulos [1], Zachary Dovey [1], Maddison Archer [1,2], Talia G. Korn [1], Kennedy E. Okhawere [1], William Nkemdirim [1], Hassan Funchess [1], Ami Rambhia [1], Nihal Mohamed [1], Steven A. Kaplan [1], Reza Mehrazin [1], Dara Lundon [1], Che-Kai Tsao [3], Ketan K. Badani [1] and Natasha Kyprianou [1,2,4,*]

1 Department of Urology, Tisch Cancer Institute, Icahn School of Medicine at Mount Sinai, New York, NY 10029, USA; meredith.mihalopoulos@icahn.mssm.edu (M.M.); zachary.dovey@mountsinai.org (Z.D.); Maddison.Archer@mountsinai.org (M.A.); Talia.korn@mountsinai.org (T.G.K.); Kennedy.Okhawere@mountsinai.org (K.E.O.); wn442@nyu.edu (W.N.); hf1031@nyu.edu (H.F.); ar6326@nyu.edu (A.R.); nihal.mohamed@mountsinai.org (N.M.); steven.kaplan@mountsinai.org (S.A.K.); reza.mehrazin@mountsinai.org (R.M.); Dara.Lundon@mountsinai.org (D.L.); ketan.badani@mountsinai.org (K.K.B.)

2 Department of Oncological Sciences, Icahn School of Medicine at Mount Sinai, New York, NY 10029, USA

3 Department of Medicine/Division of Hematology-Oncology, Icahn School of Medicine at Mount Sinai, New York, NY 10029, USA; che-kai.tsao@mssm.edu

4 Department of Pathology and Laboratory Medicine, Icahn School of Medicine at Mount Sinai, New York, NY 10029, USA

* Correspondence: natasha.kyprianou@mountsinai.org

Abstract: Renal cancer ranks twelfth in incidence among cancers worldwide. Despite improving outcomes due to better therapeutic options and strategies, prognosis for those with metastatic disease remains poor. Current systemic therapeutic approaches include inhibiting pathways of angiogenesis, immune checkpoint blockade, and mTOR inhibition, but inevitably resistance develops for those with metastatic disease, and novel treatment strategies are urgently needed. Emerging molecular and epidemiological evidence suggests that quinazoline-based α1-adrenoceptor-antagonists may have both chemopreventive and direct therapeutic actions in the treatment of urological cancers, including renal cancer. In human renal cancer cell models, quinazoline-based α1-adrenoceptor antagonists were shown to significantly reduce the invasion and metastatic potential of renal tumors by targeting focal adhesion survival signaling to induce anoikis. Mechanistically these drugs overcome anoikis resistance in tumor cells by targeting cell survival regulators AKT and FAK, disrupting integrin adhesion ($\alpha5\beta1$ and $\alpha2\beta1$) and engaging extracellular matrix (ECM)-associated tumor suppressors. In this review, we discuss the current evidence for the use of quinazoline-based α1-adrenoceptor antagonists as novel therapies for renal cell carcinoma (RCC) and highlight their potential therapeutic action through overcoming anoikis resistance of tumor epithelial and endothelial cells in metastatic RCC. These findings provide a platform for future studies that will retrospectively and prospectively test repurposing of quinazoline-based α1-adrenoceptor-antagonists for the treatment of advanced RCC and the prevention of metastasis in neoadjuvant, adjuvant, salvage and metastatic settings.

Keywords: renal tumors; prevention; α1-adrenoceptor antagonists; anoikis; vascularity

1. Introduction: The Therapeutic Challenge

Renal cancer ranks twelfth in incidence among cancers worldwide and has a lifetime risk of 1 to 63 for a given individual, with numbers estimated to be increasing at a rate of 2.4% per year [1,2].

Globally, 6 in 100,000 males and 3 in 100,000 females are diagnosed annually with renal cancer, with the incidence estimated to be increasing at a rate of 2.4% per year [1,2] with limited therapeutic management options [3–5]. In the United States alone, over 60,000 individuals were diagnosed with renal cell carcinoma (RCC) in 2018, with an estimated 14,970 deaths resulting from the illness [6]. Despite the introduction of systemic targeted therapies, five-year survival rates for locally advanced and metastatic disease remain at 70% and 12%, respectively in the year 2020 [7].

The most common genetic abnormality for clear cell RCC (ccRCC) is the chromosome 3p deletion and inactivation of the von Hippel Lindau (VHL) tumor suppressor gene, present in almost all familial and up to 60% of sporadic RCCs [8,9]. Loss of the VHL gene leads to the upregulation of hypoxia-inducible factor (HIF) and activation of vascular endothelial growth factor receptors (VEGFR) and other signaling pathways, leading to tumorigenesis with an aggressive angiogenic phenotype [8,9]. Current treatment of RCC is based on the tumor stage at diagnosis. Localized disease, with or without evidence of regional spread, is typically managed surgically alone. For those with more advanced localized or loco-regional disease after nephrectomy, treatment with adjuvant VEGFR TKI sunitinib has been approved by the Federal Drug Administration, although the modest clinical benefit and concern for the potential side effects has largely limited its clinical application to data [10].

For metastatic ccRCC, a number of approaches combining immune checkpoint inhibitors or with VEGFR-TKIs have now become the standard of care after demonstrating a definitive survival benefit in the first-line setting [11], compared to sunitinib alone [2]. However, the optimal first-line and sequence of subsequent therapies are not well defined. The current systemic therapeutic approaches include: targeting pathways of angiogenesis, immune checkpoint blockade, and mTOR inhibition. Inevitably, treatment resistance is either intrinsic or eventually develops. New mechanistic approaches are urgently needed to improve survival outcomes in this patient population.

Investigative efforts from our group and others have focused on the role of quinazoline-derived α1-adrenoreceptor antagonists in the treatment of renal cancer. By inducing smooth muscle relaxation and vasodilation, these drugs are currently used in the treatment of hypertension (HTN) and renal and ureteric stones [12,13], as well as of benign prostatic hyperplasia (BPH) [13]. More recently the potential efficacy of these drugs in the treatment of prostate cancer has been proposed, due to the ability to induce apoptosis and overcome anoikis resistance in tumor cells [14–18]. Reassuringly, in earlier clinical trials assessing their use for the treatment of BPH, they were well tolerated with only reversible adverse effects in a minority of patients, including postural hypotension (4%), asthenia or light-headedness (10%), somnolence (3%) and retrograde ejaculation (8%) [19,20].

Expression and distribution of α1-adrenoreceptors has been found in the cortex, pelvis, calyces, blood vessels and tubules of the kidney, suggesting potential effects of α1 adrenoceptor antagonists in renal pathophysiology [21–25]. Evidence at the cellular level suggests that the antitumor effect of α1-adrenoreceptor antagonists in renal tumors proceeds via reducing vascularity and impairing growth within the tumor microenvironment (via apoptosis and overcoming anoikis resistance). In this review, we outline the mechanism of α1-adrenoceptor antagonists in targeting renal cancer epithelial and endothelial cells and the potential therapeutic efficacy of using these clinically used FDA-approved drugs for the treatment of advanced RCC.

2. Mechanism of Action of α-Adrenoreceptor Antagonists in Human Disease

Adrenergic receptors (adrenoreceptors) are G-Protein coupled-receptors that are distributed throughout the body. They serve as receptors for catecholamines (noradrenaline and epinephrine) secreted from the autonomic sympathetic nervous system and play an important role in the regulation of a wide range of physiological systems in the body [23,24]. Alpha (α) receptors mediate smooth muscle contraction and vasoconstriction, while beta (β) receptors mediate vasodilation, smooth muscle relaxation, bronchodilation, and excitatory cardiac function [17,21]. The α-adrenoceptors are divided into two classes: α1 and α2, both of which are present in the renal vasculature and mediate vasoconstriction of exogenous and endogenous noradrenaline [22,24]. The α1-adrenoceptors are further sub-divided into α1A, α1B, α1D, with α1A subtype of therapeutic interest because of its location in the prostate, vas deferens, and urethra in humans [21,23–25].

Quinazoline-derived compounds blocking α1-adrenoreceptors have been found to reduce prostatic smooth muscle tone and relieve overall obstruction, as seen by their success in treating BPH [19]. This mechanism of action is also utilized in the treatment of renal and ureteric stones, as α1 blockers reduce intra-ureteral pressure and increase fluid passage [12,26–28]. Remarkably in human prostatic disease, these compounds not only target the alpha1-adrenergic-receptor mediated smooth muscle contraction [29], but they can also effectively induce apoptosis of tumor epithelial and endothelial cells [17,30,31]. It is important to note that the quinazoline-derived compounds can induce apoptosis among benign prostate epithelial cells, as well as in both androgen-dependent and castration-resistant prostate cancer cells, via α1-adrenoceptor –independent mechanisms [30–35]. This supports a strong cellular basis for their pharmacologic use in other cancer types.

The signaling mechanisms driving the intracellular antitumor action by quinazoline-based α1-adrenoceptor antagonists against prostate cancer epithelial and endothelial cells are summarized on Figure 1. (1) Smad activation of transforming growth factor (TGF)-β1 signaling, which controls cellular proliferation, differentiation, and apoptosis in human cancers cell including prostate cancer cells [3,30–32]; (2) Engaging the death receptor Fas-associated death domain (FADD)-mediated caspase-8 activation and apoptosis induction [3,32,33]; (3) Inhibition of the VEGF-mediated angiogenesis and Akt survival mechanisms navigating tumor vascularity [3,33,34]; and (4) α1-adrenoceptor antagonists have the ability to block cellular adhesion and invasion by targeting cell-cell interaction and impairing cell tight junctions (and also between epithelial and endothelial cells with the extracellular matrix; ECM), consequentially impacting epithelial–mesenchymal-transition (EMT) to mesenchymal–epithelial-transition (MET) phenotypic interconversions and increasing cellular vulnerability to anoikis (Figure 1) [3,35,36].

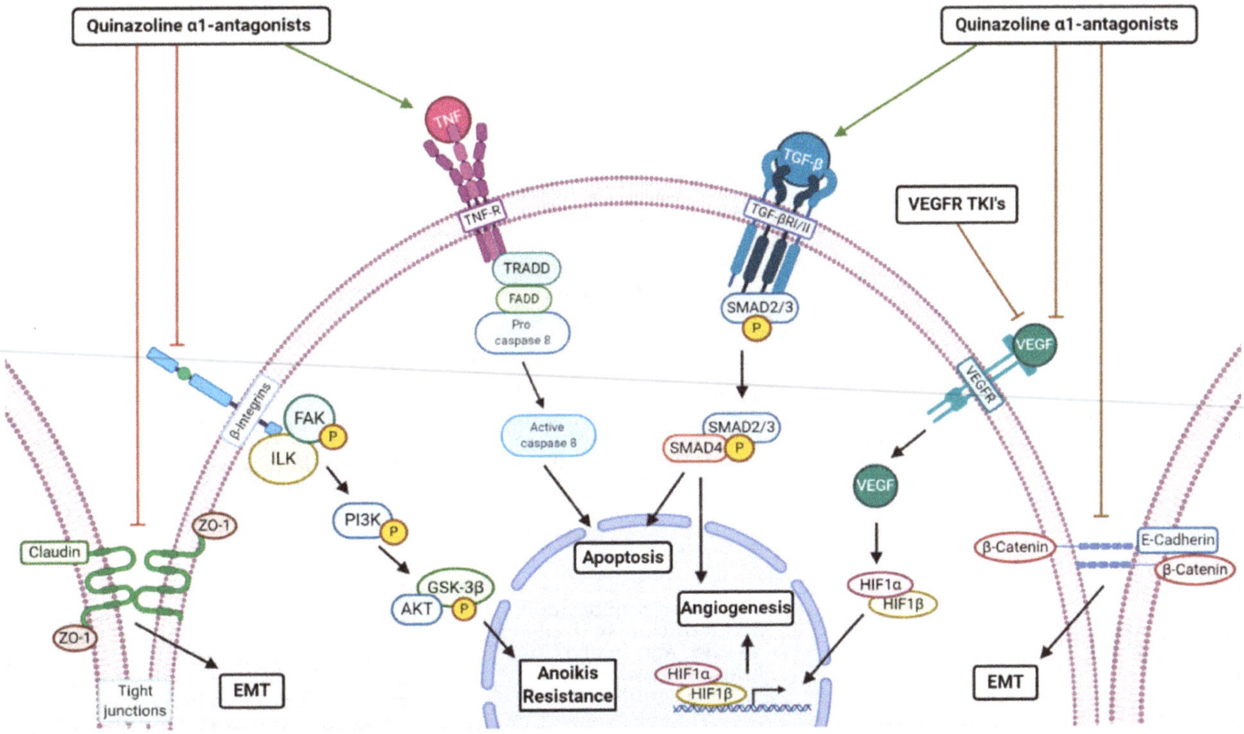

Figure 1. Biological Mechanisms of Anti-tumor Action of Quinazoline α1-Adrenoceptor Antagonists. Schematic diagram demonstrating the signaling mechanisms potentially targeted by quinazolne α1-andrenoceptor antagonists in attenuating renal tumor initiation and progression to metastasis. Quinazoline based α1-andrenoceptor antagonists influence the interconversion of epithelial–mesenchymal-transition (EMT) to mesenchymal–epithelial-transition (MET) phenotypes by targeting

tight junctions and E-cadherin-mediates cell adherence. Tumor cells succumb to anoikis by disruption of integrin-mediated cell survival via integrin-linked kinase (ILK). Quinazoline based α1-andrenoceptor antagonists induce apoptosis by either tumor necrosis factor (TNF)-mediated Fas-associated death domain (FADD)/caspase 8 activity and DNA fragmentation and/or Smad4 activation and apoptotic gene induction by transforming growth factor (TGF)-β. Angiogenesis is inhibited by vascular endothelial growth factor receptor (VEGFR)–tyrosine kinase inhibitors and quinazoline based α1-andrenoceptor antagonists can also target tumor vascularity by disruption of VEGF-mediated HIF1 transcriptional expression and potentially TGF-β signaling.

Moreover we previously established that integrin-linked kinase (ILK), a serine and threonine protein kinase, plays a key role in anoikis resistance by interacting with the cytoplasmic domains of β1-integrin and β3-integrin, which are pivotal in regulating cell adhesion, fibronectin–ECM assembly, and anchorage-dependent cell growth [34–37]. Within the tumor microenvironment (TME), ILK is activated in its phosphorylated form by focal adhesion kinase (FAK) and phosphatidylinositol 3-kinase (PI3-kinase)/Akt pathways [33,38–40]. By inhibiting ILK, quinazoline-derived α1-adrenoceptor antagonists can disrupt these cell-survival signals towards anoikis induction [3,41,42]. Considering that resistance to anoikis (and evasion of apoptosis in detached cells) is a primary contributor to cancer metastasis [43,44] and ultimately lethal disease, the ability to overcome this resistance points to a unique therapeutic value of quinazoline-derived α1-adrenoreceptor antagonists.

3. Antitumor Effects of α1-Adrenoceptor Antagonists

Table 1 summarizes the updated evidence from clinical, translational and epidemiological studies, suggesting the antitumor action of α1-adrenoceptor antagonists in human malignancies. The published work from our group and other investigators makes a strong case in support of the repurposing of the α1-adrenoceptor antagonists (with a good safety profile) and advance our current understanding of the clinical value of these therapeutic modalities for the treatment of GU-cancers including renal cancer

Table 1. Therapeutic Impact of α1-Adrenoreceptor Antagonists Use against Human Cancers.

Drug	Neoplasm	Effect	Cellular Mechanism
Naftopidil, Prazosin [14,45]	Bladder Cancer	Inhibit cell growth and viability in vitro in ACHN human cell lines	- Induce apoptosis via caspase activity
Doxazosin [46]	Colorectal Cancer	Decrease tumor numbers and size in vitro in RKO human cell lines and in vivo in mouse models	- Induce apoptosis via caspase activity
Doxazosin, Naftopidil, Prozasin, Terozasin, DZ-50 [14,17,32,35,45]	Prostate Cancer	Reduce cell viability and tumor vascularity in vitro and in vivo, including in castration-resistant prostate cancer	- G2 checkpoint arrest Inhibit cell growth Decrease microvessel density Induce apoptosis via caspase activity, Smad activation of TGF- β1 signaling *(Doxazosin)* Induce anoikis by disrupting integrin-mediated cell survival pathways *(DZ-50)*
Doxazosin, Naftodipil, DZ-50 [3,45]	RCC	Inhibit cell proliferation and reduce vascularity in vitro and in vivo in lines with and without VHL mutation	- Induce apoptosis by disabling FADD inhibitors, Smad activation of TGF-β1 signaling *(Dozazosin)* G1 cell cycle induction arrested in tumor and vascular epithelial cells *(Naftopidil)* Induce anoikis by disrupting integrin-mediated cell survival pathways *(DZ-50)*
Terazosin [46]	TCC	Reduce tumor vascularity and cell growth in vivo	- Induce apoptosis and decrease microvessel density

3.1. *Prostate Cancer*

Based on these pharmacological mechanisms of actions, α1-adrenoceptor antagonists have been shown to have efficacy in the treatment of several genitourinary cancers. There is mounting evidence of the effectiveness of quinazoline-derived α1 blockers in the clinical treatment patients with BPH and prostate tumors. Studies have shown that α1-adrenoceptor antagonists like prozasin and naftopidil inhibit cell growth, arrest cell cycling, decrease microvessel density, and induce apoptosis in human prostate cancer cells [34,35,45]. Doxazosin, a clinically used quinazoline-based α1-adrenoreceptor antagonist, reduced endothelial cell viability and suppressed tumor vascularity in prostate cancer xenografts. The drug additionally exhibited significant antitumor efficacy against models of metastatic castration-resistant prostate cancer (CRPC) [17,30]. In a retrospective observational cohort study at the VA Medical Center in Kentucky, Harris et al. (2007) found that in over a 5-year period in this clinical setting, exposure to quinazoline-based α1-adrenoreceptors antagonists, such as doxazosin and terazosin, significantly decreased the incidence of prostate cancer from 2.4% to 1.65%, corroborating the results of previous investigations [15,45]. While a case-control study of 23,320 men in the Finnish Cancer Registry and national prescription database found tamsulosin and alfuzosin did not improve the odds of developing prostate cancer, the study did discover the drugs significantly decreased the incidence of high-grade tumors in the cohort [47].

More recently, Hart et al. (2020) studied 303 prostate cancer patients to retrospectively determine if α1-blockers influenced response to radiotherapy for localized prostate cancer. The authors found that those treated with prazosin had a 3.9 lower relative risk of biochemical relapse. While not statistically significant, both tamsulosin and prazosin extended survival without recurrence by 13.15 and 9.21 months, respectively [48]. Furthermore, drug optimization efforts led to the development of the quinazoline-derived drug DZ-50. This novel α1 blocker has exerted chemoprotective qualities in vivo in BPH and prostate cancer cells through decreasing angiogenesis and increasing anoikis via inhibition of the TGF-β1 and insulin-like growth factor (IGF) pro-growth pathways [34,35].

3.2. *Bladder Cancer*

When evaluating antitumor activity of α1 blockers in terms of cell viability, cell cycle progression, competition, and apoptotic signaling in bladder cancer, Nakagawa et al. (2016) showed that naftopidil was one of the strongest antitumor α1-adrenoceptor antagonists [45]. Significantly enough, oral administration of naftopidil reduced tumor volume in a xenograft model in a concentration (10–100 μmol/L)-dependent manner, suggesting promising outcomes of α1 blockers in bladder cancer treatment [16]. To a lesser extent, prazosin has been shown to reduce survival of human bladder cancer cells at concentrations more than 30 μmol/L [14]. Terazosin, proven to induce apoptosis in prostate cancer cells, reduced tumor vascularity and induced apoptosis in transitional cell carcinoma (TCC) of the bladder in a retrospective case-control study using a pathological examination of specimens from patients undergoing radical cystectomy (Table 1) [49]. An independent retrospective observational study of 27,183 men confirmed these results and found that those treated with the quinazoline based adrenoceptor antagonists terazosin and doxazosin had a 43% lower relative risk of developing bladder cancer than unexposed men [50].

3.3. *Colorectal Cancer*

Epidemiological evidence from case-control studies enabled promising insights into the use of doxazosin as therapeutic and a chemopreventive strategy in treating colorectal cancer. An in vitro case-control study found that the α1 adrenoceptor antagonist, doxazosin significantly suppressed the proliferation of RKO colon cancer cell lines within human colorectal cancer cell assays. Recent pre-clinical studies demonstrated in vivo treatment of mice harboring colon cancer xenografts with doxazosin resulted in a significant decrease in tumor numbers and size compared to control untreated mice [46]. While limited, these results support the ongoing pursuit of the use of α1-adrenoreceptors antagonists in cancer treatment.

3.4. Adrenal Cancer

While not directly related to the genitourinary system as the other malignancies we have discussed, it is important to address the recent discoveries of the effect of α1-adrenoreceptors antagonists on adrenal cancer, specifically pheochromocytoma. While limited, there are promising preliminary results in the anti-adrenergic effects of α1-blockade in managing unchecked catecholamine production in pheochromocytoma. High circulating catecholamine levels stimulate alpha receptors on blood vessels, thereby causing vasoconstriction and increased total peripheral resistance. Thus, α-adrenergic blockade helps control blood pressure and prevent hypertensive crisis in the preoperative setting of surgical resection for metastatic pheochromocytomas [51]. While randomized controlled trials are lacking, a literature review has shown the effectiveness of doxazosin and phenoxybenzamine in the preoperative treatment of pheochromocytomas; however, further research is needed in better understanding the use of these drugs, especially in combination with β-blockers for preoperative treatment [51,52].

4. Potential Therapeutic Value in Renal Cancer

Original studies by our group provided initial translational insights into the therapeutic effects of α1-adrenoceptor antagonists in RCC preclinical models [3]. Doxazosin induces apoptosis in cancer cells through similar α1-adrenoreceptor-independent mechanisms as found in human prostate cancer cell models [3]. Molecular assays have demonstrated this quanizoline-based α1-adrenoceptor antagonist induces apoptosis in prostate cancer cells expressing C-Flip, an endogenous inhibitor of FADD-mediated activation, and subsequently cleaving caspase-8 [3]. As illustrated on Figure 1, doxazosin also induces apoptosis in renal cancer cells through activation of TGF-β1 signaling via Smad effector phosphorylation and targeting Akt survival mechanisms [31–34].

Additional cell-based evidence suggests that α1-blockers impair cancer progression to metastasis via anoikis induction at pharmacologically relevant doses, proceeding via an α1-adrenoreceptor-independent mechanism. Structural optimization studies led to the generation of a quinazoline-based derivative, of α1-adrenoreceptors antagonist, DZ-50, that was shown to overcome anoikis resistance in human renal cancer cells by disrupting integrin/FAK-mediated cell survival pathways in vitro and in vivo [3]. Doxazosin and DZ-50 were both found to exert potent antitumor action against human renal cancer cell lines 786-0 (harboring a VHL tumor-suppressor gene mutation and a highly angiogenic phenotype) and Caki cells (without a VHL mutation) [3].

DZ-50 has the chemoprotective potential to suppress angiogenesis and reverse the hypoxic nature of cancer through disrupting the tumor microenvironment [30]. The process of EMT, directed by TGF-β within the tumor microenvironment phenotypic landscape, confers acquisition of an invasive phenotype via resistance to anoikis, promoting angiogenesis, metastatic progression, and treatment failure. We first reported the ability of the novel quinazoline-derivative, DZ-50 to disrupt the ILK-1/integrin β1 complex and reduce phosphorylation of its downstream targets, AKT and GSK-3β [3]. As mentioned, this is an important mechanism in inducing anoikis in cancer cells because ILK regulates several integrin-mediated cellular processes, including cell adhesion, fibronectin-ECM assembly and anchorage-dependent cell growth [35,39]. By inhibiting ILK, DZ-50 is then able to kill tumor cells via blocking AKT and FAK phosphorylation and subsequent cell survival, disrupting integrin adhesion (α5β1 and α2β1), and engaging ECM associated tumor suppressors [3,30]. Through anoikis induction, DZ-50 has been found to significantly impair RCC metastasis in in vitro and in vivo models [3,17]. In vitro metastasis assays found that DZ-50 significantly decreased the adhesion potential of RCC to fibronectin and laminin in a time-dependent manner and subsequently suppressed the cells' migratory and invasive capabilities. Mechanistic analysis of anoikis induction (determined by Annexin V-based flow cytometry) revealed that this novel agent inactivates critical cellular survival pathways through inhibition of FAK phosphorylation, inactivation of AKT and GSK-β in the focal adhesion complex signaling cascade, and disruption of integrin-mediated focal adhesion complexes, such as FAK, ILK-1 and paxillin [3]. By interfering with this survival signaling, DZ-50 successfully reverses anoikis resistance and induces cancer cell death [3,17]. By sensitizing cells to anoikis through disruption of integrin β1-mediated focal adhesion complexes, the novel quinazoline-derived agent acquires a high therapeutic value by effectively reversing anoikis resistance in metastatic RCC tumors [3]. Temporal analysis of cell death in response to DZ-50, established that anoikis occurred prior to apoptosis [3]. Furthermore, DZ-50 exerted a more potent inhibitor effect than doxazosin on ILK-1, FAK, and paxillin binding to integrin-β1 in vivo in human renal cancer 786-0 and Caki cells [3,17,18]. In both RCC cell lines, DZ-50 led to significantly greater inhibition of tumor cell adhesion, migration and invasion than doxasozin did at pharmacologically relevant doses [3]. These findings support that the structural optimization of this particular quinazoline-based α1-adrenoreceptor antagonist has furthered a promising effect in inducing anoikis and impairing renal tumor vascularity to impair metastasis. Naftopidil has also been investigated in this context, with studies demonstrating in vitro suppression of proliferation in ACHN and Caki-2 RCC cell lines [13,53]. Fluorescence-activated cell sorting (FACS) analysis revealed that renal cancer cells treated with naftopidil underwent G_1-cell cycle arrest in vitro; the drug also decreased tumor weight and vascularity in RCC xenograft models in naftopidiol-treated excised human RCC [53]. Therefore, naftopidil provides another putative systemic therapy for the treatment and prevention of RCC that, based on this evidence, warrants further investigation.

5. The Repurposing of α1-Blockade in the Management of RCC

Drug repurposing refers to the development of new applications and uses for existing drugs. The advantage of this method is that the drugs under investigation have already been "de-risked," have been approved by the FDA, have an established safety/toxicity profile and their subsequent development timelines and costs are significantly reduced. Historically, the concept of drug repurposing has been based on incidental discoveries, but a more formal approach has been proposed internationally to realize the potential in reusing currently available drugs. Emerging recommendations for integrative platforms of data analysis to systematically synthesize results from industry drug trials for more efficient discovery of new therapeutic uses and effects of novel compounds, advance combinatorial approaches for efficacy and treatment optimization. Drug repurposing has also been accelerated by the removal of patency and regulatory barriers that may prevent clinical use and the increasing funding opportunities for drug repurposing initiatives, particularly for less common diseases [54].

Quinazoline-based α1-adrenoceptor-antagonists represent an important category of drug repurposing, having already been FDA approved, with an established safety profile and extensively prescribed for the treatment of HTN and BPH for the last 30 years. Moreover, RCC patients, who have an average age at diagnosis of 65 years, commonly suffer from comorbidities including HTN and BPH (if male), notwithstanding the common association of HTN with RCC as a paraneoplastic syndrome secondary to renin and adrenocorticotropic hormone (ACTH) secretion, parenchymal or ureteral compression, and polycythaemia or an arterio-venous fistula. This would lend itself to the use of quinazoline-α1-adrenoceptor-antagonists as a logical choice in RCC patients with HTN for a potential bimodal treatment effect. Clinicians treating patients with RCC have a strong advantage to further explore such treatment and impact patient survival.

Analogous to the observational cohort study in prostate cancer discussed earlier, epidemiology studies retrospectively exploring the use of quinazoline-based α1-adrenoceptor-antagonists for the treatment of HTN or BPH for patients who were subsequently diagnosed with RCC would allow comparisons of cumulative incidence with populations of RCC patients who were unexposed, thus providing insight into the chemopreventive effects of the drug [17,46]. In a surgical setting, retrospective analyses of patient cohorts who underwent nephrectomy for renal masses with and without extensive exposure to α1-adrenoceptors for the treatment of HTN or BPH pre-operatively, as well as patients who continued α1 blockade for a period of time post-surgery, would allow an assessment of the efficacy of neoadjuvant or adjuvant quinazoline-based α1-adrenoceptor-antagonists on long-term RCC oncological outcomes. Moreover, immunohistochemical profiling of renal tumors may establish a novel anoikis signature that could correlate with the effects of $\alpha1$ blockade on clinical outcome and survival in patients with high-risk RCC, potentially contributing to risk stratification and treatment decisions. Finally, applying translational research to further investigate the mechanisms of quinazoline-induced anoikis in RCC and its influence on both the tumor microenvironment and EMT may reveal additional actions on alternative signaling pathways and guide the development of combination regimes with other emerging targeted therapies.

6. Conclusions and Future Directions

In summary, this review accomplishes the aim of the study to investigate the effectiveness of quinazoline-based $\alpha1$-adrenoceptor antagonists in the treatment of RCC by demonstrating the translational value of quinazoline-based $\alpha1$-adrenoceptor-antagonists as anti-tumor-modalities with potential efficacy at all stages of the RCC patients' journey (neoadjuvant, adjuvant, salvage and metastatic). Retrospective epidemiological studies are underway to assess the impact of quinazoline-derived $\alpha1$ adrenoceptor antagonists as chemopreventive agents, and prospective clinical trials designed to investigate their efficacy in pre-surgical, post-surgical, and in-patient settings of metastatic disease. There is high translational significance in the repurposing of the $\alpha1$-adrenoceptor antagonists (FDA-approved drugs) to establish their therapeutic benefit as effective treatment modalities for patients with metastatic renal cell carcinoma (RCC). Our current research efforts pursue this drug repurposing at three levels: (a) the mechanistic level, by interrogating the functional exchanges between anoikis signaling and phenotypic EMT within the kidney TME to define novel mechanisms of action; (b) the translational level by directly examing precision combination therapies in pre-clinical models of RCC with and without VHL mutations; and (c). at the clinical setting by undertaking retrospective epidemiological studies to determine the impact of the use of quinazoline-derived $\alpha1$ adrenoceptor antagonists as chemopreventive agents in RCC cancan also by prospective clinical trials designed to investigate their efficacy in pre-surgical, post-surgical, and in-patient settings of RCC patients with metastatic disease [54]. If such investigative efforts demonstrate clear efficacy, RCC patients with advanced disease can therapeutically benefit from their clinical use in the near future. With the international initiatives in place encouraging the use of repurposed drugs, the introduction of new, effective RCC treatment modalities based on $\alpha1$-blockade can rapidly be integrated into clinical use and markedly improve oncological outcomes of RCC patients.

Author Contributions: Conceptualization, M.M., Z.D., K.K.B. and N.K.; methodology, M.M., Z.D., M.A., T.G.K.; software, M.A., K.E.O., W.N., H.F.; validation, M.M., A.R., N.M., and N.K.; formal analysis, M.M., Z.D., T.G.K., S.A.K., R.M., D.L., C.-K.T., K.K.B.; investigation, M.M., Z.D., K.E.O., R.M., K.K.B., N.K.; resources, S.A.K., C.-K.T., K.K.B., N.K.; data curation, Z.D., N.M., D.L., N.K.; writing—original draft preparation, M.M., Z.D., S.A.K., R.M., K.K.B., N.K.; writing—review and editing, M.M., Z.D., N.K.; visualization, M.M., M.A., T.G.K.; supervision, N.K.; project administration, K.K.B., N.K.; funding acquisition, N.K. All authors have read and agreed to the published version of the manuscript.

Acknowledgments: The authors wish to acknowledge the support of the Department of Urology and the Kidney Cancer Center of Excellence at the Icahn School of Medicine at Mount Sinai for the completion of this work.

Abbreviations

ACTH	Adrenocorticotropic Hormone
ASCO	American Society of Clinical Oncology
BPH	Benign Prostatic Hyperplasia
CRPC	Castration-Resistant Prostate Cancer
ECM	Extracellular Matrix
EMT	Epithelial–Mesenchymal Transition
MET	Mesennchymal–Epithelial-Transition
FACS	Fluorescence-activated cell sorting
FADD	Fas-Associated Death Domain
FAK	Focal Adhesion Kinase
FDA	Food and Drug Administration
HIF-α	Hypoxia-Inducible Factor-α

HTN	Hypertension
IGF	Insulin-Like Growth Factor
ILK	Integrin-Linked Kinase
PI3-K	Phosphatidylinositol 3-Kinase
RCC	Renal Cell Carcinoma
TCC	Transitional Cell Carcinoma (of the bladder)
TGF-β	Transforming Growth Factor-β
TKI	Tyrosine Kinase Inhibitors
TME	Tumor Microenvironment
TNF	Tumor Necrosis Factor
VHL	von Hippel-Lindau
VEGF	Vascular Endothelial Growth Factor
VEGFR	Vascular Endothelial Growth Factor Receptor

References

1. Saad, A.M.; Gad, M.M.; Al-Husseini, M.J.; Ruhban, I.A.; Sonbol, M.B.; Ho, T.H. Trends in Renal-Cell Carcinoma Incidence and Mortality in the United States in the Last 2 Decades: A SEER-Based Study. *Clin. Genitourin Cancer* **2019**, *17*, 46–57.e45. [CrossRef] [PubMed]
2. Ljungberg, B.; Albiges, L.; Bensalah, K.; Bex, A.; Giles, G.H.; Hora, M.; Kuczyk, M.A.; Lam, T.; Marconi, L.; Merseburger, A.S.; et al. EAU Guidelines: Renal Cell Carcinoma. Available online: http://uroweb.org/guidelines/compilations-of-all-guidelines/ (accessed on 15 June 2020).
3. Sakamoto, S.; Schwarze, S.; Kyprianou, N. Anoikis disruption of focal adhesion-Akt signaling impairs renal cell carcinoma. *Eur. Urol.* **2011**, *59*, 734–744. [CrossRef] [PubMed]
4. Gangadaran, S.G.D. Current Management Options in Metastatic Renal Cell Cancer. *Oncol. Rev.* **2017**, *11*, 339. [CrossRef] [PubMed]
5. Gandaglia, G.; Ravi, P.; Abdollah, F.; Abd-El-Barr, A.E.; Becker, A.; Popa, I.; Briganti, A.; Karakiewicz, P.I.; Trinh, Q.D.; Jewett, M.A.; et al. Contemporary incidence and mortality rates of kidney cancer in the United States. *Can. Urol. Assoc. J.* **2014**, *8*, 247–252. [CrossRef] [PubMed]
6. Siegel, R.L.; Miller, K.D.; Jemal, A. Cancer statistics, 2018. *CA Cancer J. Clin.* **2018**, *68*, 7–30. [CrossRef]
7. A.S.O.C. Kidney Cancer: Statistics. Available online: https://www.cancer.net/cancer-types/kidney-cancer/statistics (accessed on 15 June 2020).
8. Cairns, P. Renal cell carcinoma. *Cancer Biomark.* **2010**, *9*, 461–473. [CrossRef] [PubMed]
9. Chappell, J.C.; Payne, L.B.; Rathmell, W.K. Hypoxia, angiogenesis, and metabolism in the hereditary kidney cancers. *J. Clin. Investig.* **2019**, *129*, 442–451. [CrossRef]
10. Ravaud, A.; Motzer, R.J.; Pandha, H.S.; George, D.J.; Pantuck, A.J.; Patel, A.; Chang, Y.H.; Escudier, B.; Donskov, F.; Magheli, A.; et al. Adjuvant Sunitinib in High-Risk Renal-Cell Carcinoma after Nephrectomy. *N. Engl. J. Med.* **2016**, *375*, 2246–2254. [CrossRef]
11. Zhang, T.; Hwang, J.K.; George, D.J.; Pal, S.K. The landscape of contemporary clinical trials for untreated metastatic clear cell renal cell carcinoma. *Cancer Treat. Res. Commun.* **2020**, *24*, 100183. [CrossRef]
12. Campschroer, T.; Zhu, Y.; Duijvesz, D.; Grobbee, D.E.; Lock, M.T. Alpha-blockers as medical expulsive therapy for ureteral stones. *Cochrane Database Syst. Rev.* **2014**. [CrossRef]
13. Lepor, H. Landmark studies impacting the medical management of benign prostatic hyperplasia. *Rev. Urol.* **2003**, *5*, S34–S41. [PubMed]
14. Batty, M.; Pugh, R.; Rathinam, I.; Simmonds, J.; Walker, E.; Forbes, A.; Anoopkumar-Dukie, S.; McDermott, C.M.; Spencer, B.; Christie, D.; et al. The Role of α1-Adrenoceptor Antagonists in the Treatment of Prostate and Other Cancers. *Int. J. Mol. Sci.* **2016**, *17*, 1339. [CrossRef] [PubMed]
15. Harris, A.M.; Warner, B.W.; Wilson, J.M.; Becker, A.; Rowland, R.G.; Conner, W.; Lane, M.; Kimbler, K.; Durbin, E.B.; Baron, A.T.; et al. Effect of alpha1-adrenoceptor antagonist exposure on prostate cancer incidence: An observational cohort study. *J. Urol.* **2007**, *178*, 2176–2180. [CrossRef] [PubMed]
16. Gotoh, A.; Nagaya, H.; Kanno, T.; Nishizaki, T. Antitumor action of α(1)-adrenoceptor blockers on human bladder, prostate and renal cancer cells. *Pharmacology* **2012**, *90*, 242–246. [CrossRef] [PubMed]
17. Wade, C.A.; Goodwin, J.; Preston, D.; Kyprianou, N. Impact of α-adrenoceptor antagonists on prostate cancer development, progression and prevention. *Am. J. Clin. Exp. Urol.* **2019**, *7*, 46–60.
18. Bilbro, J.; Mart, M.; Kyprianou, N. Therapeutic value of quinazoline-based compounds in prostate cancer. *Anticancer Res.* **2013**, *33*, 4695–4700.

19. Lepor, H. Alpha blockers for the treatment of benign prostatic hyperplasia. *Rev. Urol.* **2007**, *9*, 181–190. [CrossRef]
20. Karabacak, O.R.; Sener, N.C.; Yilmazer, D.; Karabacak, Y.; Goktug, H.N.; Yigitbasi, O.; Alper, M. Alpha adrenergic receptors in renal pelvis and calyces: Can rat models be used? *Int. Braz. J. Urol.* **2014**, *40*, 683–689. [CrossRef]
21. Minamisawa, K.; Umemura, S.; Hirawa, N.; Hayashi, S.; Toya, Y.; Ishikawa, Y.; Yasuda, G.; Ishii, M. Characteristic localization of alpha 1- and alpha 2-adrenoceptors in the human kidney. *Clin. Exp. Pharmacol. Physiol.* **1993**, *20*, 523–526. [CrossRef]
22. Uhlén, S.; Lindblom, J.; Kindlundh, A.; Mugisha, P.; Nyberg, F. Nandrolone treatment decreases the level of rat kidney alpha(1B)-adrenoceptors. *Naunyn. Schmiedebergs Arch. Pharmacol.* **2003**, *368*, 91–98. [CrossRef]
23. Bylund, D.B. Adrenergic Receptors. In *The Adrenergic Receptors: In the 21st Century*; Perez, D.M., Ed.; Humana Press: Totowa, NJ, USA, 2006; pp. 3–21. [CrossRef]
24. Civantos Calzada, B.; Aleixandre de Artiñano, A. Alpha-adrenoceptor subtypes. *Pharmacol. Res.* **2001**, *44*, 195–208. [CrossRef] [PubMed]
25. Hesse, I.F.; Johns, E.J. An in vivo study of the alpha-adrenoreceptor subtypes on the renal vasculature of the anaesthetized rabbit. *J. Auton Pharmacol.* **1984**, *4*, 145–152. [CrossRef] [PubMed]
26. Kobayashi, S.; Tang, R.; Shapiro, E.; Lepor, H. Characterization and localization of prostatic alpha 1 adrenoceptors using radioligand receptor binding on slide-mounted tissue section. *J. Urol.* **1993**, *150*, 2002–2006. [CrossRef]
27. Marshall, I.; Burt, R.P.; Chapple, C.R. Noradrenaline contractions of human prostate mediated by alpha 1A-(alpha 1c-) adrenoceptor subtype. *Br. J. Pharmacol.* **1995**, *115*, 781–786. [CrossRef]
28. Taniguchi, N.; Ukai, Y.; Tanaka, T.; Yano, J.; Kimura, K.; Moriyama, N.; Kawabe, K. Identification of alpha1-adrenoceptor subtypes in the human prostatic urethra. *Naunyn Schmiedeberg's Arch. Pharmacol.* **1997**, *355*, 412–416. [CrossRef]
29. Forray, C.; Bard, J.A.; Wetzel, J.M.; Chiu, G.; Shapiro, E.; Tang, R.; Lepor, H.; Hartig, P.R.; Weinshank, R.L.; Branchek, T.A.; et al. The alpha 1-adrenergic receptor that mediates smooth muscle contraction in human prostate has the pharmacological properties of the cloned human alpha 1c subtype. *Mol. Pharmacol.* **1994**, *45*, 703–708.
30. Kyprianou, N.; Benning, C.M. Suppression of human prostate cancer cell growth by alpha1-adrenoceptor antagonists doxazosin and terazosin via induction of apoptosis. *Cancer Res.* **2000**, *60*, 4550–4555.
31. Anglin, I.E.; Glassman, D.T.; Kyprianou, N. Induction of prostate apoptosis by alpha1-adrenoceptor antagonists: Mechanistic significance of the quinazoline component. *Prostate Cancer Prostatic Dis.* **2002**, *5*, 88–95. [CrossRef]
32. Benning, C.M.; Kyprianou, N. Quinazoline-derived alpha1-adrenoceptor antagonists induce prostate cancer cell apoptosis via an alpha1-adrenoceptor-independent action. *Cancer Res.* **2002**, *62*, 597–602.
33. Garrison, J.B.; Kyprianou, N. Novel targeting of apoptosis pathways for prostate cancer therapy. *Curr. Cancer Drug Targets* **2004**, *4*, 85–95. [CrossRef]
34. Partin, J.V.; Anglin, I.E.; Kyprianou, N. Quinazoline-based alpha 1-adrenoceptor antagonists induce prostate cancer cell apoptosis via TGF-beta signalling and I kappa B alpha induction. *Br. J. Cancer* **2003**, *88*, 1615–1621. [CrossRef] [PubMed]
35. Keledjian, K.; Garrison, J.B.; Kyprianou, N. Doxazosin inhibits human vascular endothelial cell adhesion, migration, and invasion. *J. Cell Biochem.* **2005**, *94*, 374–388. [CrossRef] [PubMed]
36. Hannigan, G.E.; Leung-Hagesteijn, C.; Fitz-Gibbon, L.; Coppolino, M.G.; Radeva, G.; Filmus, J.; Bell, J.C.; Dedhar, S. Regulation of cell adhesion and anchorage-dependent growth by a new beta 1-integrin-linked protein kinase. *Nature* **1996**, *379*, 91–96. [CrossRef] [PubMed]
37. Li, F.; Liu, J.; Mayne, R.; Wu, C. Identification and characterization of a mouse protein kinase that is highly homologous to human integrin-linked kinase. *Biochim. Biophys. Acta* **1997**, *1358*, 215–220. [CrossRef]
38. Wu, C.; Dedhar, S. Integrin-linked kinase (ILK) and its interactors: A new paradigm for the coupling of extracellular matrix to actin cytoskeleton and signaling complexes. *J. Cell Biol.* **2001**, *155*, 505–510. [CrossRef] [PubMed]
39. Radeva, G.; Petrocelli, T.; Behrend, E.; Leung-Hagesteijn, C.; Filmus, J.; Slingerland, J.; Dedhar, S. Overexpression of the integrin-linked kinase promotes anchorage-independent cell cycle progression. *J. Biol. Chem.* **1997**, *272*, 13937–13944. [CrossRef]

40. Cieslik, K.; Zembowicz, A.; Tang, J.L.; Wu, K.K. Transcriptional regulation of endothelial nitric-oxide synthase by lysophosphatidylcholine. *J. Biol. Chem.* **1998**, *273*, 14885–14890. [CrossRef]
41. Attwell, S.; Roskelley, C.; Dedhar, S. The integrin-linked kinase (ILK) suppresses anoikis. *Oncogene* **2000**, *19*, 3811–3815. [CrossRef]
42. Fukuda, T.; Chen, K.; Shi, X.; Wu, C. PINCH-1 is an obligate partner of integrin-linked kinase (ILK) functioning in cell shape modulation, motility, and survival. *J. Biol. Chem.* **2003**, *278*, 51324–51333. [CrossRef]
43. Frisch, S.M.; Francis, H. Disruption of epithelial cell-matrix interactions induces apoptosis. *J. Cell Biol.* **1994**, *124*, 619–626. [CrossRef]
44. Frisch, S.M.; Screaton, R.A. Anoikis mechanisms. *Curr. Opin. Cell Biol.* **2001**, *13*, 555–562. [CrossRef]
45. Nakagawa, Y.U.; Nagaya, H.; Miyata, T.; Wada, Y.; Oyama, T.; Gotoh, A. Piperazine-based Alpha-1 AR Blocker, Naftopidil, Selectively Suppresses Malignant Human Bladder Cells via Induction of Apoptosis. *Anticancer Res.* **2016**, *36*, 1563–1570. [PubMed]
46. Suzuki, N.; Niikura, R.; Ihara, S.; Hikiba, Y.; Kinoshita, H.; Higashishima, N.; Hayakawa, Y.; Yamada, A.; Hirata, Y.; Nakata, R.; et al. Alpha-Blockers As Colorectal Cancer Chemopreventive: Findings from a Case-Control Study, Human Cell Cultures, and In Vivo Preclinical Testing. *Cancer Prev. Res.* **2019**, *12*, 185–194. [CrossRef] [PubMed]
47. Murtola, T.J.; Tammela, T.L.; Määttänen, L.; Ala-Opas, M.; Stenman, U.H.; Auvinen, A. Prostate cancer incidence among finasteride and alpha-blocker users in the Finnish Prostate Cancer Screening Trial. *Br. J. Cancer* **2009**, *101*, 843–848. [CrossRef] [PubMed]
48. Hart, J.; Spencer, B.; McDermott, C.M.; Chess-Williams, R.; Sellers, D.; Christie, D.; Anoopkumar-Dukie, S. A Pilot retrospective analysis of alpha-blockers on recurrence in men with localised prostate cancer treated with radiotherapy. *Sci. Rep.* **2020**, *10*, 8191. [CrossRef]
49. Tahmatzopoulos, A.; Lagrange, C.A.; Zeng, L.; Mitchell, B.L.; Conner, W.T.; Kyprianou, N. Effect of terazosin on tissue vascularity and apoptosis in transitional cell carcinoma of bladder. *Urology* **2005**, *65*, 1019–1023. [CrossRef]
50. Martin, F.M.; Harris, A.M.; Rowland, R.G.; Conner, W.; Lane, M.; Durbin, E.; Baron, A.T.; Kyprianou, N. Decreased risk of bladder cancer in men treated with quinazoline-based α1-adrenoceptor antagonists. *Gene Ther. Mol. Biol.* **2008**, *12*, 253–258.
51. Blake, M.; Sweeney, A.T.; Griffing, G. Pheochromocytoma. Available online: https://emedicine.medscape.com/article/124059-overview (accessed on 18 August 2020).
52. Van der Zee, P.; de Boer, A. Pheochromocytoma: A review on preoperative treatment with phenoxybenzamine or doxazosin. *Neth. J. Med.* **2014**, *72*, 190–201.
53. Iwamoto, Y.; Ishii, K.; Sasaki, T.; Kato, M.; Kanda, H.; Yamada, Y.; Arima, K.; Shiraishi, T.; Sugimura, Y. Oral naftopidil suppresses human renal-cell carcinoma by inducing G(1) cell-cycle arrest in tumor and vascular endothelial cells. *Cancer Prev. Res.* **2013**, *6*, 1000–1006. [CrossRef]
54. Pushpakom, S.; Iorio, F.; Eyers, P.A.; Escott, K.J.; Hopper, S.; Wells, A.; Doig, A.; Guilliams, T.; Latimer, J.; McNamee, C.; et al. Drug repurposing: Progress, challenges and recommendations. *Nat. Rev. Drug Discov.* **2019**, *18*, 41–58. [CrossRef]

Permissions

All chapters in this book were first published by MDPI; hereby published with permission under the Creative Commons Attribution License or equivalent. Every chapter published in this book has been scrutinized by our experts. Their significance has been extensively debated. The topics covered herein carry significant findings which will fuel the growth of the discipline. They may even be implemented as practical applications or may be referred to as a beginning point for another development.

The contributors of this book come from diverse backgrounds, making this book a truly international effort. This book will bring forth new frontiers with its revolutionizing research information and detailed analysis of the nascent developments around the world.

We would like to thank all the contributing authors for lending their expertise to make the book truly unique. They have played a crucial role in the development of this book. Without their invaluable contributions this book wouldn't have been possible. They have made vital efforts to compile up to date information on the varied aspects of this subject to make this book a valuable addition to the collection of many professionals and students.

This book was conceptualized with the vision of imparting up-to-date information and advanced data in this field. To ensure the same, a matchless editorial board was set up. Every individual on the board went through rigorous rounds of assessment to prove their worth. After which they invested a large part of their time researching and compiling the most relevant data for our readers.

The editorial board has been involved in producing this book since its inception. They have spent rigorous hours researching and exploring the diverse topics which have resulted in the successful publishing of this book. They have passed on their knowledge of decades through this book. To expedite this challenging task, the publisher supported the team at every step. A small team of assistant editors was also appointed to further simplify the editing procedure and attain best results for the readers.

Apart from the editorial board, the designing team has also invested a significant amount of their time in understanding the subject and creating the most relevant covers. They scrutinized every image to scout for the most suitable representation of the subject and create an appropriate cover for the book.

The publishing team has been an ardent support to the editorial, designing and production team. Their endless efforts to recruit the best for this project, has resulted in the accomplishment of this book. They are a veteran in the field of academics and their pool of knowledge is as vast as their experience in printing. Their expertise and guidance has proved useful at every step. Their uncompromising quality standards have made this book an exceptional effort. Their encouragement from time to time has been an inspiration for everyone.

The publisher and the editorial board hope that this book will prove to be a valuable piece of knowledge for researchers, students, practitioners and scholars across the globe.

List of Contributors

Yasuyoshi Miyata, Tomohiro Matsuo, Yuji Sagara, Kojiro Ohba and Hideki Sakai
Department of Urology, Nagasaki University Graduate School of Biomedical Sciences, 1-7-1 Sakamoto, Nagasaki 852-8501, Japan

Kaname Ohyama
Department of Pharmaceutical Science, Nagasaki University Graduate School of Biomedical Sciences, 1-7-1 Sakamoto, Nagasaki 852-8501, Japan

Manuela A. Hoffmann
Department of Occupational Health & Safety, Federal Ministry of Defense, 53123 Bonn, Germany
Clinic of Nuclear Medicine, Johannes Gutenberg-University, 55101 Mainz, Germany

Hans-Georg Buchholz, Matthias Miederer and Mathias Schreckenberger
Clinic of Nuclear Medicine, Johannes Gutenberg-University, 55101 Mainz, Germany

Helmut J Wieler
Clinic of Nuclear Medicine, Bundeswehr Central Hospital, 56072 Koblenz, Germany

Florian Rosar
Clinic of Nuclear Medicine, Johannes Gutenberg-University, 55101 Mainz, Germany
Department of Nuclear Medicine, Saarland University Medical Center, 66421 Homburg, Germany

Nicolas Fischer
Department of Urology, University of Cologne, 50937 Cologne, Germany

Marco Moschini
Department of Urology, Comprehensive Cancer Center, Medical University of Vienna, Vienna General Hospital, A-1090 Vienna, Austria
Department of Urology, Urological Research Institute, San Raffaele Scientific Institute, 20132 Milan, Italy
Department of Urology, Luzerner Kantonsspital, Spitalstrasse, 6000 Luzern, Switzerland

Francesco Montorsi, Alberto Briganti, Andrea Gallina and Armando Stabile
Department of Urology, Urological Research Institute, San Raffaele Scientific Institute, 20132 Milan, Italy

Stefania Zamboni, Agostino Mattei, Philipp Baumeister and Livio Mordasini
Department of Urology, Luzerner Kantonsspital, Spitalstrasse, 6000 Luzern, Switzerland

Francesco Soria
Department of Urolog
y, Comprehensive Cancer Center, Medical University of Vienna, Vienna General Hospital, A-1090 Vienna, Austria
Division of Urology, Department of Surgical Sciences, University of Studies of Torino, 10124 Turin, Italy

Romain Mathieu
Department of Urology, Comprehensive Cancer Center, Medical University of Vienna, Vienna General Hospital, A-1090 Vienna, Austria
Department of Urology, Rennes University Hospital, 35000 Rennes, France

Evanguelos Xylinas
Department of Urology Bichat Hospital, Paris Descartes University, 75877 Paris, France
Department of Urology, Hôpital Cochin, APHP, 75014 Paris, France

Wei Shen Tan and John D Kelly
Division of Surgery and Intervention Science, University College London, London WC1E 6BT, UK
Department of Uro-Oncology, University College London Hospital NHS Foundation Trust, London W1T 4EU, UK

Giuseppe Simone
Department of Urology, "Regina Elena" National Cancer Institute, 00128 Rome, Italy
Department of Urology, IRCCS Regina Elena National Cancer Institute, 00144 Rome, Italy

Anoop Meraney
Urology Division, Hartford Healthcare Medical Group, Hartford, CT 06106, USA

Suprita Krishna and Badrinath Konety
Department of Urology, University of Minnesota, Minneapolis, MN 55455, USA

Rafael Sanchez-Salas and Xavier Cathelineau
Department of Urology, L'Institut Mutualiste Montsouris, Université Paris Descartes, 75014 Paris, France

Michael Rink
Department of Urology, University Medical Center Hamburg-Eppendorf, 20251 Hamburg, Germany
Department of Urology, Medical University of Hamburg, Martinistraße 52, 20246 Hamburg, Germany

Andrea Necchi
Fondazione IRCCS Istituto Nazionale dei Tumori, 20133 Milan, Italy

Pierre I. Karakiewicz
Cancer Prognostics and Health Outcomes Unit, University of Montreal Health Centre, Montreal, QC H4A 3J1, Canada

Morgan Rouprêt
Sorbonne Université, GRC no. 5, ONCOTYPE-URO, AP-HP, Hôpital Pitié-Salpêtrière, F-75013 Paris, France

Anthony Koupparis
Bristol Urological Institute, North Bristol NHS Trust, Southmead Hospital, Bristol BS10 5NB, UK

Wassim Kassouf
Department of Urology, McGill University Health Center, Montreal, QC H4A3J1, Canada

Douglas S Scherr
Department of Urology, Weill Cornell Medical College, New York-Presbyterian Hospital, New York, NY 10038, USA

Guillaume Ploussard
Department of Urology, La Croix du sud Hospital, 314000 Toulouse, France

Stephen A. Boorjian
Department of Urology, Mayo Clinic, 200 First Street Southwest, Rochester, MN 55905, USA

Yair Lotan
Department of Urology, University of Texas Southwestern Medical Center, Dallas, TX 75390, USA

Prasanna Sooriakumaran
Department of Uro-Oncology, University College London Hospital NHS Foundation Trust, London W1T 4EU, UK
Department of Molecular Medicine and Surgery, Karolinska Institutet, 17177 Stockholm, Sweden

Douglas S. Scherr
Department of Urology, Weill Cornell Medical College, New York-Presbyterian Hospital, New York, NY 10038, USA

Mathieu Roumiguié and Bernard Malavaud
Department of Urology, Institut Universitaire du Cancer, 31059 Toulouse CEDEX 9, France

Antonin Brisuda and Marek Babjuk
Department of Urology, 2nd Faculty of Medicine, Charles University, Teaching Hospital Motol, 15006 Prague, Czech Republic

Maximillian Burger
St. Josef, Klinik für Urologie, Caritas-Krankenhaus, 93053 Regensburg, Germany

Hugh Mostafid
Department of Urology, Royal Surrey County Hospital, Surrey, Guildford GU2 7RF, UK

Marc Colombel
Department of Urology, Hôpital Edouard Herriot, 69437 Lyon, France

Joan Palou Redorta
Department of Urology, Fundacio Puigvert, 08025 Barcelona, Spain

Fred Witjes
Department of Urology, Radboud UMC, 6525 GA Nijmegen, The Netherlands

Florian Janisch
Department of Urology, Medical University of Hamburg, Martinistraße 52, 20246 Hamburg, Germany
Department of Urology, Medical University of Vienna, Währinger Gürtel 18-20, 1090 Vienna, Austria

Hang Yu, Malte W. Vetterlein, Roland Dahlem, Oliver Engel, Margit Fisch and Armin Soave
Department of Urology, Medical University of Hamburg, Martinistraße 52, 20246 Hamburg, Germany

Shahrokh F. Shariat
Department of Urology, Medical University of Vienna, Währinger Gürtel 18-20, 1090 Vienna, Austria
Institute for Urology and Reproductive Health, Sechenov University, Bolshaya Pirogovskaya str. 2-4, 119991 Moscow, Russia
Department of Urology, University of Texas Southwestern Medical Center, 5323 Harry Hines Blvd, Dallas, TX 75390, USA
Karl Landsteiner Institute of Urology and Andrology, Franziskanergasse 4, a 3100 St. Poelten, Austria
Department of Urology, Second Faculty of Medicine, Charles University, Ovocný trh 5, Prague 1-116 36, Czech Republic
Department of Urology, Comprehensive Cancer Center, Medical University of Vienna, Vienna General Hospital, A-1090 Vienna, Austria
Department of Urology, Weill Cornell Medical College, New York Presbyterian Hospital, New York, NY 10021, USA
Department of Urology, The University of Texas M.D. Anderson Cancer Center, Houston, TX 77030, USA

lNiklas Klümper
Department of Urology, University Hospital Bonn, 53127 Bonn, Germany
Center for Integrated Oncology, University Hospital Bonn, 53127 Bonn, Germany
Institute of Experimental Oncology, University Hospital Bonn, 53127 Bonn, Germany

Marthe von Danwitz, Johannes Stein, Doris Schmidt, Anja Schmidt, Manuel Ritter, Abdullah Alajati and Jörg Ellinger
Department of Urology, University Hospital Bonn, 53127 Bonn, Germany
Center for Integrated Oncology, University Hospital Bonn, 53127 Bonn, Germany

Glen Kristiansen and Michael Muders
Center for Integrated Oncology, University Hospital Bonn, 53127 Bonn, Germany
Institute of Pathology, University Hospital Bonn, 53127 Bonn, Germany

Michael Hölzel
Center for Integrated Oncology, University Hospital Bonn, 53127 Bonn, Germany
Institute of Experimental Oncology, University Hospital Bonn, 53127 Bonn, Germany

Donghyun Kim and Jin Man Kim
Department of Pathology, Chungnam National University School of Medicine, 266 Munhwa Street, Daejeon 35015, Korea
Department of Pathology, Chungnam National University Hospital, 282 Munwha-ro, Daejeon 35015, Korea

Jun-Sang Kim
Department of Radiation Oncology, Chungnam National University School of Medicine, 288 Munhwa Street, Daejeon 35015, Korea
Department of Radiation Oncology, Chungnam National University Hospital, 282 Munwha-ro, Daejeon 35015, Korea

Sup Kim
Department of Radiation Oncology, Chungnam National University Hospital, 282 Munwha-ro, Daejeon 35015, Korea

Kyung-Hee Kim
Department of Pathology, Chungnam National University School of Medicine, 266 Munhwa Street, Daejeon 35015, Korea
Department of Pathology, Chungnam National University Hospital, 282 Munwha-ro, Daejeon 35015, Korea
Department of Pathology, Chungnam National University Sejong Hospital, 20 Bodeum 7-ro, Sejongsi 30099, Korea

Carlo Cattrini
Department of Internal Medicine and Medical Specialties (DIMI), School of Medicine, University of Genoa, 16132 Genoa, Italy
Prostate Cancer Clinical Research Unit, Spanish National Cancer Research Centre (CNIO), 28029 Madrid, Spain

Davide Soldato, Elisa Zanardi, Paola Barboro and Francesco Boccardo
Department of Internal Medicine and Medical Specialties (DIMI), School of Medicine, University of Genoa, 16132 Genoa, Italy
Academic Unit of Medical Oncology, IRCCS Ospedale Policlinico San Martino, 16132 Genoa, Italy

David Olmos
Prostate Cancer Clinical Research Unit, Spanish National Cancer Research Centre (CNIO), 28029 Madrid, Spain

Alessandra Rubagotti
Academic Unit of Medical Oncology, IRCCS Ospedale Policlinico San Martino, 16132 Genoa, Italy
Department of Health Sciences (DISSAL), School of Medicine, University of Genoa, 16132 Genoa, Italy

Linda Zinoli
Academic Unit of Medical Oncology, IRCCS Ospedale Policlinico San Martino, 16132 Genoa, Italy

Carlo Messina
Department of Medical Oncology, Santa Chiara Hospital, 38122 Trento, Italy

Elena Castro
CNIO-IBIMA Genitourinary Cancer Unit, Hospitales Universitarios Virgen de la Victoria y Regional de Málaga, Instituto de Investigación Biomédica de Málaga, 29010 Malaga, Spain

Zhengqiu Zhou
Department of Molecular and Cellular Biochemistry, University of Kentucky College of Medicine, Lexington, KY 40536, USA

Connor J. Kinslow
Department of Radiation Oncology, Vagelos College of Physicians and Surgeons, Columbia University Irving Medical Center, New York, NY 10032, USA

Peng Wang
Division of Medical Oncology, Department of Internal Medicine, College of Medicine, University of Kentucky, Lexington, KY 40536, USA

Bin Huang
Department of Biostatistics, College of Public Health, University of Kentucky, Lexington, KY 40536, USA

Simon K. Cheng and Israel Deutsch
Department of Radiation Oncology, Vagelos College of Physicians and Surgeons, Columbia University Irving Medical Center, New York, NY 10032, USA
Division of Medical Oncology, Department of Internal Medicine, College of Medicine, University of Kentucky, Lexington, KY 40536, USA
Department of Biostatistics, College of Public Health, University of Kentucky, Lexington, KY 40536, USA
Herbert Irving Comprehensive Cancer Center, Vagelos College of Physicians and Surgeons, Columbia University Irving Medical Center, New York, NY 10032, USA

Matthew S. Gentry
Department of Molecular and Cellular Biochemistry, University of Kentucky College of Medicine, Lexington, KY 40536, USA
Markey Cancer Center, University of Kentucky, Lexington, KY 40536, USA

Ramon C. Sun
Markey Cancer Center, University of Kentucky, Lexington, KY 40536, USA
Department of Neuroscience, University of Kentucky College of Medicine, Lexington, KY 40536, USA

Claudia Manini
Department of Pathology, San Giovanni Bosco Hospital, 10154 Turin, Italy

José I. López
Department of Pathology, Biocruces-Bizkaia Health Research Institute, Cruces University Hospital, Barakaldo, 48903 Bizkaia, Spain

Shyama U. Tetar, Omar Bohoudi, Suresh Senan, Miguel A. Palacios, Swie S. Oei, Antoinet M. van der Wel, Berend J. Slotman, Frank J. Lagerwaard and Anna M. E. Bruynzeel
Department of Radiation Oncology, Amsterdam University Medical Centers, 1081 HZ Amsterdam, The Netherlands

R. Jeroen A. van Moorselaar
Department of Urology, Amsterdam University Medical Centers, 1081 HV Amsterdam, The Netherlands

Claudia Claroni, Marco Covotta, Giulia Torregiani, Maria Elena Marcelli and Ester Forastiere
Department of Anaesthesiology, IRCCS Regina Elena National Cancer Institute, 00144 Rome, Italy

Gabriele Tuderti
Department of Urology, IRCCS Regina Elena National Cancer Institute, 00144 Rome, Italy

Alessandra Scotto di Uccio
School of Medicine, University Hospital Center "Tor Vergata", 00133 Rome, Italy

Antonio Zinilli
IRCrES, Research Institute on Sustainable Economic Growth of the National Research Council of Italy, 00185 Rome, Italy

Sofia Karkampouna, Maria R. De Filippo, Irena Klima and Eugenio Zoni
Urology Research Laboratory, Department for BioMedical Research, University of Bern, Murtenstrasse 35, 3008 Bern, Switzerland

Charlotte K. Y. Ng
Oncogenomics Laboratory, Department for BioMedical Research, University of Bern, Murtenstrasse 40, 3008 Bern, Switzerland

Martin Spahn
Lindenhofspital Bern, Prostate Center Bern, 3012 Bern, Switzerland

Frank Stein and Per Haberkant
Proteomics Core Facility, EMBL Heidelberg, Meyerhofstraße 1, 69117 Heidelberg, Germany

George N. Thalmann and Marianna Kruithof-de Julio
Urology Research Laboratory, Department for BioMedical Research, University of Bern, Murtenstrasse 35, 3008 Bern, Switzerland
Department of Urology, Inselspital, Anna Seiler Haus, Bern University Hospital, 3010 Bern, Switzerland

Jennifer Kubon, Danijel Sikic, Angela Neumann, Bastian Keck, Bernd Wullich, Helge Taubert and Sven Wach
Department of Urology and Pediatric Urology, University Hospital Erlangen, Friedrich-Alexander Universität Erlangen-Nürnberg, 91054 Erlangen, Germany

Markus Eckstein, Veronika Weyerer, Robert Stöhr and Arndt Hartmann
Institute of Pathology, University Hospital Erlangen, Friedrich-Alexander Universität Erlangen-Nürnberg, 91054 Erlangen, Germany

Ralph M. Wirtz
STRATIFYER Molecular Pathology GmbH, 50935 Cologne, Germany

Sirin Saranyutanon, Sachin Kumar Deshmukh and Santanu Dasgupta
Cancer Biology Program, Mitchell Cancer Institute, University of South Alabama, Mobile, AL 36604, USA
Department of Medical Oncology, Mitchell Cancer Institute, University of South Alabama, Mobile, AL 36604, USA

Sachin Pai
Department of Pathology, College of Medicine, University of South Alabama, Mobile, AL 36617, USA

Seema Singh and Ajay Pratap Singh
Cancer Biology Program, Mitchell Cancer Institute, University of South Alabama, Mobile, AL 36604, USA
Department of Medical Oncology, Mitchell Cancer Institute, University of South Alabama, Mobile, AL 36604, USA
Department of Biochemistry and Molecular Biology, University of South Alabama, Mobile, AL 36688, USA

Index

www.ingramcontent.com/pod-product-compliance
Lightning Source LLC
LaVergne TN
LVHW060555210926
848485LV00005B/1317